SEXUALLY TRANSMITTED INFECTIONS

Edited by **Nancy Malla**

Sexually Transmitted Infections
Edited by Nancy Malla

Published by InTech

Janeza Trdine 9, 51000 Rijeka, Croatia

Publishing Process Manager Marina Jozipovic

Technical Editor Teodora Smiljanic

Cover Designer InTech Design Team

Additional hard copies can be obtained from orders@intechopen.com

Sexually Transmitted Infections, Edited by Nancy Malla
p. cm.
ISBN 978-593-51-0258-8

For EU product safety concerns:
IN TECH d.o.o., Prolaz Marije Krucifikse Kozulić 3, 51000 Rijeka, Croatia,
info@intechopen.com or visit our website at intechopen.com.

Meet the editor

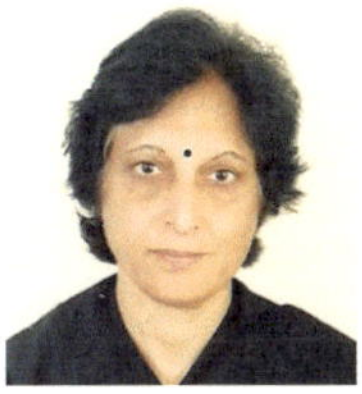

Prof. Nancy Malla was awarded Bachelor of Medicine and Bachelor of Surgery M.B.B.S. degree by Punjab University, Chandigarh, India in 1968 and received M.D. (Microbiology) degree from Postgraduate Institute of Medical Education and Research (PGIMER), Chandigarh, India in December, 1975. She worked as faculty member in the departments of Microbiology, Medical College, Srinagar, Kashmir; Medical College, Jammu; Sher-i-Kashmir Institute of Medical Sciences, Srinagar, Kashmir, and is currently holding post of Professor at PGIMER, Chandigarh, India. In recognition of her diagnostic and research capabilities, she was awarded many National level Academic Awards and British Council Fellowship. She is fellow of the Royal Society of Tropical Medicine and Hygiene; Fellow, National Academy of Medical Sciences, India and member of many National and International Academic Societies. She was presented 'Moselio Schaechter Distinguished Service Travel Award, Honorable mention' by the American Society for Microbiology in 2010.

Contents

Preface

Sexually transmitted infections (STIs) are considered as neglected diseases and are on the list of diseases targeted by WHO for control. Apart from HIV, STIs cause significant morbidity. Several STIs adversely affect outcome of pregnancy and may lead to neonatal and genital infections. Genital infection with Human papilloma virus (HPV) may lead to cervical cancer, the most common cause of cancer-related death in women worldwide. High risk group persons and women, particularly adolescents are disproportionately vulnerable to STIs, many of which remain asymptomatic favouring spread of infection. The risk of acquiring STIs is highest in urban areas, in low socioeconomic groups, in the young and in association with illicit drug users and prostitution. Prevention is the Hall mark for control of STIs. Prevention and control of STIs require a global initiative, the success of which will largely depend on the development of safe and effective vaccines. Currently, except for hepatitis B infection, no such vaccines exist. Although, there is plethora of the literature available on STIs and many books are available on the individual infections covered in this book, yet numerous advances continue to be made in understanding the different aspects of these infections.

In Tech publisher has planned to publish the book and have invited authors with their rich expertise on the topics contributed by them. The purpose of the book and approach used is an attempt made to present the historical as well as advanced reference material on different aspects of STIs. This book is essentially a collection of chapters providing novel knowledge on some of the most debated topics. The book is intended for general reference work for physicians, researchers and students interested in the subject. The strong and genuine enthusiasm of the authors is clearly visible in their respective contributions. The book does not cover all the sexually transmitted infections. In the introductory chapter, an attempt has been made to provide an overview on the STIs with special reference to syndromic approach for management as a general practitioner in the field, especially those who may not have access to specialist literature. I am sure that the information provided in this book, will stimulate the reader to understand different aspects on the topics contributed and will be of interest to health care professionals, scientists dedicated to this field as well as readers, in general.

I wish to put on record my gratitude to many colleagues for reviewing few chapters and for their time and valuable suggestions. Their ideas shaped the book and guided every step of its creation. In particular, I would like to acknowledge the help of Prof. Jane Carlton for her suggestions for the chapter on Human trichomoniasis, Prof. D.R. Arora and Dr. Neelam Taneja for chapter on Syphilis, Dr. Mini P. Singh for chapters on Human Papilloma Virus and Dr. Kusum Sharma for chapter on Chlamydia. Lastly, I would like to thank the In Tech publishers for appointing me 'Book Editor' and providing me an opportunity to review the chapters contributed in this book.

Nancy Malla
Professor and Head, Department of Parasitology,
Post Graduate Institute of Medical Education and Research
Chandigarh,
India

Part 1

Introduction

1

Sexually Transmitted Infections: An Overview

Nancy Malla and Kapil Goyal
Department of Parasitology, Postgraduate Institute of Medical Education and Research, Chandigarh India

1. Introduction

Sexually transmitted infections (STIs) are infections that are spread primarily through person-to-person sexual contact. During the past two decades, STDs have undergone a dramatic transformation. First, the change in name from venereal diseases (V.D.) to sexually transmitted diseases (STD) indicates this transformation. The term "venereal" as it relates to disease dates back to 15th century. Its root comes from the Latin *venereus* or *venus*, meaning "from sexual love or desire." Secondly, attention is now given not only to specific sexually transmitted microbial agents, but also to clinical syndromes associated with STDs as follows:

- urethral discharge
- genital ulcers
- inguinal swellings (bubo, which is a swelling in the groin)
- scrotal swelling
- vaginal discharge
- lower abdominal pain
- neonatal eye infections (conjunctivitis of the newborn).

There are more than 30 different sexually transmissible bacteria, viruses and parasites pathogenic to man. Some of the most common are listed below:

1.1 Bacteria infections

i. *Neisseria gonorrhoeae,* causes gonorrhoea or gonococcal infection
ii. *Chlamydia trachomatis,* causes chlamydial infections
iii. *Treponema pallidum,* causes syphilis
iv. *Haemophilus ducreyi,* causes chancroid
v. *Klebsiella granulomatis,* previously known as *Calymmatobacterium granulomatis* causes granuloma inguinale or donovanosis.

1.2 Viruses

i. Human immunodeficiency virus, causes AIDS
ii. Herpes simplex virus (HSV) type 1 & 2 causes genital herpes.

iii. Human papillomavirus (HPV)causes genital warts and certain subtypes lead to cervical cancer in women.
iv. Hepatitis B virus, Hepatitis C virus causes hepatitis and chronic cases may lead to cancer of the liver.
v. Molluscum contagiosum virus (member of poxvirus family), causes molluscum contagiosum virus.

1.3 Parasite

i. *Trichomonas vaginalis,* causes vaginal trichomoniasis.

1.4 Fungal agents

i. *Candida albicans,*causes vulvovaginitis in women; inflammation of the glans penis and foreskin in men.

1.5 Ectoparasites

i. *Phthirus pubis*
ii. *Sarcoptes scabiei*

Sexually transmitted diseases are divided into "traditional" or "first generation" STD (syphilis, gonorrhoea, chancroid) and "second generation" STD (Chlamydia infections and Virus infections) (Temmerman, 1992). Although many different pathogens cause STIs, some display similar or overlapping signs (what the individual or the health-care provider sees on examination) and symptoms (what the patient feels such as pain or irritation). Some of these signs and symptoms are easily recognizable and consistent, giving what is known as a syndrome that signals the presence of one or a number of pathogens. For example, a discharge from the urethra in men can be caused by gonorrhoea alone, chlamydia alone or both together. A matter of serious concern is the emergence of antimicrobial resistance to sexually transmitted microbial agents (e.g., penicillinase-producing strains of gonococci) since the late 1970s which is posing a serious barrier to patient care.

2. Significance of STI's

The true incidence of STDs is not known, because of inadequate reporting due to secrecy that surrounds these infections. The "second generation" STDs are tending to replace the first generation i.e. classical bacterial diseases (syphilis, gonorrhoea and chancroid). In many industrialized countries, the incidence of genital *C. trachomatis* infection exceeds that of gonococcal infection.

According to 2005 WHO estimates, 448 million new cases of curable STIs (syphilis, gonorrhoea, chlamydia and trichomoniasis) occur annually throughout the world in adults aged 15-49 years (WHO fact sheet 2011). This does not include HIV and other STIs which continue to adversely affect the lives of individuals and communities worldwide. In developing countries, STIs and their complications rank in the top five disease categories for which adults seek health care. Some STIs are asymptomatic and it is reported that up to 70%

of women and a significant proportion of men with gonococcal and/or chlamydial infections experience no symptoms at all. Both symptomatic and asymptomatic infections can lead to the development of serious complications, as follows.

2.1 STIs adversely affect the health of women

Untreated STIs can have critical implications for reproductive, maternal and newborn health. STIs are the main preventable cause of infertility, particularly in women. It is observed that 10 - 40% of women with untreated chlamydial infection develop symptomatic pelvic inflammatory disease. Post-infection tubal damage is responsible for 30 - 40% of cases of female infertility (Pellati et al., 2008). Furthermore, women who have had pelvic inflammatory disease are 6 - 10 times more likely to develop an ectopic (tubal) pregnancy than those who have not, and 40 - 50% of ectopic pregnancies can be attributed to previous pelvic inflammatory disease (Clark and Baranyai, 1987; Svenstrup et al., 2008). Infection with certain types of the human papillomavirus can lead to the development of genital cancers, particularly cervical cancer in women.

2.2 STIs and adverse outcomes of pregnancy

Untreated STIs are associated with congenital and perinatal infections in neonates, particularly in regions where rates of infection remain high. In pregnant women with untreated early syphilis, 25% of pregnancies result in stillbirth and 14% in neonatal death – an overall perinatal mortality of about 40%. Up to 35% of pregnancies among women with untreated gonococcal infection result in spontaneous abortions and premature deliveries, and up to 10% in perinatal deaths. In the absence of prophylaxis, 30 - 50% of infants born to mothers with untreated gonorrhoea and up to 30% of infants born to mothers with untreated chlamydial infection will develop a serious eye infection (ophthalmia neonatorum), which can lead to blindness if not treated early. Worldwide, 1000 - 4000 newborn babies become blind every year because of this condition.

2.3 STIs and HIV

The presence of untreated STIs (both those which cause ulcers or those which do not) increase the risk of both acquisition and transmission of HIV by a factor of up to 10. Prompt treatment for STIs is thus important to reduce the risk of HIV infection. Controlling STIs is important for preventing HIV infection, particularly in people with high-risk sexual behaviours.

An estimated 34 million people were living with HIV globally at the end of 2010 including 3.4 million children less than 15 (WHO, 2011). There was 2.7 million new HIV infections in 2010, including 390 000 among children less than 15. Globally, the annual number of people newly infected with HIV continues to decline, although there is stark regional variation. In sub-Saharan Africa, where most of the people newly infected with HIV live, an estimated 1.9 million people became infected in 2010. This was 16% fewer than the estimated 2.2 million people newly infected with HIV in 2001 and 27% fewer than the annual number of people newly infected between 1996 and 1998, when the incidence of HIV in sub-Saharan Africa peaked overall.

The annual number of people dying from AIDS-related causes worldwide is steadily decreasing from a peak of 2.2 million in 2005 to an estimated 1.8 million in 2010. The number of people dying from AIDS-related causes began to decline in 2005–2006 in sub-Saharan Africa, South and South-East Asia and the Caribbean and has continued subsequently. In 2010, an estimated 250 000 children less than 15 died from AIDS-related causes, 20% fewer than in 2005.

Introducing antiretroviral therapy has averted 2.5 million deaths in low- and middle-income countries globally since 1995. Sub-Saharan Africa accounts for the vast majority of the averted deaths: about 1.8 million. Providing antiretroviral prophylaxis to pregnant women living with HIV has prevented more than 350 000 children from acquiring HIV infection since 1995. Eighty-six per cent of the children who avoided infection live in sub-Saharan Africa, the region with the highest prevalence of HIV infection among women of reproductive age.

The Political Declaration on HIV/AIDS, adopted in June 2011 by the United Nations General Assembly, set ambitious targets aimed at achieving universal access and the health-related Millennium Development Goals by 2015. The WHO Global Health Sector Strategy on HIV/AIDS, 2011–2015, the UNAIDS 2011-2015 Strategy: Getting to Zero, and the UNICEF's strategic and programmatic focus on equity will help to guide national and global efforts to respond to the epidemic and move from an emergency response to a long-term, sustainable model of delivering HIV services.

2.4 STI syndromic approach

The traditional method of diagnosing STIs is by laboratory tests. However, these are often unavailable or too expensive. Since 1990 WHO has recommended a syndromic approach for the diagnosis and management of STIs in patients presenting with consistently recognized signs and symptoms of particular STIs (WHO fact sheet 2011). The syndromic approach uses flowcharts to guide diagnosis and treatment is more accurate than diagnosis based on clinical tests alone, even in experienced hands. The syndromic approach is a scientific approach and offers accessible and immediate treatment that is effective. It is also more cost-effective for some syndromes than use of laboratory tests. The pathogens causing any particular syndrome need to be determined locally and flow charts adapted accordingly. Furthermore, regular monitoring of the organisms causing each syndrome should be conducted on a regular basis to validate the treatment recommendations.

3. Genital ulcers and warts

Genital ulcers are mainly observed in the following STI's:

i. Syphilis caused by *Treponema pallidum*
ii. Chancroid caused by *Haemophilus ducreyi*
iii. Genital Herpes caused by Herpes Simplex virus
iv. Lymphogranuloma venereum (LGV) caused by *C. trachomatis*
v. Donovanosis caused by *Calymmatobacterium granulomatosis*

Genital warts are mainly observed in the following STI's

i. Human papilloma virus infection
ii. Molluscum contagiosum (caused by member of poxvirus family)

3.1 General epidemiological features

Syphilis: is a sexually transmitted disease (STD) caused by the bacterium *Treponema pallidum.* It has often been called "the great imitator" because so many of the signs and symptoms are indistinguishable from those of other diseases.

According to Centers for Disease Control and Prevention (CDC fact sheet-syphilis) estimates, in the United States, health officials reported over 36,000 cases of syphilis in 2006, including 9,756 cases of primary and secondary (P&S) syphilis. In 2006, half of all P&S syphilis cases were reported from 20 counties and 2 cities; and most P&S syphilis cases occurred in persons 20 to 39 years of age. The incidence of P&S syphilis was highest in women 20 to 24 years of age and in men 35 to 39 years of age. Reported cases of congenital syphilis in newborns increased from 2005 to 2006, with 339 new cases reported in 2005 compared to 349 cases in 2006.

Between 2005 and 2006, the number of reported P&S syphilis cases increased 11.8 percent. P&S rates have increased in males each year between 2000 and 2006 from 2.6 to 5.7 and among females between 2004 and 2006. In 2006, 64% of the reported P&S syphilis cases were among men who have sex with men (MSM).

The overall syphilis rate decreased for the first time in a decade, and is down 1.6 percent since 2009 (STD Trends US 2010). However, the rate among young black men has increased dramatically over the past five years (134 percent). There is a significant increase in syphilis among young black men who have sex with men (MSM), suggesting that new infections among MSM are driving the increase in young black men. There has also been a sharp increase in HIV infections among this population (STD Trends in the United States: 2010).

Chancroid: Since 1987, reported cases of chancroid had declined steadily until 2001. Since then, the number of cases reported has fluctuated. In 2010, a total of 24 cases of chancroid were reported in the United States. Only nine states reported one or more cases of chancroid in 2010 (CDC STD surveillance 2010). Although the overall decline in reported chancroid cases most likely reflects a decline in the incidence of this disease, these data should be interpreted with caution because *Haemophilus ducreyi*, the causative organism of chancroid, is difficult to culture, and as a result, this condition may be substantially underdiagnosed.

Genital Herpes: In US, Seroprevalence decreased from 21% in 1988–1994 to 17.0% in 1999–2004 and 16.2% in 2005–2008. These data also indicate that blacks had higher seroprevalence than whites for each survey period and age group. During 2005–2008, a survey reported a diagnosis of genital herpes was 18.9% in age group of 20–49 years . Although HSV-2 seroprevalence is decreasing, most persons with HSV-2 have were not diagnosed. An increase in the number of visits for genital herpes, may indicate increased recognition of infection.

Lymphogranuloma venereum (LGV): LGV is a rare disease in industrialised countries, but is endemic in parts of Africa, Asia, South America, and the Caribbean. Its epidemiology is poorly defined, since it cannot be distinguished clinically from other causes of genital ulceration with bubo formation—for example, chancroid, and it is difficult to diagnose with confidence in the laboratory. Clinic based series of patients with genital ulcer suggest that it is an uncommon cause of genital ulceration in Africa.(Htun et al., 1998; Behets et al., 1999) Ten per cent of patients with buboes presenting to an STD clinic in Bangkok were found to have LGV,3 and a large epidemic of LGV has been reported recently among "crack" cocaine users in the Bahamas (Bauwens et al., 2002).

Donovanosis: Even though this illness has been described for more than a century, it is frequently neglected because of its occurrence in unspecified geographical locations and with infrequent incidences. Therefore, its pathogenesis and epidemiology are not completely understood and require study (Veeranna and Raghu, 2003).

This illness is more common in Afro-Americans, in individuals with a lower socio-economic status, and among those untrained in hygiene. It is endemic in tropical and subtropical climates, such as Papua New Guinea, South Africa (provinces of KwaZulu/Natal and East Transvaal), parts of India and Indonesia, and among the aborigines of Australia. Some cases have been reported in the countries of Central America and the Caribbean, Peru (where the first cause of chronic genital ulcers in patients with immune deficiency disorder have been found), Argentina, French Guiana and Brazil. This is an illness which touches almost exclusively adults between the ages of 20 and 40 years. There are no reports of congenital infections as a result of fetal infections.(O'Farrell, 2002) However, cases have been reported in nursing and newborn babies. Cases in children are frequently associated with contact with infected adults, though not necessarily because of sexual abuse.

Human papilloma virus infection: CDC estimates in US, during 2003-2005 documented an overall high-risk HPV prevalence of 23%. Prevalence was 27% in STD clinics, 26% in family planning clinics, and 15% in primary care clinics. Prevalence by age group was 35% in women aged 14-19 years, 29% in those aged 20-29, 13% in those aged 30-39, 11% in those aged 40-49, and 6.3% in those aged 50-65 (Datta et al., 2008).

3.2 Genital ulcers

Infectious genital lesions are unique in a number of ways when compared with other infectious processes. Most are communicable and therefore are not only a clinical concern but also a public concern. Infectious genital lesion can harbour more than one pathogen at a time, making proper diagnosis and management a challenge (Dillon et al., 1997). Morphologic appearance of the ulcer or lesion itself can differ widely from one process to another and even within any single specific pathology. The unpredictable nature of lesion presentation can also make a purely clinical diagnosis unreliable. Inflammatory epithelial defects characteristic of these pathologies appear to enhance the transmission of other diseases, most importantly human immunodeficiency virus (HIV). Genital lesions may contribute substantially to the worldwide spread of this disease (Greenblatt et al., 1988). Genital ulcer disease involves a disruption of the skin and mucous membranes of the genitalia. Individuals who present with a new genital lesion and who report recent sexual activity, particularly activity with a new partner or someone with a suspected genital infection, are likely to have a sexually transmitted infection. On the other hand, certain clinical circumstances suggest non-sexually transmitted pathology, such as trauma, chemical or allergic hypersensitivity (latex allergy associated with latex condoms). A lesion that occurs proximate to sexual exposure (i.e., within hours to 1 or 2 days) may be too early to be accounted by infectious pathologies, due to variable period of incubation.

Host factors can be important historical determinants of genital lesion etiology. Patients with pre-existing psoriasis or eczema or other noninfectious dermatitides may have a genital lesion related to the underlying dermatologic pathology. Fixed drug eruption can be caused by medication such as tetracyclines or antineoplastics in a patient presenting with new genital lesion. In these cases, lesions may be characterized by pigmentation or superficial ulceration (Pandhi et al., 1984). Autoimmune diseases, such as Reiter's syndrome, Crohn's disease or Behcet's syndrome, may be associated with genital lesions (Morgan et al., 1988; Keat, 1999). The important non-infectious causes of genital ulcers have to be kept in mind in the while keeping the differential diagnosis of gential ulcers. The clinical manifestations of infectious causes of genital ulcers is described below:

3.3 Signs and symptoms

In men lesions are found on or under the prepuce, around the coronal sulcus, on the shaft of the penis, the scrotum, the perianal tissue, the inner thighs or the rectum. In the female patients, sites of involvement are equally varied. Genital lesions can appear on the mons pubis, the labia, the fourchette, anywhere in the vagina, on the cervix, the inner thighs or the perianal tissue. As a result of orogenital sex, pathogens such as HSV and syphilis can also cause orolabial lesions. Lesions of chancroid can be disseminated from the genitalia and original site of infection to distant parts, by a process of autoinoculation, although this is not common (Asin, 1952). In secondary syphilis, sometimes spirochetemia causes lesions widely dispersed from the genitalia that morphologically range from the classic papulosquamid rash of the palms and soles to the moist, raised lesions of condylomata lata (genitals) or mucous patches (orolabial area). *Neisseria gonorrhoeae,* pathogen not commonly associated with genital lesions, may disseminate and cause tender, necrotic pustules primarily on the distal extremities as part of arthritis-dermatitis syndrome (Holmes et al., 1971). Lesions associated with scabies infestation are common in the genital region as well as intertriginous areas elsewhere. Genital edema can occur after any local inflammatory process (Wright and Judson, 1979).

3.4 Pain, dysesthesias and systemic symptoms

The lesion of syphilis, lymphogranuloma venereum (LGV), scabies, and molluscum contagiosum are ordinarily painless. Granuloma inguinale (donovanosis), a genital ulcer disease seen primarily in the tropics, is caused by the bacillus *Calymmatobacterium granulomatis.* Although the lesions of this disease are often large and destructive, but it is painless. Most patients with exophytic genital warts are asymptomatic; a few may report pain or pruritus. Herpetic lesions, chancroid ulcers are typically painful. Genital lesions from immunologically mediated non-infectious causes may also be tender. Pain or other dysesthesias, including pruritis may precede the development of a recurrent disease. Pruritus is common only with ectoparasitic infestations such as scabies or lice. The pruritus associated with scabies is often described as intense and worse at night. Although pruritus may be experienced by individuals with herpes or syphilis, it is not characteristic of these conditions. Fever is occasionally seen with secondary syphilis and with primary herpes simplex infection (Brookes et al., 1992). Headache, fatigue, myalgias and malaise may also accompany these infections (Chapel, 1980). The summary of clinical features of genital ulcer disease is detailed in Table 1.

3.5 Lymphadenopathy (LAP)

Inguinal lymphadenopathy is a nonspecific finding that is characteristic of inflammatory pathology almost anywhere in the groin or either lower extremity. It often accompanies genital infection. Although the inguinal and femoral lymph nodes drain the genital region in both men and women, the inner segment of the vagina and the cervix drain into deep pelvic and perirectal lymph nodes. If these lymph are involved in inflammatory genital pathology, pelvic or rectal discomfort may be the most striking symptom.

Bilateral painless inguinal lymphadenopathy is typical in syphilis. In secondary syphilis, lymphadenopathy distant from the genital area is common. LAP associated with a herpetic genital lesion is usually bilateral and it is also tender. LGV and chancroid are characterized by expansive, tender lymph nodes called buboes. These may be unilateral or bilateral. A central area of fluctuance often develops; if left untreated. It eventually ruptures. Lymphadenitis is unusual in granuloma inguinale.

3.6 Lesion morphology

Herpes infections are characterized by vesicles that evolve into pustules and finally to shallow ulcers on an erythematous base. Multiple lesions are common which may erupt in clusters and coalesce to form a wide variety of shapes and sizes.

Syphilitic chancres are typically solitary although they may rarely occur in pairs. They are round and 1 to 2 cm in diameter, with clean margins that are indurated on palpation. The ulcer base usually lacks exudates until and unless they are super infected with other bacteria. The lesions of secondary syphilis are not chancre-like. They may start anywhere as fine, circumferential scale. In warm, moist areas such as the buttocks and genitals, unique lesions of secondary syphilis known as condylomata lata develop. These are raised, moist nodules or plaques that are teeming with treponemes. They are highly infectious.

Chancroid lesions are similar in size to syphilitic chancres but their edges are ragged and undermined. The ulcer base is necrotic with a purulent exudates. Compared with the lesions of syphilis, induration of chancroid lesions tends to be less prominent, accounting for the designation of these ulcers as "soft chancres". Despite the obvious tissue damage, adjacent inflammation is absent. Usually lesions are solitary but multiple lesions may be seen.

The lesions of granuloma inguinale start as firm subcutaneous nodules or papules that eventually ulcerate. Typically, this ulcerative process becomes hypertrophic and beefy and bleeds easily. Local tissue destruction may be extensive. Occasionally, lesions are confused with squamous cell carcinoma.

Lymphogranuloma venereum (LGV) is caused by *Chlamydia trachomatis* serovars L1, L2 and L3. At its earliest stage, LGV may cause a small papule or herpes-like ulcer. This is usually asymptomatic and resolves before recognition.

Clinically visible lesions of HPV are typically caused by viral types with low oncogenic potential (i.e. types 6 and 11). Most HPV infections are asymptomatic. Lesions may occur as flat or relatively inconspicuous papules to verrucous, pedunculated or large cauliflower like masses referred to as condylomata acuminate.

Molluscum contagiosum causes benign, wart like lesions. The etiologic agent of this condition is a member of poxvirus family.

Lesions of scabies infestation range from papules to nodules with a surrounding crust. With scratching, these lesions are often modified by excoriations or lichenification. The use of systemic or topical antimicrobial agents before clinical evaluation have a dramatic effect on lesion morphology.

3.7 Duration

Without therapy, herpes ulcers resolve within 3 weeks in cases of primary infection and recurrence resolves in 5 to 10 days. In immunocompromised patients it may persist for longer than 3 to 4 weeks. Syphilitic chancres and condylomata lata also resolve without therapy, usually between 3 and 12 weeks and usually without much scarring (Larsen et al 1995). Without therapy, the lesions of chancroid and donovanosis are slowly destructive. Scarring is typical in both these conditions. Lesions caused by HPV or molluscum contagiosum may persist unchanged for a prolonged time or they may alternate with brief periods of resolution.

3.8 Laboratory diagnosis

Laboratory tests are critical to the diagnosis and proper management of genital ulcer disease. Direct microscopic examinations e.g. dark field microscopy or direct fluorescent staining can be performed on lesion exudates or a biopsy sample, which helps in making a diagnosis. Gram staining is not usually helpful in the evaluation of genital lesions. Lesion exudates is typically laden with a variety of non-pathogenic organisms common to genitourinary and perirectal flora. Under ideal conditions, *Haemophilus ducreyi* appears as a gram negative slender rod or coccobacillus that align in a pattern referred to as "school of fish". Experienced microbiologist is required to recognize this pattern. *H. ducreyi* can be cultivated on special nutrient media using Mueller-hinton-based chocolate agar, supplemented with 1% IsoVitaleX and 3µg/mL vancomycin to inhibit the growth of other organisms (Trees and Morse, 1995). The rarity of this organism in the developed world and the expense and limited shelf life of the media make isolation of *H. ducreyi* difficult and uncommon.

Light microscopy of syphilis chancre exudates is not useful. The spirochetes are extremely thin and do not take up standard stains. Darkfield microscopy of lesion exudates from either a chancre or condylomata lata can identify spirochetes. Spirochetes appear as tightly coiled, white organisms spirally rotating against the black background of the microscopic field. To perform a proper darkfield examination, ulcers must be cleaned with gauze and saline. Exudates from the lesion is then pressed against a glass slide. The specimen should not be contaminated with too much of blood. A cover slip is then applied. Rapid examination of the specimen is essential, because desiccation reduces the viability of organisms. In vitro *T. pallidum* can not be cultured. Other diagnostic methods include direct fluorescent antibody testing and silver staining methods.

Serological testing is the most commonly used method for the diagnosis of syphilitic genital lesions. The process requires two steps: a screening test that detects serum antibodies to nontreponemal antigens (e.g., rapid plasma regain [RPR] test, Venereal Disease Research Laboratory [VDRL] test) and then a confirmatory test that detects serum antibody to specific treponemal antigens (e.g., fluorescent treponemal antibody absorbed [FTA-ABS] test, *Treponema pallidum* particle agglutination assay [TPPA]. Early after the appearance of the syphilitic chancre, only the treponemal specific test may be reactive. Repeat testing with the nontreponemal test should be considered at some time after the ulcer has formed. In rare situations, the nontreponemal test may be falsely nonreactive in secondary syphilis due to the blocking effect of excess antibody; this is known as prozone phenomenon. Repeat testing should be performed on diluted serum samples. The cardiolipin antigens used in the detection of reaginic antibodies yield a large number of false-positive tests in many conditions other than syphilis, such as viral infections or autoimmune diseases (as a result of damage in the host's tissue). False-positive reactions have also been reported in a variety of acute and chronic diseases, such as mixed connective tissue disease, autoimmune disease, diabetes mellitus, alcoholic cirrhosis, viral infections, and pregnancy (Carlsson et al., 1991). VDRL has a prognostic significance also as it becomes non reactive after the successful treatment. Ordinarily the nontreponemal serologic test reaches its highest titer in secondary disease and declines with the onset of latency or with effective treatment (Larsen et al., 1995).

Herpes simplex virus (HSV) infected genital lesions can be identified by light microscopy using Tzanck smear. In this process, epithelial cells are scraped from an ulcer base and stained with Giemsa stain. Multinucleated giant cells and intranuclear inclusions are characteristics of HSV infections. However, both the sensitivity and specificity of the Tzanck smear are poor (Solomon et al., 1986). When available, conventional cell culture provides a relatively accurate diagnosis. Though the culture is considered to be the gold standard, it has drawback due to low sensitivity and is time consuming. Fluorescent monoclonal antibodies can be used to detect the surface antigens in smears prepared from ulcer scrapings. Molecular techniques like polymerase chain reaction targeting HSV DNA polymerase, glycoprotein D encoding regions have been successfully used to diagnose the genital herpes. Serological test, detecting IgG antibodies is not useful in diagnosing acute genital lesions.

Calymmatobacterium granulomatis, the cause of granuloma inguinale or donovanosis can be identified by staining scrapings of a lesion base with either Wright's or Giemsa's stain. Surface cells alone may not harbour the organism, so biopsy is often necessary. Clusters of blue rods, with prominent polar granules and surrounded by pink capsules are seen within infected epithelial cells and are known as Donovan bodies. Cultivation is difficult.

The diagnosis of LGV is usually based on clinical criteria. Isolation by cell culture or polymerase chain reaction of *C. Trachomatis* from bubo drainage is diagnostic. The serological test like complement fixation test and microimmunofluorescence techniques are not widely available in the diagnostic laboratories outside research centres.

The lesions of HPV are diagnosed primarily by their clinical appearance and can be assessed by cytologic methods (e.g., Papanicolaou smear) or biopsy. Infestation with ectoparasites such as *Sarcoptes scabiei* is demonstrated by identification of the organism, eggs or faeces under light microscopy. This may require the unroofing of the scabies burrow bluntly with a needle or scalpel. Nucleic acid detection is an increasingly common means of diagnosing infectious diseases. Efforts have been made to apply this technology to the diagnosis of some of the more common genital lesions. Nucleic acid detection can be performed with use of hybridization techniques, amplification techniques like PCR, TMA (transcription mediated amplification), ligase chain reaction (LCR). PCR test have been developed for *H. ducreyi(Johnson et al., 1994), T. pallidum(Liu et al., 2001) and* HSV(Cone et al., 1991). These technologies have also been combined in one "multiplex" platform to aid in the clinical evaluation of genital lesions. The role of such tests in current clinical practice is undefined.

	Syphilis	Chancroid	Genital herpes	Lymphogranuloma Venereum	Donovanosis
Incubation period	Avg. 21 d Range 3-90 d	2-7 d Range 1-35 d	2-7 d	Avg. 10-14 d Range 3d - 3 wk	Variable
Number of lesions	Usually single, occasionally multiple	1-3; may be multiple	Multiple; may coalesce	Usually single	Single or multiple
Border	Sharply demarcated	Erythematous and undermined	Erythematous	Variable	Rolled and elevated
Base	Red, smooth; shiny or crusty	Yellow, gray; rough	Red, smooth	Variable	Red, rough, may be friable, beefy granulations
Induration	Firm	Rare, soft	None	None	Firm
Pain	Painless; pain may occur with secondary infection	Common	Common	Variablc	Rare
Lymphnodes	Unilateral to bilateral; nontender, firm	Usually unilateral; may suppurate	Usually bilateral; firm and tender	Unilateral or bilateral; firm tender, later indolent, may suppurate, groove sign present	Pseudo-adenopathy, inguinal swelling
Constitutional symptoms	Rare	Rare	Common in primary disease	Frequent	Rare

Table 1. Summary of clinical features of genital ulcer disease(Wilson and Sande).

3.9 Complications

All genital ulcers are prone to secondary bacterial infections with a variety of genital bacteria. Additionally, edema of the foreskin in uncircumcised men may produce phimosis. Without treatment, chancres of primary syphilis and lesions of genital herpes heal spontaneously. Patients with syphilis progress into the secondary stage, whereas those with genital herpes may later experience recurrence of their lesions. The ulcers of chancroid and LGV continue to grow slowly by local extension and can produce further tissue and organ damage. LGV may further lead to perianal abscesses and rectovaginal, rectovesical and anal fistulas and strictures. Lymphatic obstruction and edema may occur. Rectal LGV is associated with an increased incidence of rectal cancer. Complications of donovanosis scarring include urethral, vaginal and anal strictures and lymphedema of the external genitalia.

3.10 Treatment

Syphilis: Penicillin remains the treatment of choice for any stage of syphilis. For the penicillin allergic patient, doxycycline or tetracycline is treatment of choice.

Chancroid: A single dose of intramuscular ceftriaxone or oral azithromycin or 7 days of erythromycin are recommended first-line treatments. Alternative therapies include amoxicillin/clavulanic acid or ciprofloxacin. Fluctuant adenopathy may require needle aspiration or drainage.

Genital Herpes: Uncomplicated genital herpes heals spontaneously. Treatment is available to decrease viral shedding and shorten the duration of illness. For first episode genital herpes, oral acyclovir, valacyclovir or famciclovir is recommended for 10 days. For recurrent disease, any one of these regimens can be given for an additional 5 days. Suppressive therapy is recommended for patients with severe and frequent recurrent episodes of genital herpes.

4. Urethritis

Urethritis is the most common sexually transmitted disease (STD) syndrome recognized in men and is frequently seen in women with coinciding cervicitis. Cases can be of two types, gonococcal urethritis and nongonococcal urethritis (NGU), based on the presence or absence of *Neiserria gonorrhoeae*. The two forms are not mutually exclusive. Coinfection with *Neiserria gonorrhoeae and Chlamydia trachomatis or Ureaplasma urealyticum* occurs in 15-25% of heterosexual men with urethritis. Other agents which can cause NGU are *Trichomonas vaginalis*, Herpes simplex virus, *Mycoplasma genitalium, Candida spp.* NGU that occurs soon after curative therapy for gonorrhoea is called as postgonococcal urethritis (PGU).

The Centers for Disease Control and prevention estimates that NGU is 2.5-fold more prevalent than gonococcal urethritis in the United States and much of the developed world. However, gonococcal urethritis accounts for upto 80% of acute urethritis cases in certain underdeveloped regions of the world. Among people of higher socioeconomic status and college students, NGU is more common. In urban STD clinics, gonococcal urethritis is more common.

4.1 Gonococcal urethritis

N. gonorrhoeae is a gram-negative intracellular coccus that characteristically grows in pairs (diplococci). Over the last 25 years, the prevalence of penicillin and tetracycline-resistant gonococci has been increasing worldwide, requiring alternative treatment strategies. *N gonorrhoeae* may not be limited to uethritis only but coinfection of the cervix, rectum or pharynx may also be there. Some patients may also present with disseminated infection.

4.2 Non-Gonococcal Urethritis (NGU)

Nongonoccocal urethritis (NGU), which is suspected when examination findings and microscopy indicate inflammation and Gram-negative intracellular diplococci (GNID) can not be observed in stained smears and/ or culture. *C. trachomatis is the most common etiological agent leading to NGU,* in 15%-40% of cases; however, prevalence varies by age group, with a lower burden of disease occurring among older men (Bradshaw et al., 2006). Complications of NGU among males infected with *C. trachomatis*include epididymitis and Reiter's syndrome. Documentation of chlamydial infection is essential because of the need for partner referral for evaluation and treatment. In most cases of nonchlamydial NGU, no pathogen can be detected. *M. genitalium*, which appears to be sexually transmitted, is associated with both symptoms of urethritis and urethral inflammation and accounts for 15%–25% of NGU cases in the United States (Taylor-Robinson et al., 2004; Manhart et al., 2007). *T. vaginalis*, HSV, and adenovirus also can cause NGU, but data supporting other *Mycoplasma* species and *Ureaplasma* as etiologic agents are inconsistent. Diagnostic and treatment procedures for these organisms are reserved for situations in which these infections are suspected (e.g., contact with trichomoniasis, genital lesions, or severe dysuria and meatitis, which might suggest genital herpes) or when NGU is not responsive to therapy. Enteric bacteria have been identified as an uncommon cause of NGU and might be associated with insertive anal intercourse.

4.3 Diagnosis

Clinicians should attempt to obtain objective evidence of urethral inflammation. However, if clinic-based diagnostic tools (e.g., Gram-stain microscopy) are not available, patients should be treated with drug regimens effective against both gonorrhea and chlamydia. The clinically distinguishing features of gonococcal and nongonococcal urethritis are detailed in Table 2. Urethritis can be documented on the basis of any of the following signs and/ or laboratory tests:

- Mucopurulent or purulent discharge on examination.
- Gram stain of urethral secretions demonstrating ≥5 WBC per oil immersion field. The Gram stain is the preferred rapid diagnostic test for evaluating urethritis and is highly sensitive and specific for documenting both urethritis and the presence or absence of gonococcal infection. Gonococcal infection is established by documenting the presence of WBC containing gram-negative intracellular diplococci (GNID).
- Positive leukocyte esterase test on first-void urine or microscopic examination of first-void urine sediment demonstrating ≥10 WBC per high-power field.

If the urethral Gram stain is negative for gonococci, a culture should be done. *N. gonorrhoeae* is a fastidious organism requiring a selective growth medium in a carbon dioxide rich environment. Selective growth media include Thayer-Martin, Martin Lewis and New York city media. Nonculture or rapid diagnostic tests for gonococcal infection include Gonozyme, the Gen-Probe Pace 2 and the ligase chain reaction (LCR). Gonozyme is an enzyme immunoassay that can detect gonococcal antigens within urethra, cervix and urine. The gen-probe pace 2 use nonisotopic probes to detect ribosomal RNA. LCR utilizes a DNA amplification technique to detect trace amounts of organism-specific nucleic acid sequences from uretheral and endo-cervical swab specimens and urine samples.

4.4 Detection of *C. trachomatis*

Cell culture is considered to be the gold standard for chlamydial testing (Gottlieb et al., 2010). It has a sensitivity of 75-80% and a specificity approaching 100%. The addition of an enzyme immunoassay to culture increases the sensitivity to 95%. Cultures are expensive and may require 3-7 days for results. Nonculture rapid diagnostic tests, including direct fluorescence antibody (DFA) test, enzyme linked immunoassay test (EIA) and DNA probe tests, provide a more prompt diagnosis than culture with roughly an equivalent specificity (Su et al., 2011) The sensitivity is 70-90%. The Gen-Probe Pace 2 and LCR assays detect rRNA and DNA sequences, respectively of both *N. gonorrhoeae and C. trachomatis*. The sensitivity is higher than that of cell cultures without compromise in specificity.

If none of these criteria are present, testing for *N. gonorrhoeae* and *C. trachomatis* using nucleic acid amplification tests (NAATs) might identify additional infections. If the results demonstrate infection with either of these pathogens, the appropriate treatment should be given and sex partners referred for evaluation and treatment. If none of these criteria are present, empiric treatment of symptomatic males is recommended only for men at high risk for infection who are unlikely to return for a follow-up evaluation. Such patients should be treated with drug regimens effective against Gonorrhea and Chlamydia. Partners of patients treated empirically should be evaluated and treated, if indicated.

4.5 Detection of other pathogens

U. urealyticum is identified by culture. Because *U. urealyticum* can be isolated in men without urethritis, a positive culture for *U. urealyticum* may not necessarily indicate the cause of urethritis. The rapid and less expensive method for the diagnosis of trichomoniasis is the direct microscopic wet mount examination of vaginal or urethral discharge. The accuracy of the exam is based on identifying motile protozoa with characteristic morphology. The wet mount exam is routinely used to evaluate women for vaginal trichomoniasis (50-70% sensitive) but is less sensitive with urethral discharge from infected men. The gold standard for diagnosing of trichomoniasis is isolating the protozoa in culture.

4.6 Treatment

Gonococcal Urethritis: Uncomplicated urethritis can be treated with Ceftriaxone 250 mg intramuscular single dose, or Cefixime 400 mg PO single dose. In 1976, penicillin-resistant gonococci were identified and found to have acquired plasmids encoding for the production of beta-lactamase. Approximately 15% of all gonococci in the United States are now penicillin resistant. In some urban areas, the incidence is as high as 60-75%. In 1985, tetracycline-resistant gonococci were identified and also found to have plasmid encoded resistance (Johnson et al., 1988). Tetracycline resistant gonococci are responsible for upto 15% of gonococcal infections along the eastern coast of the United States. *N. gonorrhoeae* with chromosomal mutations conferring penicillin and tetracycline resistance has also been identified. Because of the increasing frequency of penicillin and tetracycline resistant gonococci, the penicillins and tetracyclines are no longer recommended. Quinolone resistant gonococci have also been identified.

Intramuscular ceftriaxone cures nearly 100% of genital infections and is effective for the treatment of gonococcal infection at all sites. Ceftriaxone is also active against incubating syphilis. Oral cefixime is nearly as active against *N. gonorrhoeae* and is less expensive. For the beta-lactam-allergic patients, oral ciprofloxacin or ofloxacin is highly effective.

Many patients who experience symptomatic relief after a single dose treatment for gonococcal urethritis develop a prompt recurrence or persistence of milder symptoms. This syndrome is called postgonococcal urethritis (PGU) and is the result of dual infection of the urethra with *N gonorrhoeae* and organism of NGU (Gaydos et al., 2009). *N gonorrhoeae* is eradicated by a single dose of the aforementioned cephalosporins and quinolones but the organisms responsible for NGU are often spared. PGU should be suspected if signs, symptoms or laboratory evidence of urethritis is found 4-7 days after a single-dose treatment for gonococcal urethritis. Unless chlamydial infection has been specifically ruled out through testing, all patients treated for gonococcal infections should also be treated for chlamydial infections.

Treatment of NGU: Azithromycin and doxycycline are highly effective for chlamydial urethritis; however, infections with *M. genitalium* respond better to azithromycin. Single-dose regimens have the advantage of improved compliance and directly observed treatment. To maximize compliance with recommended therapies, medications should be dispensed on-site in the clinic, and the first dose should be directly observed. To minimize transmission, men treated for NGU should be instructed to abstain from sexual intercourse for 7 days after single-dose therapy or until completion of a 7-day regimen, provided their symptoms have resolved. To minimize the risk for reinfection, men should be instructed to abstain from sexual intercourse until all of their sex partners are treated.

Tetracycline/doxycyline resistant *U urealyticum* exist and is the basis of for treating patients with erythromycin who fail standard therapy. Treatment of urethritis due to *Trichomonas* is usually effective with a single oral dose of metronidazole.

Persons who have been diagnosed with a new STD should testing for other infections, including syphilis and HIV.

4.7 Follow-up

Patients should be instructed to return for evaluation if symptoms persist or recur after completion of therapy. Symptoms alone, without documentation of signs or laboratory evidence of urethral inflammation, are not a sufficient basis for retreatment. Providers should be alert to the possibility of chronic prostatitis/chronic pelvic pain syndrome in male patients experiencing persistent pain (perineal, penile, or pelvic), discomfort, irritative voiding symptoms, pain during or after ejaculation, or new-onset premature ejaculation lasting for >3 months.

Unless a patient's symptoms persist or therapeutic noncompliance or reinfection is suspected by the provider, a test-of-cure (i.e., repeat testing 3–4 weeks after completing therapy) is not recommended for persons with documented chlamydia or gonococcal infections who have received treatment with recommended or alterative regimens. However, because men with documented chlamydial or gonococcal infections have a high rate of reinfection within 6 months after treatment, repeat testing of all men diagnosed with chlamydia or gonorrhea is recommended 3–6 months after treatment, regardless of whether patients believe that their sex partners were treated.

Clinical finding	Gonorrhea	NGU
Onset of symptoms	Classically abrupt 75% men develop symptoms within 4 days; 80-90% men develop symptoms within 2 weeks	Less acute onset Approx. 50% men develop symptoms within 4 days
Frankly purulent urethral discharge	75%	11-33%
Mucopurulent discharge	25%	50%
Completely clear discharge	4%	10-50%
Dysuria	73-88%	53-75%

Table 2. Summary of clinical features of gonococcal and nongonococcal urethritis (Wilson and Sande).

5. Cervicitis

The microbial agents leading to cervicitis are:

i. *N. gonorrhoeae*
ii. *C. trachomatis*
iii. *T. vaginalis*
iv. Herpes simplex virus (HSV)
v. Human papilloma virus (HPV)

Two major diagnostic signs characterize cervicitis:

1. A purulent or mucopurulent endocervical exudate visible in the endocervical canal or on an endocervical swab specimen (commonly referred to as mucopurulent cervicitis or cervicitis)
2. Sustained endocervical bleeding easily induced by gentle passage of a cotton swab through the cervical os. Either or both signs might be present. Cervicitis frequently is asymptomatic, but some women complain of an abnormal vaginal discharge and intermenstrual vaginal bleeding (e.g., after sexual intercourse). A finding of leukorrhea (>10 WBC per high-power field on microscopic examination of vaginal fluid) has been associated with chlamydial and gonococcal infection of the cervix. In the absence of inflammatory vaginitis, leukorrhea might be a sensitive indicator of cervical inflammation with a high negative predictive value. Although some specialists consider an increased number of polymorphonuclear leukocytes on endocervical Gram stain as being useful in the diagnosis of cervicitis, this criterion has not been standardized. In addition, it has a low positive-predictive value (PPV) for infection with *C. trachomatis* and *N. gonorrhoeae* and is not available in most clinical settings. Finally, although the presence of GNID on Gram stain of endocervical fluid is specific for the diagnosis of gonococcal cervical infection, it is not a sensitive indicator, because it is observed in only 50% of women with this infection.

5.1 Etiology

Mainly *C. trachomatis* or *N. gonorrhoeae are the main etiological agents in patients suspected of cervicitis.*(Hosenfeld et al., 2009) Cervicitis can also be observed in trichomoniasis and genital herpes (especially primary HSV-2 infection). However, in most cases of cervicitis, no organism is isolated, especially in women at relatively low risk for recent acquisition of these STDs (e.g., women aged >30 years). Limited data indicate that infection with *M. genitalium* and bacterial vaginosis (BV) and frequent douching might cause cervicitis. For reasons that are unclear, cervicitis can persist despite repeated courses of antimicrobial therapy, because most persistent cases of cervicitis are not caused by relapse or reinfection with *C. trachomatis* or *N. gonorrhoeae*. Other factors (e.g., persistent abnormality of vaginal flora, douching, or idiopathic inflammation in the zone of ectopy) might be involved.

5.2 Diagnosis

Cervicitis might be a sign of upper-genital-tract infection (endometritis), and thus women who seek medical treatment for a new episode of cervicitis should be assessed for signs of pelvic inflammatory disease (PID) and should be tested for *C. trachomatis* and for *N. gonorrhoeae* with the sensitive and specific tests available. Women with cervicitis also should be evaluated for the presence of Add Bacterial Vaginosis (BV) and trichomoniasis, for indicating specific treatment. The sensitivity of microscopy to detect *T. vaginalis* is relatively low (approximately 50%), symptomatic women with cervicitis and negative microscopy for trichomonads should be subjected to sensitive tests (i.e., culture or other FDA-cleared method). Although HSV-2 infection has been associated with cervicitis, the utility of specific testing (i.e., culture or serologic testing) for HSV-2 in this setting is unknown. Standardized diagnostic tests for *M. genitalium* are not commercially available.

Nucleic acid amplification technique (NAAT) should be used for diagnosing *C. trachomatis* and *N. gonorrhoeae* in women with cervicitis; this testing can be performed on either vaginal, cervical, or urine samples. A finding of >10 WBC in vaginal fluid, in the absence of trichomoniasis, might indicate endocervical inflammation caused specifically by *C. trachomatis* or *N. gonorrhoeae*.

5.3 Treatment

Several factors should affect the decision to provide presumptive therapy for cervicitis or to await the results of diagnostic tests. Treatment with antibiotics for *C. trachomatis* should be provided for those women at increased risk for this common STD (e.g., those aged ≤25 years, those with new or multiple sex partners, and those who engage in unprotected sex), especially if follow-up cannot be ensured and if a relatively insensitive diagnostic test is used in place of NAAT. Concurrent therapy for *N. gonorrhoeae* is indicated if the prevalence of this infection is >5% (those in younger age groups and those living in certain facilities).

Trichomoniasis and BV, if detected should also be treated. For women in whom any component of (or all) presumptive therapy is deferred, the results of sensitive tests for *C. trachomatis* and *N. gonorrhoeae* (e.g., NAATs) should determine the need for treatment subsequent to the initial evaluation.

5.4 Recommended regimens for presumptive treatment

Azithromycin 1 g orally in a single dose or doxycycline 100 mg orally twice a day for 7 days

Concurrent treatment for gonococcal infection should be considered, if prevalence of gonorrhea is high in the patient population under assessment.

5.5 Recurrent and persistent cervicitis

Women with persistent cervicitis should be reevaluated for possible reexposure to an STD. If relapse and/or reinfection with a specific STD has been excluded, BV is not present, and sex partners have been evaluated and treated, management options for persistent cervicitis are undefined; in addition, the utility of repeated or prolonged administration of antibiotic therapy for persistent symptomatic cervicitis remains unknown. Women who receive such therapy should be followed up post-treatment so that a determination can be made regarding whether cervicitis has resolved. Research is needed on the etiology of persistent cervicitis including the potential role of *M. genitalium*. In women with persistent symptoms that are clearly attributable to cervicitis, referral to a gynecologic specialist can be considered.

5.6 Follow up

Follow-up should be conducted as recommended for the infections for which a woman is treated. If symptoms persist, women should be instructed to return for re-evaluation because women with documented chlamydial or gonococcal infections have a high rate of reinfection within 6 months after treatment. Therefore, repeat testing of all women for Chlamydia and/ or Gonococcus is recommended 3-6 months after treatment, regardless of whether their sex partners were treated.

5.7 Management of sex partners

Management of sex partners of women treated for cervicitis should be appropriate for the identified or suspected STD. Partners should be notified and examined if Chlamydia, Gonococcus, or *T. vaginalis* was identified or suspected in the index patient; these partners should then be treated for the STDs for which the index patient received treatment. To avoid reinfection, patients and their sex partners should abstain from sexual intercourse until therapy is completed (i.e., 7 days after a single-dose regimen or after completion of a 7-day regimen). Expedited partner treatment and patient referral are alternative approaches to treating male partners of women that have Chlamydia or gonococcal infections.

6. Sexually transmitted infections characterized by vaginal discharge

Most women will have a vaginal infection, characterized by discharge, itching, or odor, during their lifetime. Obtaining a medical history alone has been shown to be insufficient for accurate diagnosis of vaginitis and can lead to the inappropriate administration of medication. Therefore, a careful history, examination, and laboratory testing to determine the etiology of vaginal complaints are warranted. Information on sexual behaviors and practices, gender of sex partners, menstrual history, vaginal hygiene practices (such as douching), and other medications should be elicited. The three diseases most frequently associated with vaginal discharge are bacterial vaginosis (BV caused by the replacement of the vaginal flora by an overgrowth of anaerobic bacteria including *Prevotella* sp., *Mobiluncus* sp., *G. vaginalis, Ureaplasma, Mycoplasma,* and numerous fastidious or uncultivated anaerobes), trichomoniasis (caused by *T. vaginalis*), and candidiasis (usually caused by *Candida albicans*). The summary of clinical features of vaginitis is depicted in Table 3. Cervicitis also can sometimes cause a vaginal discharge. Although vulvovaginal candidiasis (VVC) usually is not transmitted sexually, it is included in this chapter because it is frequently diagnosed in women who have vaginal complaints or who are being evaluated for STDs.

Various diagnostic methods are available to identify the etiology of an abnormal vaginal discharge (Khan et al., 2009). Clinical laboratory testing can identify the cause of vaginitis in most women. The cause of vaginal symptoms might be determined by pH, a potassium hydroxide (KOH) test, and microscopic examination of fresh samples of the discharge on bed side examination. The pH of the vaginal secretions can be determined by narrow-range pH paper; an elevated pH (i.e., >4.5) is common with BV or trichomoniasis. Because pH testing is not highly specific, discharge should be further examined microscopically by first diluting one sample in one to two drops of 0.9% normal saline solution on one slide and a second sample in 10% KOH solution. Cover slips are then placed on the slides, and they are examined under a microscope at low and high power. Samples that emit an amine odor immediately upon application of KOH suggest BV or trichomoniasis infection.

The saline-solution specimen might yield motile *T. vaginalis*, or clue cells (i.e., epithelial cells with borders obscured by small bacteria), which are characteristic of BV, whereas the presence of WBCs without evidence of trichomonads or yeast is suggestive of cervicitis. The KOH specimen typically is used to identify the yeast or pseudohyphae of Candida species. However, the absence of trichomonads or pseudohyphae in KOH samples does not rule out these infections, because the sensitivity of microscopy is approximately 50% compared with NAAT or culture.

In settings where pH paper, KOH, and microscopy are not available, alternative commercially available point-of-care tests or clinical laboratory testing can be used to diagnose vaginitis. The presence of objective signs of vulvar inflammation in the absence of vaginal pathogens after laboratory testing, along with a minimal amount of discharge, suggests the possibility of mechanical, chemical, allergic, or other noninfectious irritation of the vulva.

6.1 Bacterial Vaginosis (BV)

BV is a polymicrobial clinical syndrome resulting from replacement of the normal hydrogen peroxide producing *Lactobacillus sp.* in the vagina with high concentrations of anaerobic bacteria (e.g.,*Prevotella* sp. and *Mobiluncus* sp.), *G. vaginalis, Ureaplasma, Mycoplasma,* and numerous fastidious or uncultivated anaerobes (Livengood, 2009). Some women experience transient vaginal microbial changes, whereas others experience them for a longer intervals of time. Among women attending hospital for routine checkup, BV is the most prevalent cause of vaginal discharge or malodour. BV is associated with having multiple male or female partners, a new sex partner, douching, lack of condom use, and lack of vaginal lactobacilli; women who have never been sexually active can also be affected. The cause of the microbial alteration that characterizes BV is not fully understood, nor is whether BV results from acquisition of a sexually transmitted pathogen. Nonetheless, women with BV are at increased risk for the acquisition of some STDs (e.g., HIV, *N. gonorrhoeae, C. trachomatis*, and HSV), complications after gynecologic surgery, complications of pregnancy, and recurrence of BV. Treatment of male sex partners has not been beneficial in preventing the recurrence of BV.

6.2 Diagnosis

BV can be diagnosed by the use of clinical criteria (i.e., Amsel's Diagnostic Criteria) or Gram stain. A Gram stain, considered the gold standard laboratory method for diagnosing BV, is used to determine the relative concentration of lactobacilli (i.e., long Gram-positive rods), Gram-negative and Gram-variable rods and cocci (i.e., *G. vaginalis, Prevotella, Porphyromonas, and peptostreptococci*), and curved Gram-negative rods (i.e., *Mobiluncus*) characteristic of BV (Khan et al., 2009). If a Gram stain is not available, clinical criteria can be used and require three of the following symptoms or signs:

- homogeneous, thin, white discharge that smoothly coats the vaginal walls;
- presence of clue cells on microscopic examination;
- pH of vaginal fluid >4.5;
- a fishy odor of vaginal discharge before or after addition of 10% KOH (i.e., the whiff test).

Detection of three of these criteria has been correlated with results by Gram stain. Other tests, including a DNA probe-based test for high concentrations of *G. vaginalis* (Affirm VP III, Becton Dickinson, Sparks, Maryland), a proline-aminopeptidase test card (Pip Activity TestCard, Quidel, San Diego, California), and the OSOM BVBlue test have acceptable performance characteristics compared with Gram stain. Although a card test is available for the detection of elevated pH and trimethylamine, it has low sensitivity and specificity and therefore is not recommended. PCR has been used in research settings for the detection of a variety of organisms associated with BV, but evaluation of its clinical utility is uncertain. Detection of one organism or group of organisms might be predictive of BV by Gram stain. However, additional evaluations are needed to confirm these associations. Culture of *G. vaginalis* is not recommended as a diagnostic tool because it is not specific. Cervical Pap tests have no clinical utility for the diagnosis of BV because of their low sensitivity.

6.3 Treatment

Treatment is recommended for women with symptoms. The established benefits of therapy in nonpregnant women are to relieve vaginal symptoms and signs of infection. Other potential benefits to treatment include reduction in the risk for acquiring *C. trachomatis* or *N. gonorrhoeae*, HIV, and other viral STDs.

Recommended drugs: Metronidazole 500 mg orally twice a day for 7 days, Metronidazole gel 0.75%, one full applicator (5 g) intravaginally, once a day for 5 days; Clindamycin cream 2%, one full applicator (5 g) intravaginally at bedtime for 7 days.

7. Trichomoniasis

Trichomoniasis is caused by the protozoan *T. vaginalis*.(Nanda et al., 2006) Few men who are infected with *T. Vaginalis* might not have symptoms; others have NGU. Few women have symptoms characterized by a diffuse, malodorous, yellow-green vaginal discharge with vulvar irritation. However, many women have minimal or no symptoms. Because of the high prevalence of trichomoniasis in clinical and nonclinical settings, testing for *T. vaginalis* should be performed in women seeking care for vaginal discharge. Screening for *T. vaginalis* in women can be considered in those at high risk for infection (i.e., women who have new or multiple partners, have a history of STDs, indulge in sexual activity for payment, and use injection drugs).

7.1 Treatment

Metronidazole 2 g orally in a single dose or Tinidazole 2 g orally in a single dose or Metronidazole 500 mg orally twice a day for 7 days.

8. Vulvovaginal Candidiasis (VVC)

VVC is usually caused by *C.albicans*, but occasionally is caused by other *Candida* sp. or yeasts. Typical symptoms of VVC include pruritus, vaginal soreness, dyspareunia, external dysuria, and abnormal vaginal discharge. However, none of these symptoms is specific for VVC. An estimated 75% of women will have at least one episode of VVC, and 40%-45% will have two or more episodes within their lifetime. On the basis of clinical presentation, microbiology, host factors, and response to therapy, VVC can be classified as either uncomplicated or complicated. Approximately 10%-20% of women will have complicated VVC that necessitates diagnostic and therapeutic considerations.

8.1 Uncomplicated VVC

Diagnostic Considerations: A diagnosis of *Candida* vaginitis is suggested clinically by the presence of external dysuria and vulvar pruritus, pain, swelling, and redness. Signs include vulvar edema, fissures, excoriations, or thick, curdy vaginal discharge. The diagnosis can be made in a woman who has signs and symptoms of vaginitis when either 1) a wet preparation (saline, 10% KOH) or Gram stain of vaginal discharge demonstrates yeasts, hyphae, or pseudohyphae or 2) a culture or other test yields a yeast species. *Candida* vaginitis is associated with a normal vaginal pH (<4.5), and therefore, pH testing is not a useful diagnostic tool. Use of 10% KOH in wet preparations improves the visualization of yeast and mycelia by disrupting cellular material that might obscure the yeast or pseudohyphae. Examination of a wet mount with KOH preparation should be performed for all women with symptoms or signs of VVC, and women with a positive result should receive treatment. For women with negative wet mounts who are symptomatic, vaginal cultures for *Candida* should be considered. If the wet mount is negative and *Candida* cultures cannot be done, empiric treatment can be considered for symptomatic women with any sign of VVC on examination. Identifying *Candida* by culture in the absence of symptoms or signs is not an indication for treatment, because approximately 10%-20% of women harbor *Candida* sp. and other yeasts in the vagina. VVC can occur concomitantly with STDs. Most healthy women with uncomplicated VVC have no identifiable precipitating factors.

8.2 Treatment

Short-course topical formulations e.g. Butoconazole 2% cream, Clotrimazole 2% cream, Miconazole 2% cream (i.e., single dose and regimens of 1-3 days) effectively treat uncomplicated VVC. The topically applied azole drugs are more effective than nystatin. Treatment with azoles results in relief of symptoms and negative cultures in 80%-90% of patients who complete therapy.

8.3 Complicated VVC

Recurrent Vulvovaginal Candidiasis (RVVC)

RVVC, usually defined as four or more episodes of symptomatic VVC in 1 year, affects a small percentage of women (<5%).(STD guidelines 2010) The pathogenesis of RVVC is poorly understood, and most women with RVVC have no apparent predisposing or underlying conditions. Vaginal cultures should be obtained from patients with RVVC to confirm the clinical diagnosis and to identify unusual species (including nonalbicans species), particularly *Candida glabrata*. Although *C. glabrata* and other nonalbicans *Candidia* species are observed in 10%-20% of patients with RVVC conventional antimycotic therapies are not as effective against these species as they are against *C. albicans*.

8.4 Treatment

Each individual episode of RVVC caused by *C. albicans* responds well to short-duration oral or topical azole therapy. However, to maintain clinical and mycologic control, some specialists recommend a longer duration of initial therapy (e.g., 7-14 days of topical therapy or a 100-mg, 150-mg, or 200-mg oral dose of fluconazole every third day for a total of 3 doses [day 1, 4, and 7]) to attempt mycologic remission before initiating a maintenance antifungal regimen.

Maintenance Regimens: Oral fluconazole (i.e., 100-mg, 150-mg, or 200-mg dose) weekly for 6 months is the first line of treatment. If this regimen is not feasible, topical treatments used intermittently as a maintenance regimen can be considered. Suppressive maintenance antifungal therapies are effective in reducing RVVC. However, 30%-50% of women will have recurrent disease after maintenance therapy is discontinued. Routine treatment of sex partners is controversial. *C. albicans* azole resistance is rare in vaginal isolates, and susceptibility testing is usually not warranted for individual treatment guidance.

Non albicans VVC

The optimal treatment of nonalbicans VVC remains unknown. Options include longer duration of therapy (7-14 days) with a nonfluconazole azole drug (oral or topical) as first-line therapy. If recurrence occurs, 600 mg of boric acid in a gelatin capsule is recommended, administered vaginally once daily for 2 weeks. This regimen has clinical and mycologic eradication rates of approximately 70%. If symptoms recur, referral to a specialist is advised.

	Normal	Vulvovaginal candidiasis	Trichomoniasis	Bacterial Vaginosis
Symptoms	None	Pruritis Soreness Dyspareunia	Soreness Dyspareunia Often asymptomatic	Often asymptomatic Occasional abdominal pain
Discharge **Amount** **Color** **Consistency**	Variable Clear/white Nonhomogenous floccular	Scant/moderate White Clumped, adherent	Profuse Green-yellow Homogenous, frothy	Moderate White/gray Homogenous adherent
Vaginal fluid pH	4.0-4.5	4.0-4.5	5.0-6.0	>4.5
Amine test (Fish odour)	None	None	Usually positive	Positive
Microscopy **Saline**	PMN:EC ratio <1 Lactobacilli predominate	PMN:EC ratio <1 Pseudohyphae (~40%)	PMN:EC ratio >1 Motile trichomonads PMNs predominate	PMN:EC ratio <1 Clue cells Coccobacilli
10% KOH	Negative	Pseudohyphae (~70%)	Negative	Negative

Table 3. Summary of clinical features of vaginitis (Wilson and Sande).

9. Pelvic Inflammatory Disease (PID)

PID comprises a spectrum of inflammatory disorders of the upper female genital tract, including any combination of endometritis, salpingitis, tubo-ovarian abscess, and pelvic peritonitis. Sexually transmitted organisms, especially *N. gonorrhoeae* and *C. trachomatis,* are implicated in many cases; however, microorganisms that comprise the vaginal flora e.g., anaerobes, *G. vaginalis, Haemophilus influenzae,* enteric Gram-negative rods, and *Streptococcus agalactiae,* also have been associated with PID. In addition, *M. hominis, U. urealyticum,* and *M. genitalium* might be associated with some cases of PID. All women who have acute PID should be tested for *N. gonorrhoeae* and *C. trachomatis* and should be screened for HIV infection. Symptoms of PID include abnormal cervical or vaginal discharge, abdominal pain and fever. On examination there may be cervical motion and adnexal and lower abdominal tenderness. It is important to diagnose and treat PID as early as possible. For patients requiring hospitalization, intravenous cefoxitin or cefotetan plus doxycyline (i/v or oral) can be given. Alternatively clindamycin plus gentamicin can be given followed by oral doxycycline. Outpatient treatments include oral ofloxacin plus metronidazole or ceftriaxone (or cefixitin and oral probenecid) plus oral doxycycline. Duration of intravenous treatment is dependent on the severity of the clinical presentation (Romanowski, 1993).

10. Epididymitis

In men under age 35, the most common pathogens are *N. gonorrhoeae* and *C. trachomatis(Trojian et al., 2009).* Homosexual men may have enteric pathogens from rectal intercourse. Unilateral testicular pain and tenderness are common. There is usually palpable swelling of the epididymis. The evaluation and diagnostic tests are the same as those for urethritis. Treatment includes ceftriaxone plus doxycyline or ofloxacin (Berger, 1991).

11. Proctitis

Proctitis acquired through receptive anal intercourse can be caused by *N. gonorrhoeae, C. trachomatis* (including LGV serovars), *T. pallidum* (syphilis) and HSV. Treatment includes ceftriaxone plus doxycyline.

12. Prevention

The most effective means to avoid becoming infected with or transmitting a sexually transmitted infection is to have sexual intercourse only within a long-term, mutually monogamous relationship with an uninfected partner and to abstain from sexual intercourse (i.e., oral, vaginal, or anal sex) with multiple partners. Male latex condoms, when used consistently and correctly, are highly effective in reducing the transmission of HIV and other sexually transmitted infections, including gonorrhoea, chlamydial infection and trichomoniasis. Prompt diagnosis and treatment of both the partners is the key for an effective management.

13. References

Asin, J. (1952). Chancroid; a report of 1,402 cases. Am J Syph Gonorrhea Vener Dis. 36(5), 483-7.

Bauwens, J. E., H. Orlander, M. P. Gomez, M. Lampe, S. Morse, W. E. Stamm, et al. (2002). Epidemic Lymphogranuloma venereum during epidemics of crack cocaine use and HIV infection in the Bahamas. Sex Transm Dis. 29(5), 253-9.

Behets, F. M., J. Andriamiadana, D. Randrianasolo, R. Randriamanga, D. Rasamilalao, C. Y. Chen, et al. (1999). Chancroid, primary syphilis, genital herpes, and lymphogranuloma venereum in Antananarivo, Madagascar. J Infect Dis. 180(4), 1382-5.

Berger, R. E. (1991). Acute epididymitis: etiology and therapy. Semin Urol. 9(1), 28-31.

Bradshaw, C. S., S. N. Tabrizi, T. R. Read, S. M. Garland, C. A. Hopkins, L. M. Moss, et al. (2006). Etiologies of nongonococcal urethritis: bacteria, viruses, and the association with orogenital exposure. J Infect Dis. 193(3), 336-45.

Brookes, J. L., S. Haywood and J. Green (1992). Prodromal symptoms in genital herpes simplex infection. Genitourin Med. 68(5), 347-8.

Carlsson, B., H. S. Hanson, J. Wasserman and A. Brauner (1991). Evaluation of the fluorescent treponemal antibody-absorption (FTA-Abs) test specificity. Acta Derm Venereol. 71(4), 306-11.

CDC fact sheet-syphilis: available at: http://www.cdc.gov/std/syphilis/STDFact-Syphilis.htm.

CDC Sexually transmitted surveillance 2010. Available at: http://www.cdc.gov/std/stats10/other.htm

Chapel, T. A. (1980). The signs and symptoms of secondary syphilis. Sex Transm Dis. 7(4), 161-4.

Clark, K. and J. Baranyai (1987). Pelvic infection and the pathogenesis of tubal ectopic pregnancy. Aust N Z J Obstet Gynaecol. 27(1), 57-60.

Cone, R. W., A. C. Hobson, J. Palmer, M. Remington and L. Corey (1991). Extended duration of herpes simplex virus DNA in genital lesions detected by the polymerase chain reaction. J Infect Dis. 164(4), 757-60.

Datta, S. D., L. A. Koutsky, S. Ratelle, E. R. Unger, J. Shlay, T. McClain, et al. (2008). Human papillomavirus infection and cervical cytology in women screened for cervical cancer in the United States, 2003-2005. Ann Intern Med. 148(7), 493-500.

Dillon, S. M., M. Cummings, S. Rajagopalan and W. C. McCormack (1997). Prospective analysis of genital ulcer disease in Brooklyn, New York. Clin Infect Dis. 24(5), 945-50.

Gaydos, C., N. E. Maldeis, A. Hardick, J. Hardick and T. C. Quinn (2009). Mycoplasma genitalium compared to chlamydia, gonorrhoea and trichomonas as an aetiological agent of urethritis in men attending STD clinics. Sex Transm Infect. 85(6), 438-40.

Gottlieb, S. L., S. M. Berman and N. Low (2010). Screening and treatment to prevent sequelae in women with *Chlamydia trachomatis* genital infection: how much do we know? J Infect Dis. 15;(201 Suppl 2):S168-77.

Greenblatt, R. M., S. A. Lukehart, F. A. Plummer, T. C. Quinn, C. W. Critchlow, R. L. Ashley, et al. (1988). Genital ulceration as a risk factor for human immunodeficiency virus infection. Aids. 2(1), 47-50.

Holmes, K. K., P. J. Weisner and A. H. Pedersen (1971). The gonococcal arthritis-dermatitis syndrome. Ann Intern Med. 75(3), 470-1.

Hosenfeld, C. B., K. A. Workowski, S. Berman, A. Zaidi, J. Dyson, D. Mosure, et al. (2009). Repeat infection with Chlamydia and gonorrhea among females: a systematic review of the literature. Sex Transm Dis.36(8),478-89.

Htun, Y., S. A. Morse, Y. Dangor, G. Fehler, F. Radebe, D. L. Trees, et al. (1998). Comparison of clinically directed, disease specific, and syndromic protocols for the management of genital ulcer disease in Lesotho. Sex Transm Infect. 74 Suppl 1S23-8.

Johnson, S. R., D. H. Martin, C. Cammarata and S. A. Morse (1994). Development of a polymerase chain reaction assay for the detection of Haemophilus ducreyi. Sex Transm Dis. 21(1), 13-23.

Johnson, S. R. and S. A. Morse (1988). Antibiotic resistance in Neisseria gonorrhoeae: genetics and mechanisms of resistance. Sex Transm Dis. 15(4):217-24.

Keat, A. (1999). Reactive arthritis. Adv Exp Med Biol. 455:201-6.

Khan, S. A., F. Amir, S. Altaf and R. Tanveer (2009). Evaluation of common organisms causing vaginal discharge. J Ayub Med Coll Abbottabad. 21(2), 90-3.

Larsen, S. A., B. M. Steiner and A. H. Rudolph (1995). Laboratory diagnosis and interpretation of tests for syphilis. Clin Microbiol Rev. 8(1), 1-21.

Liu, H., B. Rodes, C. Y. Chen and B. Steiner (2001). New tests for syphilis: rational design of a PCR method for detection of Treponema pallidum in clinical specimens using unique regions of the DNA polymerase I gene. J Clin Microbiol. 39(5), 1941-6.

Livengood, C. H. (2009). Bacterial vaginosis: an overview for 2009. Rev Obstet Gynecol. 2(1), 28-37.

Manhart, L. E., K. K. Holmes, J. P. Hughes, L. S. Houston and P. A. Totten (2007). Mycoplasma genitalium among young adults in the United States: an emerging sexually transmitted infection. Am J Public Health. 97(6), 1118-25.

Morgan, E. D., J. D. Laszlo and P. G. Stumpf (1988). Incomplete Behcet's syndrome in the differential diagnosis of genital ulceration and postcoital bleeding. A case report. J Reprod Med. 33(10), 844-6.

Nanda N, Michel RG, Kurdgelashvili G, Wendel KA (2006). Trichomoniasis and its treatment. Expert Rev Anti Infect Ther. 4(1):125-35.

O'Farrell, N. (2002). Donovanosis. Sex Transm Infect. 78(6), 452-7.

Pandhi, R. K., A. S. Kumar, D. A. Satish and L. K. Bhutani (1984). Fixed drug eruptions on male genitalia: clinical and etiologic study. Sex Transm Dis. 11(3), 164-6.

Pellati, D., I. Mylonakis, G. Bertoloni, C. Fiore, A. Andrisani, G. Ambrosini, et al. (2008). Genital tract infections and infertility. Eur J Obstet Gynecol Reprod Biol. 140(1), 3-11.

Romanowski, B. (1993). Pelvic inflammatory disease. Current approaches. Can Fam Physician. 39346-9.

Solomon, A. R., J. E. Rasmussen and J. S. Weiss (1986). A comparison of the Tzanck smear and viral isolation in varicella and herpes zoster. Arch Dermatol. 122(3), 282-5.

STD Trends in the United States: 2010 National Data for Gonorrhea, Chlamydia, and Syphilis. Available at: http://www.cdc.gov/std/stats10/trends.htm

STD guidelines 2010: Diseases characterized by vaginal discharge. Available at: http://www.cdc.gov/std/treatment/2010/vaginal-discharge.htm#a3

Su, W. H., T. S. Tsou, C. S. Chen, T. Y. Ho, W. L. Lee, Y. Y. Yu, et al. (2011). Diagnosis of Chlamydia infection in women. Taiwan J Obstet Gynecol. 50(3),261-7.

Svenstrup, H. F., J. Fedder, S. E. Kristoffersen, B. Trolle, S. Birkelund and G. Christiansen (2008). Mycoplasma genitalium, Chlamydia trachomatis, and tubal factor infertility--a prospective study. Fertil Steril. 90(3), 513-20.

Taylor-Robinson, D., C. B. Gilroy, B. J. Thomas and P. E. Hay (2004). Mycoplasma genitalium in chronic non-gonococcal urethritis. Int J STD AIDS. 15(1), 21-5.

Temmerman, M. (1992). Sexually transmitted diseases and reproductive health. Prog Hum Reprod Res. (21), 6-7.

Trees, D. L. and S. A. Morse (1995). Chancroid and Haemophilus ducreyi: an update. Clin Microbiol Rev. 8(3), 357-75.

Trojian, T. H., T. S. Lishnak and D. Heiman (2009). Epididymitis and orchitis: an overview. Am Fam Physician. 79(7), 583-7.

Veeranna, S. and T. Y. Raghu (2003). A clinical and investigational study of donovanosis. Indian J Dermatol Venereol Leprol. 69(2), 159-62.

(WHO fact sheet 2011). available at http://www.who.int/mediacentre/factsheets/fs110/en/.

WHO (2011). http://www.who.int/hiv/pub/progress_report2011/summary_en.pdf.

Wilson, W. R. and M. A. Sande Current diagnosis and treatment in infectious diseases. United States of America: The McGraw-Hill Companies; 2001. Chapter 15, Sexually Transmitted Diseases; p.203-19.

Wright, R. A. and F. N. Judson (1979). Penile veneral edema. Jama. 241(2), 157-8.

Part 2

Bacterial Infections

2

Chlamydia trachomatis Infections of the Adults

Sabina Mahmutovic Vranic
School of Medicine, University of Sarajevo/Department of Microbiology
Bosnia and Herzegovina

1. Introduction

Chlamydiae are obligate intracellular bacteria and consist of four species, including *Chlamydia trachomatis, C. pneumoniae, C. psittaci* and *C. pecorum,* which cause many types of diseases. The word chlamys is Greek for „cloaked" or „draped", descriptive of the intracytoplasmic inclusion bodies that are „draped" around the host cell nucleus.

C. trachomatis is a Gram-negative bacteria, therefore its cell wall components retain the counter-stain safranin and appear pink under a light microscope. Identified in 1907, *C. trachomatis* was the first chlamydial agent discovered in humans.

Chlamydia trachomatis (CT) is one of the major bacterial agent of the sexually transmitted diseases (STDs) worldwide. It is a causative agent of urogenital, ocular and pneumonic infections, causing annually 92 million new infections worldwide. It is responsible for a wide range of infections, including trachoma (a chronic conjuctivitis, which is the leading preventable cause of blidness worldwide), newborn conjuctivitis, and genital infections in women and men. CT has a unique life cycle, dependent on the host cell's adenosine triphosphate (ATP) production, which differentiates it from all other microorganisms.

Chlamydial genital infection is the most frequently reported infectious disease in the United States, and prevalence is highest in persons aged ≤25 years (Centers for Disease Control and Prevention [CDC], 2009).

Asymptomatic infection is common among both, women and men. The fact is that as many as 70 to 80% of women and up to 50% of men who are infected do not experience any symptoms. The most serious sequelae as the CT infection in women include pelvic inflammatory disease- PID, tubal infertility, chronic pelvic pain and ectopic pregnancy.

In pregnant women, CT infection is associated with preterm birth and other complications such as stillbirth, premature rupture of membranes, and post-partum endometritis.

Since chlamydial infections first become a reportable disease in the United States in 1986, the number of reported cases in both men and women has increased each year. It is currently estimated that about 4 million new chlamydial infections occur each year in the United States at an estimated annual cost exceeding $ 2.4 billion (CDC, 2003).

Worldwide, it is estimated that there are more than 50 million new cases CT infection annually (CDC, 2003).

The prevalence of CT infection in sexually active adolescent women, the population considered most at risk, generally exceeds 10%, and in some adolescent and STD clinic populations of women, the prevalence can reach 40%.

The incidence of asymptomatic infection, it's impact on individuals, and it's influence on the prevalence of disease in the community has led multiple professional organizations to recommend that all sexually active women aged 25 years and younger and all asymptomatic women at risk infection be screened for CT genital infection. Chlamydial infections may increase susceptibility to and transmission of human immunodeficiency virus-HIV in both women and men (Westrom et al., 1999).

As far as Central and Eastern European ("CEE") countries are concerned, the epidemiological picture of chlamydial genital infections cannot be reliably estimated since there is no systematic registration, prevalence studies are sporadic and methodologically hardly comparable, and prevention programs focusing on asymptomatic population are scarce.

The incidence of chlamydial genital infections in CEE is estimated to be 21 to 276 cases per 100,000 inhabitants. The public health importance of chlamydial genital infections lies in the fact that their prevalence is the highest in young population, that they are mostly asymptomatic and that, if left untreated, they may later result in chronic pelvic infl ammatory disease, sterility or ectopic pregnancy.

Unfortunately, symptoms of genital infection are often completely absent or very mild among infected patients, especially women, creating a large reservoir of infected persons who continue transmission to new sexual partners. Because these infections are easy to diagnose and curable with a single dose of oral antibiotics, early detection and treatment are an important component of efforts to reduce the disease burden.

Chlamydia is often found as a co-infection with gonorrhea in both women and men. Between 30 and 50% of patients who have gonococcal infections also have infection with *C. trachomatis*. However, because the background incidence of gonorrhea is so much lower (<0.5%), it is far less likely that a person infected with *C. trachomatis* will also have gonoccocal infection. In the National Longitudinal Study, only 0.3% of young adults were co-infected (Miller et al., 2004). Although screening for *C. trachomatis* is widely recommended among young adult women, little information is available regarding the prevalence of chlamydial infections in the general young adult population. Screening programs have been demonstrated to reduce both the prevalence of *C. trachomatis* infection and rates of PID in women (Scholes et al., 1996).

Today chlamydial infections are diagnosed by simple, reliable and non-invasive tests, and the therapy of choice is a single dose of 1 g azithromycin, which has proven to be safe and effective, especially in acute infections. Azithromycin also proved to be the drug of choice in the treatment of chronic infections, chlamydial prostatitis, and in the treatment of major complications, such as pelvic inflammatory disease.

1.1 Facts

1. Chlamydia is the most commonly reported bacterial infection, with an estimated four million new cases each year.
2. Adolescents and adults are most commonly infected with *C. trachomatis.*
3. Asymptomatic infection is common among both, women and men.
4. Untreated chlamydial infections may lead to PID, ectopic pregnancy, and infertility.
5. The purpose of at least annually screening all sexually active women aged 25 years and younger is to reduce the incidence of upper tract infection.

2. Etiology

Because of their unique developmental life cycle, all chlamydiae were placed into their own order, *Chlamydiales,* family *Chlamydiaceae,* within one genus, *Chlamydia* (Pudjitamoko et al., 1997, as cited in Int J Syst Bacteriol, 1984). *C. trachomatis* is one of the four recognized species of the genus *Chlamydia,* with *C. pneumoniae, C. psittaci* and *C. pecorum. Chlamydia* species are readily identified and distinguished from other chlamydial species using DNA-based tests and on the basis unique growth cycle. *Chlamydia psitaci* is a common pathogen of avian species and domestic mammals, but only involves humans as a zoonosis. *Chlaymdia pneumoniae* is a common respiratory pathogen of humans that has been implicated as a possible cause of coronary artery disease. *Chlamydia pecorum* is a pathogen of domestic animals. Some *C. psitacci* strains are sexually transmitted in their natural hosts, and one-the guinea pig inclusion conjuctivitis (GPIC) agent -may offer a potenitially useful animal model for the study of sexually transmitted chlamydial infections. Molecular techniques such as PCR or DNA hybridization or the use of monoclonal antibodies are required to differentiate the species.

There are 15 serovars of *C. trachomatis,* which are divided into the trachoma serotypes A, B, Ba, and C, the oculogenital serovars, D-K, and the lymphogranuloma venereum (LGV) serovars L1-L3 (table 1.). Most strains of *C. trachomatis* are recognized by monoclonal antibodies (mAbs) to epitopes in the VS4 region of MOMP (major outer membrane protein). Serovars can be distinguished by serological typing using monoclonal antibodies or by molecular gene typing methods. Typing is useful for epidemiological studies, which focus on transmission and geographical differences. In the developed world, the oculogenital strains are predominantly the strains that are routinely prevalent, while trachoma is a sequelae of ocular disease in developing countries and countinues to be a leading cause of preventable blidness. LGV is sporadic in North America and Europe, and endemic in Africa, India, Southeast Asia, South America, and the Caribbean. Occasional cases or clusters of cases suggest ongoing low-level transmission in these areas. Few countries require official notification of LGV cases, and the lack of standard diagnostic criteria renders reported cases somewhat suspect. Likeother sexually transmitted diseases LGV is more common in urban than in rural areas, among the sexually active, and among the lower socioeconomic groups. Much of the reported epidemiology on LGV was based on cases diagnosed using clinical criteria or the results of serologic tests and/or Frei skin tests that were not specific for the disease.

Urogenital chlamydial infections occur primarily among young sexually active persons. Prevalence rates encompass all socioeconomic groups and geographical areas, and may range from 5-20% in various groups of young adults (Eng & Butler, 1997).

Disease/Syndrome	Biovar	Most frequent serovars
Trachoma	trachoma	A, B, Ba, C
Inclusion conjunctivits	trachoma	D, Da, E, F, G, H, I, Ia, J, K
Urethritis, cervicitis, salpingitis (pharyngitis, otitis media)	trachoma	B, C, D, E, F, G, H, I, K, L3
Lymphogranuloma venereum (syn. Lymphogranuloma inguinale, lymphopathia venerea, Favre-Durand-Nicolas disease)	lymphogranuloma venereum	L1, L2, L2a, L3

Table 1. Human infections caused by *Chlamydia trachomatis.*

3. Chlamydial biological cycle

Chlamydiae are obligate cell parasites and cannot be cultured on arteficial media. They have the ability to establish long-term associations with host cells. They are also restricted to an intracellular life style because chlamydiae lack the ability to synthesize high-energy compounds. When an infected host cell is starved for various nutrients such as amino acids (tryptophan) iron, or vitamins, this has a negative consequence for *Chlamydiae* since the organism is dependent on the host cell for these nutrients. They depend on the host cell to supply them with ATP and necessary nutrients.

It is developmental cycle of chlamydiae that sets them apart form all other bacteria. There are some differences in inclusion morphology within the chlamydiae, but all species appear to have essentially identical developmental cycles.

They go through two stages in their reproductive cycle; the elementary bodies (EBs) are optimized to survive outside of host cells. In the form of the reticular bodies (RBs), the chlamydiae reproduce inside the host cells. This cycle involves an alternation between two highly specialized morphologic forms, one adopted to an intracellular and the other to an extra cellular environment.

The cycle may be divided into several steps: (1) initial attachment of the infectious particle, or elementary body, to the host cell; (2) entry into the cell; (3) morphological change to the reticulate particle, with intracellular growth and replication; (4) morphologic change of reticulate particles to Ebs; and finally (5) release of the infectious particles (figure 1.).

The entire cycle takes place within a chlamydia -modified intracellular vacuole, which undergoes a large increase in size.

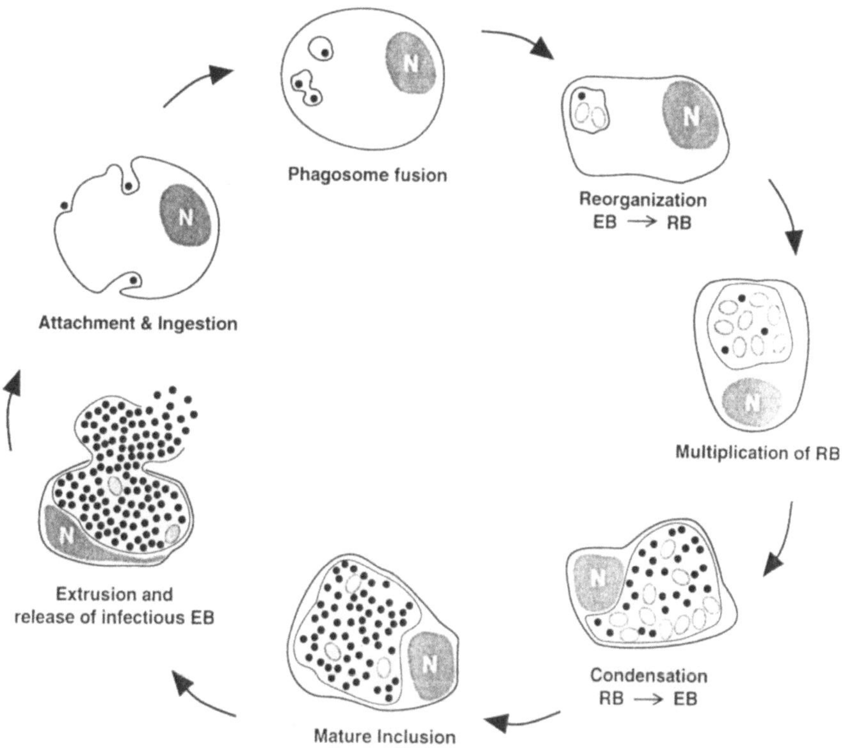

Fig. 1. Chlamydial Biological Cycle (Jones et al.,1994).

3.1 Elementary bodies

The round to oval, optically dense elementary bodies have a diameter 300 nm. Infection begins when EBs attach to specific receptors found on nonciliated columnar or cuboidal epithelium of the host. This type of epithelium is located in the endocervix, endometrium, fallopian tube, and urethra, making those sites vulnerable to infection.

3.2 Reticulate bodies

After phagocytosis, the EB exists within a cytoplasmic vacuole or phagosome, where it is protected from host defense systems. Within the phagosome, the EB transforms into a reticulate body in order to myltiply. It has a diameter of aproximately 1000 nm. At the end of the life cycle, RBs are transformed back into EBs. The cell breaks open and releases the EBs to continue the cycle by attaching themselves to new host cells.

4. Prevalence and Incidence

Chlamydial genital infection is the most frequently reported infectious disease in the United States, and prevalence is highest in persons aged ≤25 years (CDC, 2009). The Centers for Diseases Control and Prevention (CDC), Atlanta, GA, has not changed its age cutoff, and thus continues to recommend annual chlamydia screening of sexually active women aged ≤25 years. The CDC estimates that 2.8 million new cases occur in the United States each year

(CDC, 2005). Nearly 75% of cases occur in the 15-to 24-year-old age group (Grosecloseet et al., 1999). The World Heath Organization (WHO) estimated that 92 million new infections with *C. trachomatis* occured worldwide in 1999 (WHO, 2001). The prevalence of active infection in sexually active, asymptomatic, non-pregnant women in the general population is between 3 and 5% (Sweet & Gibbs, 2002). The highest age-specific rates were reported in women age 15-26. In the general population, men have the same prevalence of chalmydial infections as women (3-5%). Among men, the highest rates occurs in 20- to 24- year-old (CDC, 2005). However, accurate time trends in the incidence of chlamydia are difficult to define because of changes in reporting, increased detection due to improved laboratory tests and increasing laboratory surveillance. Gerbes et al. (Gerbes et al., 1998) estimated that the average annual incidence rates for people aged 15 to 49 years were similar in North America, Western Europe and Australasia at 2146/100,000 for males and 3073/100,000 for females in 1995.

Chlamydia causes more than 250,000 cases of epididymitis in the U.S. each year. Chlamydia causes 250,000 to 500,000 cases of PID every year in the United States. Women infected with chlamydia are up to five times more likely to become infected with human immunodeficiency virus (HIV), if exposed.

5. Risk factors

The risk factors for chlamydial infection include: age younger than 26, low socioeconomic status, minority group member, contraceptive use, age at first intercourse, multiple sexual partners and new partners, and other risk factors as well.

Younger age is shown consistently to be associated with increased risk of chlaymdial infection among the sexually active population. Age is an important risk factor because *C. trachomatis* typically infects the columnar cells of the cervix; in younger women, columnar cells are more likely to be on the ectocervix (ectopy), where they can be exposed to semen carrying the organism. As women age, the columnar cells are located higher in the cervical canal. Combination hormonal contraceptive use apparently increases cervical ectopy and has been a proposed risk factor for chlamydial infection (Jocobson et al., 2000). The highest incidence rates of infection are reported in adolescents and young adults in Canada and the United States. Differences in the prevalence of infection between adolescents and adults are also often attributed to differences in sexual behaviours.

Race/ethnicity and socioeconomic status are often considered together because they are strongly interrealted (van de Hoek, 1999). Only 10 of 23 studies in females and one of four studies in males indicated a higher risk of chlamydial infection in nonwhite people compared with white people in multivariate analysis. Socioeconomic status was not associate with chlamydia in multivariate analysis using any measure for males and females, including employment status income level of parents education use of Medicaid or occupation.

Multiple partnerships may increase the likelihood of encountering a sexually transmitted pathogen through the increased probability of choosing a partner with infection, while having new or casual sexual contacts may be related to increased risk because of a reduced familiarity between partners.

The relationship between the use of condoms and other barrier contraceptives (diaphragm), and genital chlamydial infection is inconsistent across the studies. Use of a barrier method was shown to be associated with reduced risk of infection compared with the use of other methods of contraception in two of five studies in females.

Age at first intercourse may be casually related to sexually transmitted infections through the biological mechanisms affecting adolescents that and also be an indicator of other aspects of sexual activity that will directly increase risk, including multiple partnerships and the recruitment of nonregular partners.

6. Pathogenesis, infectivity and transmission

Although the pathologic consequences of infection are well established, the mechanism of chlamydia-induced tissue damage are not fully understood. Emerging knowledge of the immune response to infection suggests that many of the complications of chlamydial infection are accompanied by important alterations in immunoregulation; both antibody-mediated and cell-mediated immune effectors may be significant in eliminatory or limiting chlamydial infection.

The ways of spreading are different; sexually, perinatal, although are not exclusive the other ways of transmission through the chloride water of swimming pool, wet towel as well as the possibility of intrahospital infections, by gynecological exam, are not keep the necessary protection measures. It is supposed, statistically, that about 10% percent of women in reproductive age are infected with *C. trachomatis*.

C. trachomatis is the most common sexually transmitted bacterial agent, which infects only humans. The single exposure male-to-female transmission rate has been estimated to be 40%, and the female-to-male transmission rate has been estimated to be 32% (Sweet & Gibbs, 2002). Other investigators have found that transmission rates between sexes are equivalent (Quinn et al., 1996).

Vertical transmission of *C. trachomatis* is more efficient than horizontal transmission. More than 60% of newborns who delivered through a chlamydia-infected cervix will aquire the infection (Sweet & Gibbs, 2002).

As well as the infection with human papilloma virus, chlamydial infection is very important promoter of cervical intraepithelial neoplasm, which result with bad Papanicolaou test, with salpingitis with consequently opturation tuba incompletely or completely, which finally results as extrauterine pregnancy and sterility. During pregnancy, *C. trachomatis* causes disorders and ruptures of the fertile membranes with consequent delayed spontaneous abortion or the earlier delivery.

7. Clinical manifestations

Genital infections caused by *C. trachomatis* closely parallel those due to *N. gonorrhoeae* in terms of clinical manifestations. Both preferentially infect columnar or transitional epithelium of the urethra, with extension to the epididymis; the endocervix, with extension to the endometrium, salpinx, and peritoneum; and the rectum. *C. trachomatis* are naturally found living only inside human cells. Chlamydia can be transmitted during vaginal, anal, or oral sex, and can be passed from an infected mother to her baby during vaginal childbirth. Between half and three-quarters of all women who have a chlamydia infection of the neck of the womb (cervicitis) have no symptoms and do not know that they are infected.

C. trachomatis serovars A, B, Ba, and C are associated with endemic trachoma, the most common preventable form of blidness, while serovars L1, L2, and L3 are associated with LGV. Serovars D through K are the major causes of nongonococcal urethritis and epididymitis in men and may induce Reiter's syndrome, proctitis, and conjuctivitis in both men and women and cervicitis, urethritis, endometritis, with salpingitis with tubal obstruction which could be complete or incomplete, and perihepatitis in women. During pregnancy CT can cause „premature" rupture of membranes, spontaneous abortions and preterm delivery.

7.1 Trachoma

Trachoma is a follicular keratoconjuctivitis. The disease occurs in all climatic zones, although it is more frequent in warmer, less-developed countries. The pathogen is transmitted by direct contact and indirectly via objects in daily use. Untreated, the initially acute inflammation could develop a chronic course lasting months or years and leading to formation of a corneal scar, which can than cause blidness.

The laboratory diagnostics procedure involves detection of *C. trachomatis* in conjuctival smears using direct immunofluorescence microscopy. The fluorochrome-marked monoclonal antibodies are directed against the MOMP of *C. trachomatis*.

The pathogen can also be grown in cell cultures. The therapeutic method of choice is systemic and local application of tetracyclines over a period of several weeks.

Chlamydia conjunctivitis or trachoma is a common cause of blindness worldwide. The WHO estimates that it accounted for 15% of blindness cases in 1995, but only 3.6% in 2002 (WHO, 2002).

7.2 Inclusion conjuctivitis

This is an acute, purulent papillary conjuctivits that may affect neonates, children, and adults (swiming-pool conjuctivitis). Newborn children are infected during birth by pathogenes colonizing the birth canal. Untreated, a pannus may form as in trachoma, followed by corneal scarring. Laboratory diagnosis and therapy as in trachoma.

7.3 Genital infections

Chlamydial infections of the genital tract have a worldwide distribution and are prevalent both in the industrialized countries and in the developing world. *C. trachomatis* as the bacterial agent is responsible for the huge number of genital infections, which is spreading especially among younger (table 2.). Adults are defined as persons between 15 and 49 years of age. Almost four million new cases of chlamydial infections on genital plane are registrated every year in the United States, and three million in Europe (CDC, 1997). Epidemiological investigations of a large number of women in the United States and Scandinavia confirm chlamydiae as the most prevalent STDs for developed countries. Considered the prevalence infections, hard consequences and huge bills for the treatment in the United States is implement screening methods, which include persons with high risk:

- Persons with anamnestic history of STDs;
- Young persons sexually active;
- Promiscuity persons;
- Male with lymphogranuloma infection;
- Newborns,
- Reiter was diagnosed in younger males.

Women		
Cervicitis	Perihepatitis	Preterm labor
Urethritis	Conjunctivitis	Preterm delivery
Acute urethral syndrome	Ectopic pregnancy	Premature rupture of membranes
Proctitis	Infertility	Postpartum endometritis
Endometritis	Chronic pelvic pain	
Salpingitis	Reiter' s syndrome	
Men		
Urethritis	Proctitis	
Epididymitis	Infertility	
Prostatitis	Conjunctivitis	
Reiter' s syndrome		
Newborns		
Conjunctivitis	Pneumonia	
Otitis media		

Table 2. Clinical manifestations of *Chlamydia trachomatis.*

In women, *C. trachomatis* can cause urethritis, proctitis, or infections of the genital organs. It has even been known to cause pelvioperitonitis and perihepatitis. Massive perinatal infection of a neonate may lead to an interstitial chlamydial pneumonia.

C. trachomatis is responsible for 30 to 60% of cases of nongonococcal urethritis (NGU) in men. Possible complications include prostatitis and epididymitis. The pathogens are communicated by venereal transmission. The source of infection is the female sexual partner, who often shows no clinical symptoms.

Urogenital chlamydial infections occur primarily among young sexually active persons. Prevalence rates encompass all socioeconomic groups and geographical areas, and more range from 5-20% in various groups of young adults (Eng & Butler, 1997; Tamm, 1999). Because symptoms are absent in most infected individuals, the prevalence in population groups may be severely underestimated. So, widespread screening of individuals at greatest risk, e.g. those individuals who are young, sexually active, and have new or multiple partners, has been recommended.

7.3.1 Genital infections in women

Genital infections caused by the *C. trachomatis* is the most frequently reported STD's worldwide, with the highest prevalence in aged category of ≤25 years (CDC, 2009). In women, *C. trachomatis* has been shown to cause both lower and upper genital tract infections. Untreated, chlamydial infection can lead to severe reproductive complications. Chlamydia is known as the "silent epidemic" because in women, it may not cause any symptoms in 75% of cases, and can linger for months or years before being discovered. Symptoms that may occur include unusual vaginal bleeding or discharge, pain in the abdomen, painful sexual intercourse (dyspareunia), fever, painful urination or the urge to urinate more frequently than usual (urinary urgency).

C trachomatis is an important causal agent in pelvic inflammatory disease, with sequelae including infertility, ectopic pregnancy, and chronic pelvic pain. Up to two thirds of cases of tubal-factor infertility and one third of cases of ectopic pregnancy may be attributable to *C. trachomatis* infection.

Chlamydial infection during pregnancy is associated with a number of adverse outcomes of pregnancy including preterm labor, premature rupture of the membranes, low birth weight, neonatal death, and postpartum endometritis. Chlamydial infection during pregnancy may be transmitted to the infant during delivery.

An infant born to a mother with active infection has a risk of acquiring infection at any anatomical site of 50 to 75%. Approximately 30 to 50% of infants born to chlamydia-positive mothers will have conjunctivitis, and at least 50 percent of infants with chlamydial conjunctivitis will also have nasopharyngeal infection. Chlamydial pneumonia develops in about 30% of infants with nasopharyngeal infection.

7.3.2 Genital infections in men

In men, the most common clinical manifestation of *C. trachomatis* infection is nongonococcal urethritis. In fact, *C. trachomatis* causes approximately 35 to 50 % of all cases of nongonococcal urethritis in heterosexual men. Symptoms of nongonococcal urethritis may develop after an incubation period of 7 to 21 days and include dysuria and mild-to-moderate whitish or clear urethral discharge. In most cases, physical examination reveals no abnormalities other than the discharge. Other clinical syndromes in men include acute epididymitis, acute proctitis, acute proctocolitis, conjunctivitis, and Reiter's syndrome. Male infertility, chronic prostatitis, and urethral strictures are possible results of infection. Both Reiter's syndrome (urethritis, conjunctivitis, arthritis, and mucocutaneous lesions) and reactive tenosynovitis or arthritis (without the other components of Reiter's syndrome) have been associated with genital *C. trachomatis* infection. Infection with *C. trachomatis* is also believed to be a cofactor for the transmission of human immunodeficiency virus in both men and women (Nelson & Helfand, 2001).

If left untreated, it is possible for chlamydia in men to spread to the testicles causing epididymitis, which in rare cases can cause sterility if not treated within 6 to 8 weeks. Chlamydia is also a potential cause of prostatitis in men, although the exact relevance in prostatitis is difficult to ascertain due to possible contamination from urethritis.

7.4 Lymphogranuloma venereum

Lymphogranuloma venereum-LGV is distinct venereal disease caused by three serotypes of *C. trachomatis* that are not associated with other chlamydial infections.

Lymphogranuloma venereum is frequently observed in the inhabitants of warm climatic zones and occurs principally in South America and Africa. The disease is uncommon in

North America, but outbreaks have occurred. A herpetiform primary lesion develops at the site of invasion in the genital area, which then becomes an ulcus with accompanying lymphadenitis. Laboratory diagnosis is based on isolating the proliferating pathogen in cell cultures from purulent material obtained from the ulcus or from matted lymph nodes. The antibodies can be identified using the complement binding reaction or the microimmunofluorescence test.

Tetracyclines and macrolides are the potentially useful antibiotic types.

8. Laboratory diagnostics of *Chlamydia trachomatis*

C. trachomatis is a biosafety level 2 agent and should be handled appropriately, although it is not considered a particularly dangerous pathogen. *C. trachomatis* urogenital infection in women can be diagnosed by testing urine or by collecting swab specimens from the endocervix or vagina. Diagnosis of *C. trachomatis* urethral infection in men can be made by testing a urethral swab or urine specimen. Rectal *C. trachomatis* infections in persons that engage in receptive anal intercourse can be diagnosed by testing a rectal swab specimen.

Today, culture-independent tests have revolutionized chlamydia diagnostics. Comercially available antigen detection methods and nucleic acid hybridization tests, when introduced in the 1980s, largely replaced the technically more demanding isolation procedures (table 3.).

8.1 Culture

Although originally chlamydia was grown in embroyonated chicken eggs, growth and detection of chlamydia is now accomplished by staining of chlamydial inclusions grown in tissue culture cells. The cell line the most commonly used is McCoy cells. The other cell lines have been used as well as monkey kidney, HeLa, and HEp-2. It is confirmed that the culture is technically difficult and has been shown to be not as sensitive as previously thought. Recent studies have indicated that culture sensitivity compared to molecular techniques can range from 50-100%, while specificity is considered to be nearly 100% (Van Der Pol et al., 2001).

8.2 Non-culture diagnostic test

Other non-culture diagnostic tests include: direct cytological examination, direct fluorescent antibody (DFA) test and antigen detection using the enzyme immunoassay (EIA).

Cytology was used to detect chlamydial infections before more sensitive tests were developed. Specimens obtained from the genital tract were diagnosed for the presence/absence of inclusion bodies. The sensitivity of cytology testing is very low with only 20% cases being detected.

DFA using commercial monoclonal antibodies which detect the major outer membrane protein (MOMP) of *C. trachomatis*, which stains only this organism. The test involves the specimen swab being rolled onto a glass slide air dried and fixed with methanol. Fluorescein-conjugated monoclonal antibody is applied to the slide, which after incubation is mounted in mounting medium, coverslipped and read for the presence of EBs with a fluorescent microscope under 1,000 x. The test requires the experience of a trained microscopist and has a sensitivity of 80-85% with specificity of 98-99% compared to culture (Mahoney &Chernesky, 2003).

Diagnostic method	Sensitivity	Specificity
Tissue Culture	70-85%	100%
Direct Fluorescence Assay	80-85%	>99%
Enzyme Immunoassay	53-76%	95%
Hybridization (Pace 2)	65-83%	99%
Ligase Chain Reaction		
Cervical	94.4-96.4%	99.5-100%
Female Urine	93-98%	99-100%
Male Urine	96.4%	94-100%
Polymerase Chain Reaction (COBAS)		
Cervical	89.7%	99.4%
Female Urine	89.2%	99.0%
Male Urine	90.3%	98.4%
Strand Displacement Amplification		
Cervical	92.8%	98.1%
Female Urine	80.5%	98.4%
Male Urine	93.1%	93.8%
Transcriptional Mediated Amplification		
Cervical	94.2%	97.6%
Female Urine	94.7%	98.9%
Male Urine	97%	99.1%
Male Urethral	95.2%	98.2%

Table 3. Sensitivity and specificity of diagnostic tests for the detection of *Chlamydia trachomatis*.

EIA was the one of the earliest non-culture developed tests. EIA was widely used before the advent of molecular tests and is still used as the most prevalent non-culture detection test for chlamydia (Gaydos et al., 1990).There are several EIAs commercially available using either polyclonal or monoclonal antibodies to detect chlamydia LPS. The sensitivity of the EIAs range from approximately 53-76%, with specificities of about 95%, especially when antibody blocking confirmatory assays is used to confirm the positive EIA result.

Because older non-culture tests, such as DFA and EIA, were traditionally compared to culture as a gold standard, the sensitivities reported in the older literature can no longer be viewed as accurate. The antigen detection techniques are generally less expensive and easier to perform than newer molecular tests.

8.3 Serology

The microimmunofluorescence test (MIF) has been the gold standard test for the detection of antibody for Chlamydia (Wang et al., 1985). The assay is useful for population studies but is not useful for the diagnosis of active *C. trachomatis* ocular or urogenital disease.

8.4 New molecular diagnostic tests for detection of *C. trachomatis*

The diagnosis of genital chlamydial infections evolved rapidly from the 1990s. The most important advance came from the introduction of nucleic acid amplification tests (NAATs), such as polymerase chain reaction (PCR), transcription mediated amplification (TMA), and the DNA strand displacement amplification (SDA). NAATs for chlamydia may be performed on swab specimens collected from the cervix (women) or urethra (men), on self-collected vaginal swabs, or on voided urine. Urine and self-collected swab testing facilitates the performance of screening tests in settings where genital examination is impractical. At present, the NAATs have regulatory approval only for testing urogenital specimens, although rapidly evolving research indicates that they may give reliable results on rectal specimens.The most sensitive and accurate of the non-culture tests are the NAATs and are highly specific, as well. Because they can be used with noninvasively collected specimens such as first catch urines from either sex, or vaginal swabs, NAATs are well suited for screening as well as diagnosis. There are several types of NAATs. The two most commonly used tests are the PCR and LCR tests. These tests offer greatly expanded sensitivities of detection, usually well above 90%, while maintaining very high specificity. Choice of test is mainly dependent upon cost and preference of the laboratory, as all of these NAATs are closely comparable in sensitivity and specificity (Gaydos et al., 2004).

Because NAATs detect DNA and RNA targets, they do not require viable organisms to detect infection.

9. Diagnosis and treatment

Chlamydial infections are often asymptomatic, so diagnosis generally requires chlamydia-specific laboratory test identification or confirmation. Treating infected patients prevents sexual transmission of the disease, and treating all sexual partners of those testing positive for Chlamydia can prevent reinfection of the index patient and infection of other partners. There is no universally accepted protocol for testing the antibiotic susceptibility of *C. trachomatis*. Because of the unique intracellular characteristics of *C. trachomatis*, only certain antibiotics are effective in treatment. The CDC treatment guidelines for chlamydial infections are summarized in tables 4. and 5. (CDC, 2009).

Recommended Regimens
Azithromycin 1 g orally in a single dose
or
Doxycycline 100 mg orally twice a day for 7 days
Alternative Regimens
Erythromycin base 500 mg orally four times a day for 7 days
Or
Erythromycin ethylsuccinate 800 mg orally four times a day for 7 days
Or
Levofloxacin 500 mg orally once a day for 7 days
Or
Ofloxacin 300 mg orally twice a day for 7 days

Table 4. Recommended regimens (CDC, 2009).

Recommended regimens
Azithromycin 1 g orally in a single dose
Or
Amoxicillin 500 mg orally three times a doa for 7 days
Alternative regimens
Erythromycin base 500 mg orally four times a day for 7 days
Or
Erythromycin base 250 mg orally four times a day for 14 days
Or
Erythromycin ethylsuccinate 800 mg orally four times a day for 7 daysbase 500 mg orally four times a day for 7 days
Or
Erythromycin ethylsuccinate 400 mg orally four times a day for 14 days

Table 5. Recommended regimens in pregnancy (CDC, 2009).

10. Follow-up

The validity of chlamydial diagnostic testing at <3 weeks after completion of therapy has not been established. False-negative results might occur in the presence of persistent infections involving limited numbers of chlamydial organisms, as well as false-positive results because of the continued presence of nonviable organisms.

In addition, NAATs conducted at <3 weeks after completion of therapy in persons who were treated successfully could yield false-positive results because oh the continued presence of nonviable organisms (CDC, 2009). Routine repeat testing is also encouraged at every other examination done 3-12 months after treatment regardless of whether the patient believes that her sex partner(s) was treated.

11. Recommendations for chlamydial screening and re-screening

In the United States, the CDC recommends that all sexually active adolescent women should be screened for chlamydia infection at least annually, even if symptoms are not present. Also recommended is annually screening of sexually active women 20-25 years of age and older women with risk factors such as a new sex partner or multiple sex partners.

Since the risk of re-infections is very high, especially in women, the CDC recommends that previously infected women are at a high risk and constitute a priority for repeat testing and should be re-screened 3-4 months after treatment.

12. Conclusion

Chlamydia trachomatis has been recognized as a genital pathogen responsible for an increasing variety of clinical syndromes. CT infection is the STD most strongly associated with adolescents. Adolescents, young women and men are consistently at higher risk of being infected with chlamydia than others. The high level of asymptomaticity and the low levels of testing among females and males make an important reservoir for chlamydial infection. Immunity induced by chlamydial infection is not well understood.

It is clear that single infections will not result in solid immunity to reinfection. Multiple infections, homo- or heterotypic, are common.

Unfortunately, the natural infection is not readily quantifiable in terms of inoculum size, and thus relative degrees of immunity may exist which are overcome with a sufficiently large challenge.

In screening studies, younger women are found to have higher cervical infection rates than older women, who often have higher antibody levels. In addition, many isolate-negative individuals attending STD clinics have IgM to the organism. This antibody may result from recent exposure and rapid resolution of the infection or its ablation by an immune response.

Having in mind that many chlamydial infections are asymptomatic, it has become clear that effective control must involve periodic testing of individuals at risk.

13. References

Centers for Disease Control and Prevention. (1997). Chlamydia trachomatis, In: *Genital Infection*-United States. MMWR, Vol.46, No.9, pp.193-198.

Centers for Disease Control and Prevention.(2002*). Sexually Transmitted Disease Treatment Guidelines.* MMWR,Vol. 51, No.RR-6, pp.:1-78.

Centers for Diseases Control and Prevention. (2004). Trends in reportable sexually transmitted diseases in the United States, 2004: *National surveillance data for Chlamydia, gonorrhoea and syphilis*. Atlanta, GA: Centers for Disease Control and Prevention, 2005. Available from: http://www.cdc.gov/std/stats. Accessed Nov, 24,2006

Centers for Diseases Control and Prevention. (2008). *Sexually Transmitted Diseases Surveillance.*

Atlanta, GA: US Department of Health and Human Services, CDC; 2009.

Eng, TR. & Butler, WT. (1997). The neglected health and economic impact of STDs, In: *The Hidden Epidemic, Confronting Sexually transmitted Diseases*, (Ed.), 28-68, National Academy Press, Washington, D.C.

Gaydos, CA.; Reichart, C. & Long, J. (1990). Evaluation of syva enzyme immunoassay for detection of Chlamydia trachomatis in genital specimens. *J Clin Microbiol*, Vol. 28, pp.1541-1544.

Gaydos, CA.; Theodore, M. & Dalesio, N. (2004). Comparison of three nucleic acid amplification tests for detection of Chlamydia trachomatis in urine specimens. *J Clin Microbiol*, Vol. 42, pp. 3041-3045.

Gerbes, AC.; Rowley, JT. & Heymann DHL. (1996). Global prevalence and incidence estimates of selected curable STDs. *Sex Transm Infect*, Vol.74, pp.S12-S16.

Groseclose, SL.; Zaidi, AA. & DeLisle, SJ. (1996). Estimated Incidence and prevalence of genital Chlamydia trachomatis infections in the United States. *Sex Transm Dis*, Vol 26, pp.339-344.

Jocobson, DL.; Peralta, L.& Graham, NM. (2000). Histologic development of cervical ectopy: relationship to reproductive hormones. *Sex Transm Dis* , Vol. 27, pp. 252-258.

Jones, RB. (1995). Chlamydia trachomatis (trachoma, perinatal infections, lymphogranuloma venereum and other genital infections), In: V: Mandel, GL.; Bennet, JE., & Dolin, R. ur. *Principles and practise of Infections diseases*, pp. 1679-1693. New York. Churchill Livingstone

Mahoney, JB. & Chernesky, MA. (2003). *Chlamydia and Chalymydophila*, In: Murray, PR., Barron, EJ. & Jorgensen, JH. *Manual of Clinical microbiology*, (Ed.), 991-1004, ASM Press, Washington, DC.

Miller, WC. ; Ford, CA.& Morris, M. (2004). Prevalence of chlamydial and gonococcal infections among young adults in the United States. *JAMA*, Vol. 291, pp. 2229-2236

Nelson, HD.& Helfand, M. (2001). Screening for chlamydial infection. *Am J Prev Med*, Vol. 20, pp. 95-107.

Pudjitamoko, H., Fukushi, Y. & Ochiai, Y. (1997). Phylogenetic analysis of the genus Chlamydia based on 16S rRNA gene sequences. *Int J Syst Bacteriol*, Vol.47, pp. 425-431.

Quinn, TC. ; Gaydos, C.& Shepard, L. (1996). Epidemiologic and microbiologic correlates of Chlamydia trachomatis infection in sexual partners. *JAMA*, Vol. 276, pp.1737-1742.

Scholes, D.; Stergachis, A.& Heindrich, FE. (1996). Prevention of pelvic inflammatory disease by screening for cervical chlamydial infection. *N Engl J Med*, Vol.334, pp. 1362-6.

Stamm WE. (1999). Chlamydia trachomatis infections of the adult, In: KK Holmes, KK., Sparling, PF. & Mardh, PA. *Sexually Transmitted Diseases*, (Ed.), 407-422, Mc-Graw-Hill, New York

Sweet ,WC.& Gibbs, RS. (2002). Chlamydial infections. In: Sweet, RL., Gibbs, RS., *Infectious Diseases of the Female Genital Tract,* (4 th Ed.), 57-100, Philadelphia, PA: Lippincott Williams & Wilkins

Van de Hoek, A. (1999). STDs, HIV/AIDS, ethnicity, and migrant populations. In: Aral, SO., Sparling, PF.& Mardh, PA. *Sexually Transmitted Diseases,* (Ed.), 163-70, New York:McGraw-Hill

Van Der Pol, BD., Ferrero, L. & Buck-Barrington, E. (2001). Multicenter evaluation of the BD ProbeTec ET System for the detection of Chlamydia trachomatis and Neisseria gonorrhoeae in urine specimens, female endocervical swabs, and male urethral swabs. *J Clin Microbiol*, Vol.39, pp. 108-1016.

Wang, SP., Kuo, CC & *Barnes RC. (1985). Immunotyping of Chlamydia trachomatis with monoclonal antibodies. J infect Dis*, Vol. 152, pp. 791-800.

Westrom, L.& Eschenbach, D. (1999). Pelvic inflammatory disease. In: Holmes, KK., Mardh, PA. & Sparling, PF.*Sexually Transmitted Diseases*., (3rd ed.), 783-809, New York, NY: McGrow-Hill

World Health Organization. (2001). *Global prevalence and incidence of selected curable sexually transmitted infections: overview and estimates*. Geneva: World Health Organization

World Health Organization. (2002). "Global data on visual impairment in the year 2002". *Bull World Health Organ,* Vol. 82, pp. 844–851.Geneva: World Health Organization

3

Gonorrhea in Men Sex Men and Heterosexual Men

Ángela María Rosa Famiglietti and Susana Diana García
Faculty of Pharmacy and Biochemistry
University of Buenos Aires
Argentina

1. Introduction

Gonorrhea is a sexually transmitted infectious disease known since ancient times, with biblical (Old Testament) references. The etiologic agent is *Neisseria gonorrhoeae,* commonly called gonococcus. *N. gonorrhoeae* has accumulated mechanisms of antimicrobial resistance so that from the year 2007 it joined the list of multi-resistant, informally called "Superbugs" (Shafer *in Neisseria* Molecular Mechanisms of Pathogenesis, 2010).

1.1 General description

Neisseria gonorrhoeae was described by Neisser in 1879 and first cultivated in 1882 by Leistikow and Loeffler. At this time, members of the genus *Neisseria* are classified in the family *Neisseriaceae* with the genera *Kingella, Eikenella, Simonsiella,* and *Alysiella.* This family is now placed in the β-subgroup of the Phylum *Proteobacteria* (Janda and Gaydos *in* Manual of Clinical Microbiology, 2007).

N. gonorrhoeae is a gram-negative diplococci with adjacent sides flattened, like coffee beans, do not form spores, oxidizes dimethil or tetramethil-phenylenediamine (oxidase test positive) and catalase positive (superoxol test with 30% H_2O_2); not to reduce nitrites. It may grow optimally at 35-37ºC, but it's unable to grow at low temperature (22ºC). The most of gonococcus have an obligate requirement for CO_2 (5%) and humidity of 70-80%, it does not tolerate drying out. Clinical specimens should be collected with Dacron or rayon swabs. These swabs should be inoculated immediately on appropriate media. Calcium alginate may have inhibitory effect and cotton swabs contain fatty acids that inhibit the growth of gonococci. *N. gonorrhoeae* grows on selective media, modified Thayer Martin, as *Neisseria meningitidis.* Cysteine is an essential aminoacid for their growth. Some strains have specific requirements of certain amino acids, pyrimidines and purines as a result of defective or altered biosynthetic pathways. These particular nutritional requirements form the basis for a typing method for gonococci called auxotyping. *N. gonorrhoeae* differs from other species of the genus by oxidizing glucose and do not use maltose, sucrose, lactose or fructose in cysteine-tryptic digest semisolid agar-base medium (CTA) containing 1% carbohydrate and a phenol red pH indicator, or rapid carbohydrate test; not to reduce nitrites and their inability to grow at low temperatures (22ºC).

The use of enzyme substrates that demonstrate the presence of prolyl-hydroxyprolyl aminopeptidase and the abscense of β-galactosidase and γ-glutamyl aminopeptidase also to confirm the identification. Currently there are commercially available rapid tests to confirm the isolation of *N. gonorrhoeae* such as immune reactions by using fluorescent monoclonal antibodies or coagglutination tests, as well as molecular techniques using specific probes or specific primers (Janda and Gaydos *in* Manual of Clinical Microbiology, 2007).

1.2 Transmission and clinical manifestations

N. gonorrhoeae is an exclusive human pathogen and this is their only reservoir. The transmission is from person to person through sexual intercourse, so the primary infection in adults is installed in the genital area, anal and/ or pharynx, where there is susceptible epithelium: cubic or cylindrical not stratified.

In males, *N. gonorrhoeae* causes an acute urethritis with dysuria and urethral discharge. The incubation period averages 2 to 7 days. About 2.5 to 5 % of men are asyntomatic. Complications of untreated gonococcal urethritis are: epididymitis, periurethral abscesses, infections of the Tyson's glands and Cowper's glands, orchitis and prostatitis (Janda and Gaydos *in* Manual of Clinical Microbiology, 2007). In women, gonococcal infections cause cervicitis, only approximately half of which occur with symptoms and which can go on to cause pelvic inflammatory disease, ectopic pregnancies, and infertility. In addition, in both men and women exposed orally or anally, gonococcal infections can cause a predominantly asyntomatic pharyngitis or proctitis. Less commonly, *N. gonorrhoeae* can cause conjunctivitis, endocarditis, tenosynovitis, arthritis, meningitis, inflammation of the liver capsule and disseminated blood stream infections (Barry, 2009).

Conjunctival infection occurs in adult and neonatal by accidental inoculation or contamination in the birth canal and causes ophthalmia neonatorum, which if not treated properly can lead to blindness (Marrazo *in* Principle and Practice of Infections Disease, 2010).

Asymptomatic infection in women has been linked to the biofilm production, which includes nature complex mixes of exopolysaccharides, proteins and DNA. Bacteria living in biofilms are more resistant to biocides and antimicrobial agents. Also, the horizontal transfer of resistance genes is more likely and increases the spread of resistance genes (Apicella *in Neisseria* Molecular Mechanisms of Pathogenesis, 2010). Gonococcal infection may facilite transmission of human immunodeficiency virus (HIV), increasing the number of target cells for HIV in the inflammatory exudate present in symptomatic patients (Bala, 2010)

1.3 Diagnosis of gonococcal infections

Diagnosis of gonococcal infection has historically been a combination of clinical signs and symptoms plus the microbiologic study. The diagnosis of urethritis in men can be made by observing gram-negative intracellular diplococci associated with polymorphonuclear leukocites on a smear prepared from the urethral discharge. The Gram stain has a sensitivity of 90 to 95% and specificity of 95 to 100% for diagnosing genital gonorrhea in symptomatic men. In cervicitis, the sensitivity of this test is less than 50%, when compared with properly performed culture. Culture on selective media, modified Thayer Martin, it allows recovery of *N. gonorrhoeae* from body sites harboring an endogenous bacterial flora.

At the last years, nucleic acid detection techniques allow direct detection of *N. gonorrheae* in clinical samples and do not require viable organisms. The assay may be divided into three types: (i) direct detection probe hybridization to the target nucleic acid with direct detection of the hybrid; (ii) nucleic acid amplification tests (NAATs); and (iii) amplified-signal probe test, which hybridize with nucleic acid and then amplify the signal of the probe. These assays are generally much more sensitive that culture and are highly specific for urogenital infections, however, depending on the assay used (e.g. PCR) some concerns have arisen about the specificity of these tests from other anatomic sites. The advantages of the test are specimens may be transportes from geographically distant areas and stored for several days prior to testing. The NAATs also allow use non-invasive specimen types such as urine and vaginal swabs. The disadvantages of using nonculture nucleic acid probe or amplification tests include unavailability of a viable isolate for antimicrobial susceptibility testing and the possibility of a positive test after treatment, since nucleic acids from organism may persist for a period of time after successful therapy (Barry, 2009).

1.4 Epidemiology of gonococcal infections

Gonococcal infection is more common among young persons, particularly those aged 15-24 years, persons with lower socio-economic status, men who have sex with men (MSM), illicit drug users, commercial workers an racial/ethnic minority groups (Barry, 2009).

Gonococcal infections are among the most common reportable infections around the World. In the Unite Stated, gonorrhea is consistently the second-most frequently reported notifiable infection with more than 350,000 reported in 2006 (Barry, 2009; CDC, 2006).

In the United States, some European countries and Australia, the incidence of gonorrhea decreased at the end of the 1.980s to mid of 1.990s it was mainly attributed to changes in sexual behaviour produced after the appearance of HIV and the introduction of fluoroquinolone treatment (Famiglietti, 2000; Griemberg, 1997; Trotter *in Neisseria* Molecular Mechanisms of Pathogenesis, 2010).

Gonococcal infection has increased over previous years, although not consistently in all countries. In the United States the incidence of gonorrhea in recent years shows an upward trend, while the rate of gonorrhea in 2009 decreased 10.5% respect 2008 (Diez, 2011).

The World Health Organization (WHO) estimated that, globally, there were 62 million new cases of gonorrhea in 1999, with 27 million (44%) in South and South-East Asia, 17 million (27%) in Sub-Saharan Africa and 7.5 million (12%) in Latin America and the Caribbean (WHO, 2001).

2. Currents problems

2.1 *Neisseria gonorrhoeae*: Antimicrobial resistance and clinic impact

The penicillin introduction by the end of 1940s led to the eradication of *N. gonorrhoeae* sulfonamides resistant and it was the antimicrobial agent that kept its effectiveness for nearly forty years (approximately 1945-1985), although it required increasing the dose in response to the emergence of chromosomal resistance and the use of alternative drugs for the treatment of isolates penicillinase producers (PPNG), since its appearance in 1976 (Ashford, 1976). In the mid of 1980s the prevalence of these strains exceeded 40% for what should no longer be used for empiric treatment of gonorrhea. At that time, the percentage of isolates tetracycline resistant was high, greater than 50% (Famiglietti, 2001). To the high prevalence of isolates with chromosomal resistance to tetracycline (CMRNG), originated in 1970, joined the plasmid resistance (TRNG) which is mediated by the *tetM* determinant in conjugative plasmid that confers high level resistance (Morse, 1986).

The market introduction of fluoroquinolones in the middle of 1980s, was the ideal replacement of penicillin, not only be used as a single-dose and would be highly effective, but also has advantage on the route of administration of drug and fewer adverse effects.

In the United States, due to increased resistance to penicillin and tetracycline, the Centers for Disease Control and Prevention (CDC) recommended the use of extended- spectrum cephalosporin or a fluoroquinolone as firt line treatment for the uncomplicated gonococcal infection (CDC, 1993).

The use of highly effective fluoroquinolone against PPNG helped limit rapid spread of these strains (Janda and Gaydos *in* Manual of Clinical Microbiology, 2007). However, in 1986 resistance to enoxacin was reported in Netherlands and the first treatment failures to fluorquinolones were documented in Japan in 1.994. (Tapsall, 1992; Deguchi, 2010). Such isolates emerged in Argentina in 2000 (Fiorito, 2001).

At the last years, the emergence of *N. gonorrhoeae* resistant to fluoroquinolones reintated the global problem of the treatment and control of gonorrhea (Update CDC, 2007). The increase followed a kinetics up more often affecting men who have sex with men (MSM), but then also was extended to heterosexuals men (HET) Figure 1 (CDC,2004; García 2008). MSM constitute the most important sources of transmission to sexual contacts from extragenital infections (rectum and pharynx), which are often asymptomatic. The high incidence of these strains forced a change in the empirical treatment of gonorrhea by cephalosporins, initially in MSM and their contacts, and later in the heterosexual men (CDC, 2006, 2010).

About macrolides, since its introduction in 1952, erythromycin was used for the treatment of various infections with an acceptable degree of adverse effects. In 1975 it was recommended as treatment for gonorrhoea in pregnant women allergic to penicillin (U.S. Public Health Service, 1975). In 1977, it was observed a decline in the drug effectiveness (Brown, 1977).

Azithromycin is an azalide, structurally and pharmacologically related with erythromycin. It was recommended for the treatment of infection caused by *Chlamydia trachomatis*, a single dose of 1 g orally, while for gonorrhea is used in a higher dose (2g) (CDC, 2002).

Given that *N. gonorrhoeae*, easily develops resistance to antimicrobial agents and its rapid spread, the WHO and CDC recommend changing the treatment regimen when the prevalence of antimicrobial resistance is> 5% (WHO, 2003).

Currently, the CDC recommends for the treatment of uncomplicated gonorrhea and infections located in the cervix, urethra and rectum, ceftriaxone 250 mg IM in one dose or cefixime 400 mg associated with azithromycin 1g VO or doxycycline 100 mg / day for 7 days , VO (CDC, 2010). However there are regions where resistance to cefixime does not allow its use (Barry, 2009).

Azithromycin and doxycycline are intended to cover the presence of *Chlamydia trachomatis* non gonococcal urethritis . The recommended dose of azithromycin for treatment of gonorrhea is 2g VO to prevent the emergence of resistance (CDC, 2010).

About the antimicrobial agents which are recommended by the CDC, there were treatment failures with azithromycin when it was given in a single dose of 1g VO for uncomplicated gonorrhea, with isolates had MICs between 0.125 and 0.5 μg / ml (Zarantonelli , 1999; Ehret, 1996). Recently, in several countries are emerging of high-level resistance to azithromycin strains (Galarza 2009; Palmer, 2008; Chisholm, 2009; Starnino, 2009).

Ceftriaxone (third-generation cephalosporin, parenteral) retains its activity against *N. gonorrhoeae*, but recently have been appearing isolates with decreased sensitivity in various regions of the world (Martin, 2006; Barry, 2009, Tapsall, 2009; Chisholm, 2010; Deguchi, 2010; Garcia, 2010a).

3. Present study with review of literature

3.1 Incidence of gonorrhea

The STD Program of the National Hospital of Clinics, "José de San Martín" University of Buenos Aires, Argentina, deals with 80% patients from the city and 20% from the suburban areas. In a period of 10 years (2000-2009), was investigated the presence of *Neisseria gonorrhoeae* in 4273 male patients (52% MSM and 48% HET).

The average age of MSM was 33 years (range 14-75 years) and HET was 34 years (range 15-82 years). The incidence of gonorrhea was 10.3% and 9.5% in MSM and HET respectively ($p > 0.05$) and it was more frequent in men between 20 and 29 years old in both groups of patients.

In MSM urethral location was the most frequent (70%), followed by rectal (34%) and lastly the pharynx (17%). This increase in the incidence of gonorrhea in HET in 2008 and 2009 compared to 2007, was significant ($p < 0.05$) and has also been reported by other authors (Velicko, 2009). It could be due to increased in this population of *N. gonorrhoeae* fluoroquinolone resistant in this population, since it was initially installed in the MSM.

Fluctuations were observed in the annual incidence of gonorrhea in MSM and heterosexual men between 1995 and 2009, with a decrease at the end of the 1990s and beginning of the new millennium but then it continued to increase slowly in recent years, specially among heterosexual men.

The analysis of results was divided into two periods: 2000-04 (first period), the emergence of *N. gonorrhoeae* fluoroquinolone resistant in 2005 in our Hospital pointed the beginning of the second period: 2005-09 (second period). The Table 1 shows the incidence of *N. gonorrhoeae* from clinical specimens according to patient's sex habits.

The National Health Surveillance of the Ministry of Health of Argentina (SNVS) had registered 28.517 and 17.017 cases of gonorrhea in the periods 2000-4 and 2005-09 respectively.

Period	Heterosexual men			MSM				
	N°		Location	N°		Location		
	Patients	Positive (%)	Urethra	Patients	Positive (%)	Urethra	Rectum	Pharinx
2000-04	1259	100 (7.9)	100	1143	117 (10.2)	78	45	15
2005-09	802	95 (11.8)	94 Joined (1)	1069	111 (10.4)	81	33	24
Total	2061	195 (9.5)	195	2212	228 (10.3)	159	78	39

Table 1. Number and percentaje of gonorrhea cases in males according their sexual habits and location sites.

3.2 Antimicrobial resistance

All isolates were tested for beta lactamase by chromogenic cephalosporin Nitrocefin method (Cefinase BBL. Beckton Dickinson). Over 324 isolates of *N. gonorrhoeae* was determined the minimum inhibitory concentration (MIC) of several antimicrobial agents by the agar dilution method according to the recommendation of Clinical Laboratory Standard Iinternational (CLSI, 2009).

3.2.1 Penicillin

The mechanisms of resistance to penicillin are the production of β-lactamase (penicillinase), chromosomal resistance by altering PBP1 and 2, reduced income and increased efflux.

During periods 2000-04 and 2005-09 the global prevalence of *N. gonorrhoeae* β- Lactamase positive (PPNG) was 8.3% and 12.6%, and chromosomal resistance (CMRNG) was 4.2% and 23.7% respectively. A significant increase of *N. gonorrhoeae* with chromosomal resistance to penicillin was observed for both groups of patients ($p<0.05$) in the second period, the results are showed in table 2.

Period/SH	total N° isolates	CMRNG%	PPNG%
2000-04			
MSM	117	6.8	10.2
HET	100	1.0	6
Total	**217**	**4.2**	**8.3**
2005-09			
MSM	111	33.3	7.2
HET	95	12.6	18.9
Total	**206**	**23.7**	**12.6**

Table 2. Prevalence of *Neisseria gonorrhoeae* resistant to penicillin

Whereas the number of isolates β- lactamase positive (PPNG) among MSM decreased ($p> 0.05$) between first and second periods, the prevalence of chromocomal resistance (CMRNG) to penicillin was significantly higher than HET ($p<0.05$). It could be related to the rectal location, since the environment is rich in fatty acids and hydrophobic molecules that can act as a positive selection factor favoring the emergence of resistant strains (Mtr phenotype) (García, 2011).

Resistance to penicillin founded is within the range of Argentine national data (Galarza, 2010).

3.2.2 Tetracycline

Plasmid tetracycline resistance is mediated by the *tet M* determinant (MIC ≥ 16 µg/ml) while chromosome type resistance involves the modification of ribosomal protein (S10-Val 57) (MIC ≥2 µg/ml) (Shaffer *in Neisseria* Molecular mechanisms of Pathogenesis, 2010).

The resistance was higher in the second period for both groups ($p>0.05$) (figure 1).

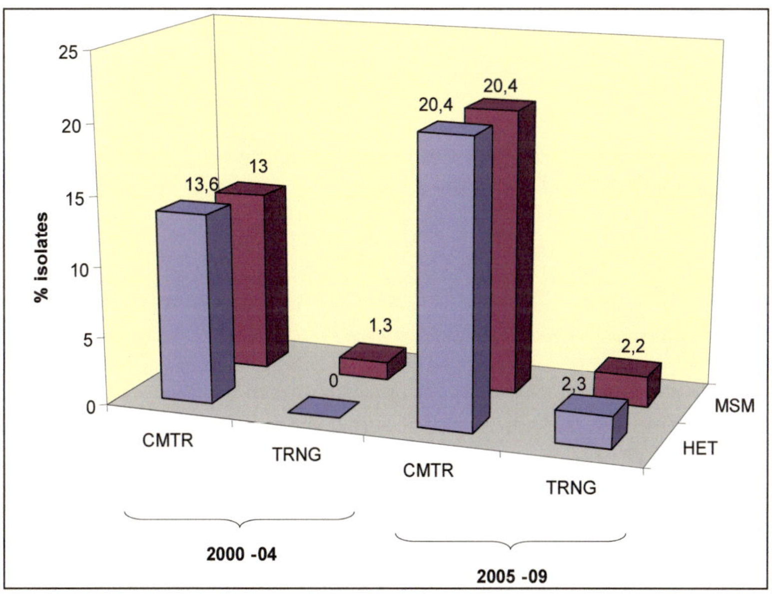

Fig. 1. Percentage of chromosomal and plasmid resistance to tetracycline.

Isolates with low-level resistance to tetracycline (MIC <16 μg / ml) had no cross-resistance to minocycline (CIM: 0062-4 μg / ml) (García, 2010a, 2011)

Tetracycline showed little activity. The plasmid resistance was uncommon (5 / 324), as in other regions of Argentina (Galarza, 2010b).

In figure 1 are shown the plasmid and chromosomal resistance to tetracycline in both groups of patients.

3.2.3 Spectinomycin

In 2005-09 period a 11% of the isolates showed intermediate sensitivity to spectinomycin (MIC = 64 μg / ml), 80% of cases from MSM (García, 2010a, 2011). However, the Argentina national data showing 100% sensitivity, but in South Africa was found 33.4% resistance to this antimicrobial (Govender, 2006).

Spectinomycin is effective for the treatment of anogenital gonorrhea but is not useful for pharyngeal infection. Besides *N. gonorrhoeae* can rapidly develop resistance of high-level resistance by a single mutation, it was documented in the U.S., Korea and United Kingdom (Reyn, 1973; Ashford, 1981; Barry, 2009).

3.2.4 Emerging of antimicrobial resistance

The emerging resistance of *N. gonorrhoeae* in the last decade is to erythromycin, azithromycin, fluoroquinolones and decreased sensitivity to ceftriaxone.

In *N. gonorrhoeae* were identified four efflux pumps: MtrCDE, FarAB, MacAB, and NorM that belong to the families RND, MF, ABC and MATE respectively. Only a few gonococci *mef* gene was detected (Shafer *in Neisseria* Molecular Mechanisms of Pathogenesis, 2010).

3.2.4.1 Resistance to erythromycin and azithromycin

Resistance to macrolides and azalides in *N. gonorrhoeae* may be due to different mechanisms: overexpression of efflux pumps, alteration of the target site, decreased outer membrane permeability and inactivation of the drug.

Of the efflux pumps, MtrCDE, MacAB and NorM recognized relevant antibiotics to treat gonorrhea. Protein efflux pump encoded by the *mef* gene can also recognize macrolides. The *mef* gene is located on a conjugative transposon, but has been found in a limited number of gonococci (Luna, 2002).

The MtrCDE-efflux pump can export erythromycin, tetracycline, penicillin, and hydrophobic compounds including fatty acids, bile salts, steroids and antibacterial peptides (Morse, 1982, Hagman, 1995), while the pump NorM exports quinolones (Rouquette-Loughlin, 2003) and MacAB pump exports macrolides (Rouquette-Loughlin, 2005)

The expression of genes encoding the bacterial efflux depends of several regulatory levels. The loss of regulatory systems can result in high levels of antimicrobial resistance.

The *mtrCDE* operon has three genes encoding each of the proteins that make up this bomb: MtrC (fusion protein) and MtrR (cytoplasmic membrane protein), MtrE (outer membrane protein).

The complex of genes *mtrCDE* represents a transcriptional unit is located 250 bp upstream and divergently transcribed respect to *mtrR* gene, which is the gene that encodes a regulatory protein MtrR (repressor) of *mtrCDE* transcription (Lucas, 1997).

The MtrR protein negatively regulates transcription of the *mtrCDE* operon, it binds to DNA in the region of 250 bp separating the genes *mtrR* and *mtrC*, a region where is the promoter of the operon transcription. In clinical isolates were found *mtrR* mutations that alter the repressor protein and its binding to DNA, resulting in decreased repression of the *mtrCDE* operon (Lucas, 1997).

These mutations are found in the region between residues 32 and 53 that make up the domain helix-turn-helix protein in the DNA binding and mutations "missense" causing A39T amino acid replacement (replacement of alanine by threonine in position 39) or G45D (replacement of glycine by aspartic acid at position 45) can increase the resistance to hydrophobic antimicrobial presumably because avoid the binding of the MtrR repressor protein to DNA up stream on *mtrCDE* . Another mutation described in clinical isolates is one that occurs in the middle of the coding sequence of *mtrR*: H105Y

(Replacement of histidine by tyrosine at position 105) or in the C-terminal domain that can impact the function of MtrR probably by altering the formation of multimer MtrR (Shafer, 1995; Warner, 2008).

There are differences in the level of resistance conferred by mutations, the "missense" mutations in the coding sequence typically result in low to intermediate level of resistance while mutations in the promoter are associated with high level of resistance (Warner, 2008).

Another mechanism of regulation of this efflux system is exercised by a region of inverted repeats of 13 bp in the *mtrR* gene promoter, it has a function as a transcriptional control element cis type. In laboratory mutants and clinical isolates was found that the deletion of one base pair A: T in this region causes an increased expression of *mtrCDE* operon and repression of *mtrR* gene transcription, it confers low-level resistance to tetracycline , erythromycin, penicillin and hydrophobic agents such as crystal violet, fecal lipids, bile salts, detergents (Eg: Triton X-100, nonoxynol-9) (Hagman, 1995) In these cases, erythromycin and azithromycin MICs were up to 2 μg / ml and 0.5 μg / ml respectively (Zarantorelli, 2001, Cousin, 2003).

Previous studies indicate that isolates of *N. gonorrhoeae* from MSM were more resistant compared to inhibition by a variety of structurally different hydrophobic compounds, including fecal lipids, bile salts, detergents (eg, Triton X-100) and hydrophobic antibiotics (eg: erythromycin). It has been attributed to mutations in the efflux system of multiple transferable resistance(Mtr) resistance to erythromycin and Triton X-100, it can serve as a phenotypic marker for resistance mediated by Mtr in *N. gonorrhoeae* (Morse, 1982; Zarantonelli, 1999).

There is clinical evidence to suggest that efflux pumps increase the capacity of gonococci to survive during human infection. First, *mtrR* mutants are isolated frequently from rectum of infected patients presumably because it environment is rich in hydrophobic compounds such as long chain fatty acids (Morse, 1982).

Another mechanism is described in gonococcal is the ribosomal rRNA methylation by methylases, thereby blocks the binding site of macrolides by methylation in 23 S rRNA in an adenosine residue at position 2058 (in *E.coli*), it site is the domain of the peptidyl transferase (Leclerq and Courvalin, 1991).

In *N. gonorrhoeae* have been identified enzymes rRNA methylases encoded by the genes *ermB, ermC, ermF* and recently *ermA* (Roberts, 1999; Chen, 2010).

The genes encoding rRNA methylase may be in conjugative transposons and they may confer to gonococci highly level of resistance to erythromycin (4-16 µg / ml) or decreased sensitivity to azithromycin (1 - 4 µg / ml) without mutations in *mtrR* (Roberts, 1999; Shafer, *in Neisseria* Molecular Mechanisms of Pathogenesis, 2010)

In recent years the study of strains highly resistant to azithromycin revealed another mechanism of resistance due to mutations in the gene encoding the "loop" domain V of 23S rRNA peptidyl transferase in the 50S subunit of the ribosome (Chisholm, 2010; Galarza, 2010a).

The outer membrane of gram-negative represents a significant permeability barrier to antibiotics, particularly hydrophobic compounds. Different degrees of truncation of LPS oligosaccharides (known as lipooligosaccharides [LOS] in *Neisseria*) can alter the entry of hydrophobic molecules (Lucas, 1995).

There was not agreement between the diffusion and dilution methods for erythromycin and azithromycin, which is why we could not recommend break points for diffusion test.

In our study, erythromycin resistance increased statistically significantly from first to second period for MSM 20.8% and 39.8% respectively ($p < 0.05$), while for the HET the difference was not significant, 22.9% and 25.0% respectively;($p > 0.05$).

The difference between MSM and HET was not statistically significant ($p > 0.05$). The activity of azithromycin was superior to erythromycin.

In the second period two isolates of *N. gonorrhoeae* with erythromycin MICs = 256 µg / ml were associated with azithromycin MICs of 4 and 16 µg / ml, the second strain also was resistant to tetracycline, penicillin and ciprofloxacin. These findings are consistent with those of other regions of Argentina and other countries (Galarza, 2009; Palmer, 2008; Starnino, 2009, Chisholm, 2010) and point to the emergence of high-level resistance to azithromycin, it has impact public health and would limit the drug as a treatment option for gonorrhea.

In the isolates with Mtr phenotype (MIC of Triton-X100> 2000 µg/ml), the most frequently mutation found was a deletion of a base pair A:T in the region of inverted repeats of 13 bp in the promoter region and mutations in the coding region of *mtrR* gene which could be associated with overexpression of MtrCDE pump efflux and subsequent macrolide resistance as other authors have shown (Morse, 1982; Zantorelli, 2001). It was the only mechanism of macrolide resistant found in these isolates (García, 2011).

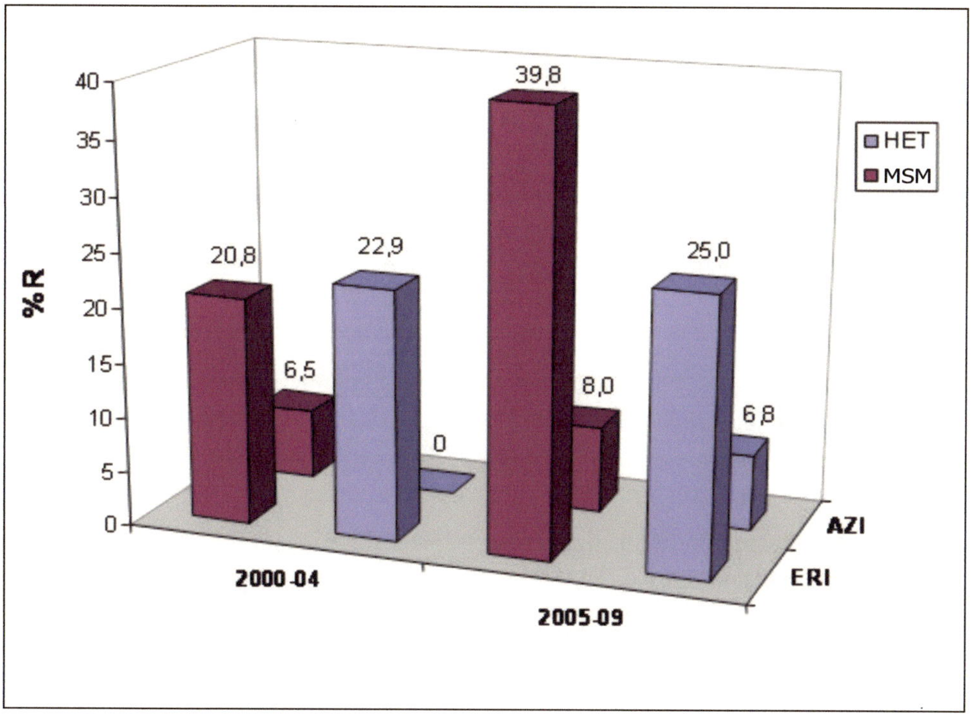

Fig. 2. Percentage of *N. gonrrhoeae* resistant to erythromycin and azithromycin.

In recent years there were communications about the finding of gonococci with high level of resistance to azithromycin (MIC ≥ 256 µg / ml) in many countries. The first isolation came from Argentina in 2001 (Galarza, 2009), and then in Europe: Scotland, 2004, England, Wales and Italy 2007 (Chisholm, 2009, 2010, Stamino, 2009).

The argentine isolate had a MIC > 2048 µg / ml and A2143G mutation was detected in the 4 allele. This mutation corresponds to A2059G, described previously in *Escherichia coli* but not in gonococci (Galarza, 2010).

The use of subtherapeutic doses of azithromycin may be the cause of the emergence of strains of *N. gonorrhoeae* resistant to the antimicrobial agents.

3.2.4.2 Resistance to fluoroquinolones

In gonococci the most frequently found mechanism is the alteration of the target site of fluoroquinolones: mutations in QRDR regions (Quinolone Resistance Determining Region) of genes *gyrA, gyrB, parC* and *parE* encoding topoisomerase enzymes that translate in changes in the amino acids sequence in GyrA and GyrB, subunits of topoisomerase II (DNA gyrase) and ParC, subunit of topoisomerase IV. Mutations in *gyrB* have little significance, since low-level confer resistance to nalidixic acid only, whereas, mutations in *gyrA* and *parC* genes, confer clinical resistance to the fluoroquinolones. Mutations in *parC* occur only in isolates that had at least one mutation in *gyrA* (Otero, 2002). Mutations in *parE* is not related to high-level resistance to quinolones.

Another mechanism is related to the decrease in cytoplasmic concentration of the drug, it can occur by overexpression of efflux pumps and reduced permeability.

The *mtrCDE* overexpression can confer low-level resistance to fluoroquinolones and hydrophobic compounds (Hagman, 1995).

Other efflux system detected in *N. gonorrhoeae* , like NorM of Vibrio parahaemolyticus tht belonged to the MATE transporter superfamily, it recognizes cationic compounds resulting in increased gonococci resistance to norfloxacin and ciprofloxacin (Rouquette-Loughlin, 2003).

The phenotype of low resistance may be due to decreased penetration of antibiotic through the bacterial cell membrane. The routes of penetration of quinolones through the bacterial cell wall are not completely defined, but hydrophilic molecules seem to diffuse through the outer membrane of gram-negative porin-type channels (Hooper *in* Infectious Diseases Principles and Practice, 2010).

In the Hospital of Clinics of the University of Buenos Aires were detected the first isolates fluoroquinolone resistant (QRNG) in 2005 and its frequency was increasing in the coming years especially in the MSM, this forced a change in empirical therapy later extended to heterosexual men (Garcia, 2008). We couldn't demonstrate epidemiological link among cases, excepting two. The percentage of QRNG according to the patient's sexual habits are shown in Figure 3.

Resistance to ciprofloxacin is extensive to other fluoroquinolone (norfloxacin, ofloxacin, gatifloxacin and lomefloxacin).

The resistance to fluoroquinolones was associated to multidrug resistance (García 2010b)

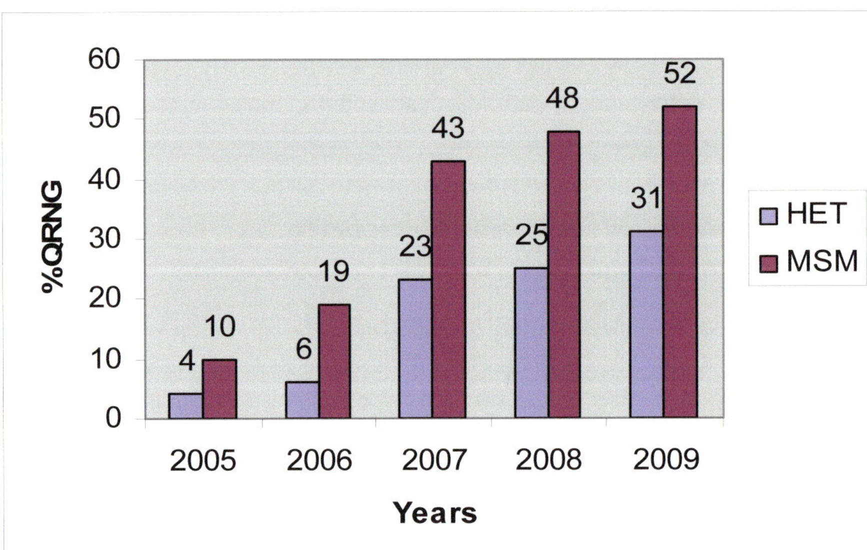

Fig. 3. *N. gonorrhoeae* fluoroquinolone resistant along the years.

In the QRNG the mechanism found was mutations in topoisomerases (subunits GyrA and ParC) (García, 2011).

3.2.4.3 Ceftriaxone decreased sensitivity

The genetic mechanisms that increase resistance to third generation cephalosporins in *N. gonorrhoeae* have not been fully elucidated, but much of that resistance is due to mosaic *penA* alleles and probably require alterations in PBP, decreased membrane permeability barrier and overexpression of efflux pumps.

N. gonorrhoeae has three PBPs, named 1, 2 and 3. The PBP2 has a 10 times higher affinity for penicillin G that PBP1 and is believed to be the site of increased binding to cephalosporins.

Some alterations in PBP2 were associated with resistance to β-lactams including cephalosporins. The most common mechanism associated with resistance to cefixime is altered PBP2 (Ameyama, 2002). Recently, *penA* alleles different from previously known strains appeared in increased resistance to third generation cephalosporins such as cefixime and ceftriaxone. These alleles encode at least 60 mutations in PBP2 compared to the wild strain and they have a mosaic gene organization appears to have been caused by recombination with commensal *Neisseria* genes such as *N. perflava, N. sicca, N. cinerea or N. flavescens* (Ameyama, 2002; Tanaka, 2006).

It was reported the isolation of *N. gonorrhoeae* with ceftriaxone MIC = 0.5 μg / ml had the mosaic PBP2, but also mutations in *ponA* (L421P), *penB* (A120 and A121) and *mtrR*. They hypothesized that the L421P substitution in the gene encoding PBP1 *ponA* may be important in conferring resistance to ceftriaxone. The possible importance of ponA L421P was subsequently supported by data Takahata in which strains with the substitution L421P was associated with increased cephalosporin MICs, compared with only transformants that had the mosaic PBP2 (Takahata, 2006). However, Nicholas found neither the presence or absence of *ponA* affected the MICs of cephalosporins (Nicholas, 2008).

This indicates that the mosaic is important but not worth enough to generate the high level of resistance to cefixime (Barry, 2009).

penB mutations, in the "loop" of the gene, reduces the permeability to hydrophilic antibiotics and is considered related to chromosomal resistance to penicillin, cephalosporins, tetracyclines and fluoroquinolones (Tanaka, 2006).

In our experience, ceftriaxone proved to be more active, however there is an emergence of strains with decreased sensitivity (0.125 to 0.25 μg / ml) and the increase of such isolates was notable especially in the year 2009. A 100% of the isolates were susceptible to ceftriaxone, but the 7.7% showed reduced susceptibility (MIC: 0.125 to 0.25 μg / ml) and did not express extended spectrum beta lactamase (βLEE) (García, 2010b)

This situation is similar to other countries, in Australia (2005) 1% of the isolates of *N. gonorrhoeae* had MIC ≥ 0.062 μg / ml; 12.1% in Amsterdam in 2008; 3% in Russia (2004) and elsewhere (Tanaka, 2006; Barry, 2009; Martin, 2006).

In Japan, cefixime therapy failures date back to 2000, it stopped to be used in 2006 and it was replaced by ceftriaxone and spectinomycin which are used as first-line drugs for empirical treatment of uncomplicated gonorrhea (Barry, 2009). In China, Hong Kong and

Taiwan were detected isolates with decreased sensitivity to ceftriaxone and treatment failures with ceftibuten. In Vietnam, Thailand and the Philippines have been isolated sporadically *N. gonorrhoeae* with ceftriaxone MICs of ≥ 0.5 μg / ml. In Europe and the U.S. were also found isolates of *N. gonorrhoeae* with ceftriaxone MIC ≥ 0.125 μg / ml. (Barry, 2009, Martin 2006).

In Argentina, the first report of isolates of *N. gonorrhoeae* with decreased sensitivity to ceftriaxone came from in the Hospital of Clinics, "José de San Martín", Universiy of Buenos Aires. The emergence of strains with reduced sensitivity to ceftriaxone is an alert to the possibility of treatment failure in a short period of time.

The combination of different mechanisms of resistance in the same strain, or affectation of multiple antimicrobial for developing a type of mechanism leads to the emergence of strains resistant to several antimicrobial agents simultaneously. Tapsall (2009) defined *N. gonorrhoeae* multi drug resistant (MDR-NG) when the isolate has resistance to a class of antimicrobial listed in category I: parenteral Cephalosporins / oral cephalosporins / Spectinomycin, plus the resistance of two or more classes of antimicrobial in category II:

penicillins/ fluoroquinolones/azithromycin/aminoglycosides/carbapenems.

Extensively-drug resistant *N. gonorrhoeae* (XDR-NG) include those resistant to two or more of the antibiotic classes in category I and three or more in category II.

In our study 4.3% (14/324) isolates of *N. gonorrhoeae* were categorized as multiresistant and 0.3% (1 / 324) resistant gonococci extensively according to the definitions of Tapsall (2009) (García, 2011).

4. Genetic relationship of isolates of *N. gonorrhoeae* ciprofloxacin resistant

The characterization of different isolates of *N. gonorrhoeae* provides the information necessary to understand the strains circulating in a community, identify chains of transmission, the temporal changes that may occur and the emergence and spread of antimicrobial resistance (Rahman, 2001).

The first methods used were based on phenotypic characteristics, the auxotipificación and serotyping; also the profile of antimicrobial resistance and type of plasmids contribute to the characterization of strains, but they do so limited, these techniques have less discrimination index for delineate strains of a species that genotyping assays.

Several molecular techniques have been applied to the study of *N. gonorrhoeae*, ribotyping, AP-PCR, REP-PCR, ARDRA, PCR-RFLP, sequencing of the genes *opa*, *TbpB*, NG-MAST, MLST. Pulsed-field gel electrophoresis (PFGE) is a standard technique for studying populations of many bacteria, but it would not be discriminating enough to distinguish the great diversity of genotypes expected in a recombinant nonclonal population as *N. gonorrhoeae* (O'Rourke, 1995).

However, in a study by Van Looveren, 1999, was found that the discriminative power of some typing methods for *N. gonorrhoeae*, defined as the method's ability to differentiate unrelated strains (Simpson Index) was higher for PFGE (SI:0.997).

The election of the technique depends of objective early or late evolution.

The most discriminative techniques are multilocus sequence typing (MLST), multiantigen sequence typing (NG-MAST), *porB*-based DNA sequence analysis and PCR-RFLP *opa.* To study isolates during short time periods in order to detected transmission chains, identify circulating strains community epidemics, e.g. the elected methods are *porB* sequence analysis and NG-MAST. Furthermore, isolates with identicalDNA sequencing types may be further subdivided by using bother high-resolution methods, such as PFGE and Opa typing.

The family of *opa* genes evolve rapidly in order to distinguish genetically unrelated strains and to demonstrate sexual contacts, as well as the persistence of strains in the community present in asymptomatic individuals.

opa gene analysis is sufficiently discriminative to detect short chains of transmission (García, 2011).

The analysis of different genotypes of *N. gonorrhoeae* over the years, in the population stutied, let we conclude that the increase in quinolone resistance was not due to the spread of a single strain.

Other molecular technique applicable for this purpose to *N. gonorrhoeae* are MLST and NG-MAST with discriminatory indices exceeding 0.9 (Tazi, 2010; Morris, 2009).

5. Conclusion

In conclusion, selective pressure exerted by antibiotics and the inappropriate use of them reflects the high number of *N. gonorrhoeae* fluoroquinolone resistant is circulating in our program area, resistance to erythromycin and azithromycin and the findings of decreased susceptibility to ceftriaxone and especinomicina.

An increase of *N. gonorrhoeae* fluoroquinolone resistant was detected initially in the MSM population that later spread to the HET and based the modification of empiric treatment of gonorrhea by ceftriaxone. Be alert to the emergence of gonococci with decreased susceptibility to ceftriaxone, which also presented simultaneous resistance to other agents and its association with MSM population.

Currently exist a large number of resistant strains of *N. gonorrhoeae* fluoroquinolone resistant circulating and most of them are not shared between HET and MSM.

6. Future perspectives

In view of the widespread emergence of resistant isolates and the multidrug resistance profile of *N. gonorrhoeae* also to emphasize or intensify prevention campaigns among young people should be evaluated strategies that can be applied in case of emergence of resistance to ceftriaxone. One of them is not yet tested other antibiotics prescribed for the treatment of gonorrhea in order to search for drugs up in case of emerging resistance to third generation parenteral cephalosporins. There is limited experience in the treatment of gonococcal infections with aminoglycosides, these drugs have been used in Asia and Africa. No kanamycin resistance was detected but it developed resistance to gentamicin when it is used in Malawi (Barry, 2009). In a surveillance study of resistance of *N.*

gonorrhoeae in Europe, 95% of 1366 isolates showed MIC of gentamicin in a narrow range: 4-8 ug / ml (Chisholm, 2010).

The frequency of tetracycline resistance is very high and resistance to azithromycin is more than 5% and circulating strains with high resistance, so that these drugs would not be appropriate to empirical treatment of gonorrhea.

Spectinomycin, is an aminocyclitol that shows good activity and appear to be among the possible treatment in case of resistance to ceftriaxone, but there are gonococci with intermediate sensitivity (Garcia, 2010; Barry, 2009). Furthermore, mutations in a single step are able to quickly generate resistance and it was checked when spectinomycin was used as treatment against PPNG strains. We should also take into account the lack of eradication of throat infection (Barry, 2009).

Tigecycline, glycylcycline derivative of tetracycline, showed in vitro activity against *N. gonorrhoeae* resistant to tetracycline, but there have been no clinical trials for infections caused by this organism. Rifampin may be an alternative but quickly generates resistance (Barry, 2009).

Other drugs that could be tested are Lactivicinas (LTV) that inhibits PBPs but their structure does not contain the β-lactam ring and thus is resistant to the action of β-lactamases, are active against clinical isolates of *Streptococcus pneumoniae* resistant to penicillin (Macheboeuf, 2007).

Medicinal plants like Ocimum sanctum were investigated as possible source of new active drugs against *N. gonorrhoeae,* after extraction and purification of its active ingredient "eugenol" tested its activity against *N. gonorrhoeae* and shown to have antimicrobial activity, in view of its efficacy and low toxicity can be a potential molecule to be developed for clinical application (Shoken, 2008).

Some authors suggest the design of drugs to site of action of efflux pumps as they are responsible for simultaneous resistance to several antimicrobial (Shafer *in Neisseria* Molecular Mechanisms of Pathogenesis, 2010).

Other strategies to use would be: I) Increase the dose of cephalosporin, ii) multi-dose cephalosporin regimens; III) microbiologically directed treatment, IV) association of antimicrobial agents, V) Rotate empirical treatments (Chisolmon, 2010).

The development a vaccine for *N. gonorrhoeae* would be effective tool to act from prevention, however attempts at developing it were difficult because of the antigenic diversity and variability, and the lack of an animal model. Research in these areas will play a large rol in the future.

On the other hand, is not only important to detect carriers but also testing antimicrobial susceptibility against the isolation of *N. gonorrhoeae* from each sites of infection.

7. Acknowledgment

We thank UBACyT B108 Project of University of Buenos Aires. Argentina.

8. References

Ameyama S, Onodera S, Takahata M, Minami S, Maki N, Endo K, Suzuki H & Oishi Y.(2002). Mosaic-like structure of penicillin-binding proteína 2 Gene (*pen*A) in clinical isolates of *Neisseria gonorrhoeae* with reduced susceptibility to cefixime. *Antimicrob Agents Chemother*, Vol. 46, N° 12, (December, 2002), pp. 3744-3749, ISSN: 0066-4804.

Apicella MA, Falsetta M, Neil R & Steichen C. (2010). Gonococcal Biofilms, In: *Neisseria Molecular Mechanisms of Pathogenesis*, Attardo Genco C & Wetzler L, editors, pp. 55-60, Caister Academic Press Boston MA. USA, ISBN: 978-1-904455-51-6, Boston MA. USA.

Ashford WA, Golash RG & Henning VG. (1976). Penicillinase producing *Neisseria gonorrhoeae. Lancet*, Vol. 2, pp.:657-658, ISSN: 0140-6736.

Ashford WA, Potts DW & Adams HJU. (1981). Spectinomycin- resistant penicillinase-producing *Neisseria gonorrhoeae. Lancet*, Vol. 2, pp. 1035-1037, ISSN: 0140-6736.

Bala M & Sood Seema. (2010). Cephalosporin Resistance in *Neisseria gonorrhoeae. J Glob Infect Dis*, Vol. 2, N° 3. pp. 284-290, ISSN: Print- 0974-777X.

Barry PM & Klausner J. (2009). The use of cephalosporins for gonorrhea: The impending problem of resistance. *Expert Opin Pharmacother*, Vol. 10, N° 4, (March, 2009), pp. 555-577, ISSN: 1465-6566.

Brown ST, Pedersen IIB & Holmes KK. (1977). Comparison of erythromycin base and escolate in gonococcal urethritis. *Jama*, Vol. 238 (13), pp. 1371-1373, ISSN: 0098-7484.

Centers for Disease Control and Prevention. (1993). Sexually transmited disease treatment Guidelines. *Morb Mortal Weekly Rep*, Vol. 42, N° (RR-14), pp. 1-101, ISSN: 0149-2195.

Centers for Disease Control and Prevention. (2002). Increases in fluorquinolone- resistant *Neisseria gonorrhoeae* - Hawaii and California 2001. *Morb Mortal Weekly Rep*, Vol. 51, pp. 1041-1044 , ISSN: 0149-2195.

Centers for Disease Control and Prevention. (2004). Increases in fluorquilonolone resistance *Neisseria gonorrhoeae* among men who have sex with men- US, 2003 and revised recomendations for gonorrhea treatment. *Morb Mortal Weekly Rep*, Vol. 53, N° 16 pp.335-338, ISSN: 0149-2195.

Centers for Disease Control and Prevention (CDC). (2006). Sexually Transmitted Diseases Treatment Guidelines. *Morb Mortal Weekly Rep*, Vol. 55, N° (RR-11), pp. 364-366, ISSN: 1545-8601.

Centers for Disease Control and Prevention. (2010). Sexually transmitted Diseases Treatment Guidelines. *Morb Mortal Weekly Rep*, Vol. 59, N° (RR-12), (December, 2010), pp. 49-55, ISSN: 1545-8601.

Chen PL, Lee HC, Yan JJ, Hsieh YH, Lee NY, Ko NY, Lin CW, Chang CM & Wu CJ. (2010). High Prevalence of Mutations in Quinolone- resistance- determining Regions and *mtr*R Loci in Polyclonal *Neisseria gonorrhoeae* Isolates at Tertiary Hospital in Southern Taiwan. *J Formos Med Assoc*, Vol. 109, N° 2, pp.120-127, ISSN: 0929-6646.

Chilsholm SA, Neal TJ, Alawattegama AB, Birley HDL, Howe RA & Ison CA. (2009). Emergence of high-level azithromycin resistance in *Neisseria gonorrhoeae* in England and Wales. *J Antimicrob Chemother*, Vol. 64, N° 2, (May 2009), pp. 353-358, ISSN: 0305-7453.

Chisholm SA, Dave J & Iso C. (2010). High-Level azithromycin resistance occurs in *Neisseria gonorrhoeae* as a result of a single point mutation in the 23S rRNA genes. *Antimicrob Agents Chemother*, Vol.54, N° 9, (September, 2010), pp. 3812-3816, ISSN: 0066-4804.

Clinical Laboratory Standards Institute. (CLSI). 2009. *Methods for dilution antimicrobial susceptibility test for bacteria that grow aerobically*, 19th Informational Suplement M07-A8, Vol. 29, N° 3, (January 2009), pp.68-71. Wayne, Pa, USA, ISBN: 1—56238-690-5; ISSN: 0273-3099.

Cousin SL, Whittington WL & Roberts MC. (2003). Acquired macrolide resistance genes and the 1 bp deletion in the *mtrR* promoter in *Neisseria gonorrhoeae*. *J. Antimicrob Chemother*, Vol. 51, N° 12 pp.131-133, ISSN: 0305-7453

Deguchi T, Nakane K, Yasuda M & Maeda S. (2010). Emergence and Spread of Drug Resistant *Neisseria gonorrhoeae*. *J Urol*, Vol. 184, (September, 2010), pp. 851-858, ISSN: 0066-4804.

Diez M & Díaz A. (2011). Infecciones de transmisión sexual: epidemiología y control. *Rev Esp Sanid Penit*, Vol 13; pp. 58-66, ISSN: 1575-0620.

Ehret JM, Nims LJ & Judson FN. (1996). A clinical isolation of *Nesisseria gonorrhoeae* with in vitro resistance to erytromycin and decreased susceptibility to azithromycin. *Sex Transm Dis*, Vol. 23, N° 4, (July- August, 1996), pp. 270-272, ISSN: 0148-5717.

Famiglietti A, García S, de Mier C, Casco R, Vay C& de Torres R. (2000). *Neisseria gonorrhoeae* Drug Susceptibility in Buenos Aires, Argentina. *APUA Newsletter*, Vol. 18, N° 4, pp. 1-4, ISSN: 1524-1424.

Famiglietti A, García S, de Mier C, Casco R, Belli L, Marcenac F, Vay C& de Torres R. (2001). Evolución of *Neisseria gonorrhoeae* drug susceptibility in Buenos Aires, Argentina 1985 1999. *Sex Transm Infect*, Vol. 77, N° 2, (April, 2001), pp. 142 - 143, ISSN: 1368-4973.

Fiorito S, Galarza P, Pagano I, Oviedo C, Lanza A, Smayevsky J, Weltman G, Buscemi L & Sanjuán E .(2001). Emergence of high level ciprofloxacin resistant *Neisseria gonorrhoeae* strain in Buenos Aires, Argentina. *Sex Transm Dis*, Vol. 77, pp. 77, ISSN: 0148-5717.

Galarza PG, Alcalá B, SalcedoC, Fernández Canigia L, Buscemi L, Pagano I, Oviedo C& Vázquez JA. (2009). Emergence of high level azithromycin- resistant *Neisseria gonorrhoeae* strain isolated in Argentina. *Sex Transm Dis*, Vol. 36c, pp. 787-788, ISSN: 1368-4973.

Galarza PG, Abad R, Fernández Canigia L, Buscemi L, Pagano I & Oviedo C. (2010a). New Mutation in 23S rRNA Gene Associated with Level of Azithromycin resistance in *Neisseria gonorrhoeae*. *Antimicrob Agents Chemother*, Vol. 54, N° 4, (April, 2010) pp. 1652-1653.

Galarza P, Pagano I, Oviedo C, Reggiane S & RED ITS. (2010b). Vigilancia de la sensibilidad antimicrobiana de *Neisseria gonorrhoeae* en Argentina- PROVSAG 2009. XII Congreso Argentino de Microbiología, Resumen 28058. *Rev Argent Microbiol*, Vol. 42 (Supl 1), (October, 2010), pp. 256, ISSN: 0325-7541.

García S, Casco R, Perazzi B, De Mier C, Vay C & Famiglietti A. (2008). Resistencia de *Neisseria gonorrhoeae* a ciprofloxacina según hábitos sexuales. *Medicina (B. Aires)*, Vol. 68, pp. 358-362, ISSN: 0025-7680.

García SD, Casco R, De Mier C, Perazzi B, Yaya J, Vay C & Famiglietti A. (2010a). Vigilancia epidemiológica de las resistencias emergentes en *Neisseria gonorrhoeae*. Análisis de 5 años (2005-2009). 9° Congreso Internacional de Medicina Interna del Hospital de Clínicas. Resumen 64. *Medicina (B. Aires)* , Vol. 70 (Supl 1), (August, 2010), pp. 27, ISSN: 0025-7680.

García S, Casco R, Perazzi B, de Mier C, Yaya J, Vay C & Famiglietti A. (2010b). *Neisseria gonorrhoeae*: La era de la multiresistencia? XII Congreso Argentino de Microbiología. Resumen 625. *Rev Argent Microbiol*, Vol. 42 (Supl 1), (October, 2010), pp. 257, ISSN: 0325-7541.

García SD. (2011). Epidemiología y bases moleculares de la resistencia a los antimicrobianos en *Neisseria gonorrhoeae*. Doctoral Thesis. Faculty of Pharmacy and Biochemist, University of Buenos Aires. Buenos Aires, Argentina. 248 pp.

Govender S, Lebani T & Nell R. (2006). Antibiotic susceptibility patterns of *Neisseria gonorrhoeae* isolates in Porth Elizabeth. *S Afr Med J*, Vol. 96, N°3; pp. 225-226, ISSN: 0256-9574.

Griemberg G, Pizzimenti MC, Famiglietti AMR, Belli L, Vay C, Garcia S, Cardinalli A, Costa M, Marcenac F& Casco R. (1997). El impacto del HIV sobre la incidencia de sífilis y gonorrea en un Hospital Universitario (1985 - 1994). *Medicina (B. Aires)*, Vol. 57, N° 11, pp. 1-6, ISSN: 0025-7680.

Hagman KF, Pan W, Spratt BG, Balthazar JT, Judd RC& Shafer WM. (1995). Resistance of *Neisseria gonorrhoeae* to antimicrobial hydrophobic agents is modulated by the *mtrRCDE* efflux system. *Microbiol*, Vol. 141, N° 3, (November, 1994), pp. 611-622.

Hooper DC& Strahilelevitz. (2010). Quinolones, In: *Principles and Practice if Infectious Diseases*, Mandell G, Bennett JE & Dolin R (Eds.) 7th ed, Churchill Livingston, Elsevier Philadelphia PA, pp. 451-470, ISBN: 978-0-4430-6839-3.

Janda WM & Gaydos CA. (2007). *Neisseria*, In: *Manual of Clinical Microbiology*, 9th , Murray PR, Baron EJ, Jorgensen JH, Landry ML& Pfaller MA (Eds), pp. 601-620, Ed. Washington D. C., ASM Press, ISBN:-10:1-55581-371-2; ISBN: -13: 978-1-55581-371-0, Phiadelphia PA.

Leclercq R & Courvalin P. (1991). Bacterial resistance to macrolide, lincosamide and streptogramin antibiotics by target modification. *Antimicrob Agents Chemother*, Vol. 35, pp. 1267-1272, ISSN: 0066-4804.

Lucas CE, Hagman KE, Levin JC, Stein DC & Shafer WM. (1995). Importance of lipooligosaccharide structure in determining gonococcal resistance to hydrophobic antimicrobial agents resulting from the *mtr* efflux system. *Mol Microbiol*, Vol. 16, N° 5, (June 1995), pp. 1001-1009, ISSN: 0305-7453.

Lucas CE, Balthazar JT, Hagman KE & Shafer WM. (1997). The MtrR repressor binds the DNA sequence between the *mtrR* and *mtrC* genes of *Neisseria gonorrhoeae*. *J Bacteriol*, Vol.179, N° 13, (July, 1997), pp. 4123-4128, ISSN: 0021-9193.

Luna VA, Heiken M, Judge K, Ulep C, Van Kirk N, Luis H, Bernardo M, Leitao J & Roberts MC. (2002). Distribution of mef(A) in gram-positive bacteria from healthy Portuguese children. *Antimicrob Agents Chemother*, Vol. 46, N° 8; pp. 2513-2517

Macheboeuf P, Fischer DS, Brown T, Zervosen A, Luxen A, Joris B, Dessen A & Schofield CJ. (2007). Structural and mechanistic basis of penicillin- binding protein inhibition by lactivicins. *Nature Chemical Biology*, Vol. 3, N° 9, (September, 2007), pp. 565-569, ISSN: 1552-4450.

Martin IM, Hoffman S & Ison CA. (2006). European Surveillance of Sexually Transmitted Infections (ESSTI): The first combined antimicrobial susceptibility data for *Neisseria gonorrhoeae* in Western Europe. *J Antimicrob Chemother,* Vol. 58, N° 3, (July,2006), pp. 587-593, ISSN: 0305-7453.

Marrazo JM, Handsfield H H& Sparling PF. (2010). *Neisseria gonorrhoeae,* In: *Principle and Practice of Infections Disease* 7 th ed, Mandell G, Bennett JE & Dolin R (Eds.) , Churchill Livingston, Elsevier, pp. 2242-2258, ISBN: 978-0-4430-6839-3, Philadelphia PA.

Morse SA, Lysko PG, Mc Farland L, Knapp JS, Sandstrom E, Critchlow C & Holmes KK. (1982).Gonococcal strains from homosexual men have outer membrane with reduced permeability to hydrophobic molecules. *Infect Inmun,* Vol. 37, N° 2, (August, 1982) pp. 432-438.

Morse SA, Johnson SR, Biddle JW & Roberts MC. (1986). High -level tetracycline resistance in *Neisseria gonorrhoeae* is result of acquisition of streptococcal *tet M* determinant. *Antimicrob Agents Chemother,* Vol. 30, pp. 664-670.

Morris SR, Moore DF, Hannah PB, Wang SA, Wolfe J, Trees DL, Bolan G & Bauer HM. (2009). Strain Typing and Antimicrobial Resistance of Fluoroquinolone- Resistant *Neisseria gonorrhoeae* Causing a California Infection Outbreak. *J Clin Microbiol,* Vol. 47, N° 9, (September, 2009), pp. 2944-2949.

Nicholas RA, Zhao S, Tomberg J, Unemo M & Davies C. (2008). Genetics of intermediate resistance to expanded-spectrum cephalosporins in *Neisseria gonorrhoeae,* Abstract P054. 16th International Pathogenic Neisseria Conference; Sep, Rotterdam, The Netherlands; pp.133. Available at: http://www.ipnc2008.org/

O'Rourker M, Ison CA, Renton AM & Spratt BG. (1995). Opa-typing: a high-resolution tool for studying the epidemiology of gonorrhoea. *Mol Microbiol* , Vol: 17, N° 5, pp.865-875.

Otero L, Villar H, Vázquez JA & Vázquez F. (2002). *Neisseria gonorrhoeae* resistente a quinolonas: Un nuevo problema de salud pública en España. *Enferm Infecc Microbiol Clin,* Vol. 20, N° 3. pp. 123-126, ISSN: 0213-005X.

Palmer HM, Young H, Winter A & Dave J. (2008). Emergence and spread of azithromycin-resistant *Neisseria gonorrhoeae* in Scotland. *J Antimicrob Chemother,* Vol. 62, N° 3, (June,2008), pp. 490-494, ISSN: 0305-7453.

Rahman M, Alam A, Nessa K, Nahar S, Dutta DK, Yasmin L, Monira S, Sultan Z, Khan SA & Albert MJ. (2001). Treatment Failure with the Use of Ciprofloxacin for Gonorrhea Correlates with the Prevalence of Fluoroquinolone-Resistant *Neisseria gonorrhoeae* Strains in Bangladesh. *Clin Infect Dis,* Vol. 32, N° 6, pp. 884-889, ISSN: 1058-4838.

Reyn A, Schmith H, Trier M & Bentzon MW. (1973). Spectinomycin hydrochloride Trobicin in the treatment of gonorrhea. Observation of resistant strains of *Neisseria gonorrhoeae. Br J Vener Dis,* Vol. 49, N°1, pp. 54- 59.

Roberts MC, Chung WO, Roe D, Xia M, Marquez C, Borthagaray G, Whittington W & Holmes KK. (1999). Erythromycin-Resistant *Neisseria gonorrhoeae* and Oral Commensal *Neisseria* spp. Carry Know rRNA Methylase Genes. *Antimicrob Agents Chemother,* Vol. 43, N° 6, (June, 1999) pp. 1367-1372, ISSN: 0162-0134.

Rouquette-Loughlin C, Dunham SA, Kuhn M, Balthazar JT & Shafer WM. (2003). The Nor M efflux pump of *Neisseria gonorrhoeae* and *Neisseria meningitidis* recognizes antimicrobial cationic compounds. *J. Bacteriol*, Vol. 185, N° 3, (February, 2003), pp. 1101-1106, ISSN: 0305-7453.

Rouquette-Loughlin CE, Balthazar JT & Shafer WM. (2005). Characterization of the MacA-MacB efflux system in *Neisseria gonorrhoeae. J Antimicrob Chemother*, Vol. 56, (September, 2005), pp. 856-860, ISSN: 0021-9193.

Shafer WM, Balthazar JT, Hagman KE & Morse SA. (1995). Missense mutations that alter the DNA- binding domain of the MtrR protein occur frecuently in rectal isolates of *Neisseria gonorrhoeae* that are resistant to faecal lipids. *Microbiol*, Vol. 41, pp. 907-911.

Shafer WM, Folster JP & Nicholas RA. (2010). Molecular Mechanisms of Antibiotic Resistance Expressed by the Pathogenic *Neisseriae*, In: *Neisseria* Molecular Mechanisms of Pathogenesis, Genco CA, Wetzler L(Eds), pp. 245-268, Caister Academic Press, ISBN: 978-1-904455-51-6, Boston, MA. USA,

Starnino S, Stefanelli P & on behalf of the *Neisseria gonorrhoeae* Italian Study Group. (2009). Azithromycin- resistant *Neisseria gonorrhoeae* strains recentjy isolated in Italy. *J Antimicrob Chemother*, Vol. 63, N° 6, (April, 2009), pp. 1200-04, ISSN: 0305-7453.

Shokeen P, Bala M, Singh M & Tandon V. (2008). In vitro activity of eugenol, an active component from Ocimum sanctum, against multiresistant and susceptible strains of *Neisseria gonorrhoeae. Int J Antimicrob Agents*, Vol. 32, (August, 2008), pp. 174-179, ISSN: 0924-8579.

Takahata S, Senju N, Osaki Y, Yoshida T & Ida T. (2006). Amino acid substitutions in mosaic penicillin-binding proteína 2 associated with reduced susceptibility to cefixime in clinical isolates of *Neisseria gonorrhoeae. Antimicrob Agents Chemother*, Vol. 50, N° 11, (November, 2006) pp. 3638-3645, ISSN: 0305-7453.

Tanaka M, Nakayama H, Huruya K, Konomi I, Irie S, Kanamaya A, Saika T & Kobayashi T. (2006). Analysis of mutations within multiple genes associated with resistance in a clinical isolate of *Neisseria gonorrhoeae* with reduced ceftriaxone susceptibility thatshows a multidrug-resistant phenotype. *Int J Antimicrob. Agents*, Vol. 27, pp. 20-26.

Tapsall JW, Schultz RR, Lovett R, Munro R. (1992). Failure of 500 mg ciprofloxacin therapy in male urethral gonorrhea. *Med J* Aust, Vol. 156, pp.143, ISSN: 1058-4838.

Tapsall JW (2009) *Neisseria gonorrhoeae* and emerging resistance to extended spectrum cephalosporins. Curr *Opin Infect Dis*, Vol. 22, N° 1, (February, 2009) pp. 87-91.

Tazi L, Pérez-Losada M, Gu W, Yang Y, Xue L, Crandall KA & Viscidi RP. (2010). Population dynamics of *Neisseria gonorrhoeae* in Shanghai, China: a comparative study. *BMC Infect Dis* , Vol. 10, N° 1, pp. 13, ISSN: 14712334.

Trotter C, Hughes G & Ison C. (2010). Epidemiology in the Vaccine Era. In: *Neisseria Molecular Mechanisms of Pathogenesis*, Attardo Genco C & Wetzler L, editors, pp. 227-243, Caister Academic Press Boston MA. USA, ISBN: 978-1-904455-51-6, Boston MA. USA.

Unemo M, Dillon JR. (2011). Review and International Recommendation of Methods for Typing *Neissseria gonorrhoeae* Isolates and Their Implications for Improved Knowledge of Gonococcal Epidemiology, treatment, and Biology. Clin Microbiol Rev, Vol 24, pp. 447-458

Update to CDC's sexually transmitted diseases treatment guidelines, 2006: Fluoroquinolones no longer recommend for treatment of gonococcal infections. (2007). *Mortal Weekly Rep*, Vol. 56, N° 14, pp. 332-336, ISSN: 1545-861X.

US Public Health Service. (1975). Gonorrhea recommended treatment schedules. *Ann Intern Med*, Vol. 82, pp. 230-233.

Van Looveren M, Ison CA, Ieven M, Vandamme P, Martin IM, Vermeulen K, Renton A & Goosens H. (1999). Evaluation of the Discriminatory Power of Typing Methods for *Neisseria gonorrhoeae*. *J Clin Microbiol*, Vol. 37, N° 7, pp.2183-2188.

Velicko I & Unemo M. (2009). Increase in reported gonorrhea cases in Sweden, 2001-2008. *Euro Surveill*, Vol. 14, N° 34, pp24.

Warner DM, Shafer WM & Jerse AE. (2008). Clinically relevant mutations that cause derepression of the *Neisseria gonorrhoeae* MtrC MtrD-MtrE efflux pump system confer different levels of antimicrobial resistance and in vivo fitness. *Mol – Microbiol*, Vol. 70, N° 2, (October, 2008), pp. 462-478, ISSN: 0305-7453.

World Health Organization (WHO). (2001). Global prevalence and incidence of selected curable sexually transmitted infections: overview and estimates. (WHO/HIV_AIDS/2001.02, WHO/CDC/CSR/EDC/2001.10), pp. 1-43.

World Health Organization (WHO) (2003) Guidelines for the management of sexually transmitted infections. Geneva, Switzerland. Available at: http://www.who.int/hiv/pub/sti/en/STIGuidelines2003.pdf.

Zarantonelli L, Borthagaray G, Lee EH & Shafer WM. (1999). Decreased azithromycin susceptibility of *Neisseria gonorhoeae* due to mtrR mutatins. *Antimicrob Agents Chemother,* Vol. 43, N° 10, (October, 1999), pp. 2468-2472, ISSN: 0305-7453.

Zarantonelli L, Borthagaray G, Lee E H, Veal W & Shafer WM. (2001). Decreased susceptibility to azithromycin and erythromycin mediated by a novel *mtr*(R) promoter mutation in *Neisseria gonorrhoeae*. *J Antimicrob Chemother*,Vol. 47, pp. 651-654, ISSN: 0305-7453.

4

Mucosal Immunity and Evasion Strategies of *Neisseria gonorrhoeae*

Mónica Imarai[1], Claudio Acuña[1], Alejandro Escobar[2], Kevin Maisey[1] and Sebastián Reyes-Cerpa[1]
[1]*Department of Biology, Faculty of Chemistry and Biology, Universidad de Santiago de Chile*
[2]*Department of Basic Sciences, Faculty of Dentistry, University of Chile*
[1,2]*Chile*

1. Introduction

Neisseria gonorrhoeae, the gonococcus, is a gram-negative diplococcus which causes the sexually transmitted disease gonorrhea (Figure 1). The contagious nature of gonococcal infection remains a major global health problem and represents 88 million new cases every year (WHO, 2011). *N. gonorrhoeae* is transmitted by human to human contact and is highly adapted to the genital tract, surviving poorly outside the human body. However, gonococcus develops resistance to antimicrobials, antigenic variability and mechanisms of immune evasion by which it evades host defenses, thus persisting and often causing undetected asymptomatic infection (Tapsall, 2001).

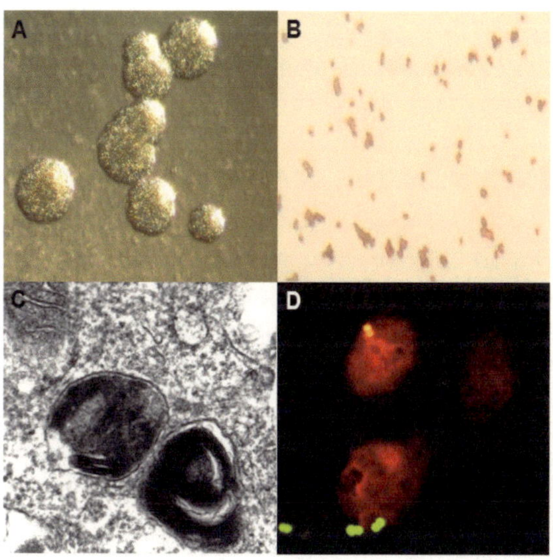

Fig. 1. *Neisseria gonorrhoeae*. (A) Colonies on agar, (B) Gram-staining, (C) Transmission electron microscopy, (D) Confocal microscopy of the bacteria (in green).

The symptoms of gonorrhoea are similar to those caused by other agents, most notably *Chlamydia trachomatis*. *N. gonorrhoeae* causes infections mainly of the urethra in men and the endocervix in women, although it may also infect extragenital mucosal sites, including the oropharynx and anorectum. Ocular infections also occur, and in neonates could cause blindness (Tapsall, 2001). Genital infection in men usually causes urethritis and epididimitis with purulent urethral exudates (Apicella et al., 1996), however an important proportion of infected men never develop symptoms and more than half of infected women develop an asymptomatic silent infection (Farley et al., 2003; Handsfield et al., 1974; John and Donald, 1978). Genital tract gonorrhea gives rise to well recognized complications including upper reproductive tract infections in women, such as pelvic inflammatory disease (PID), a condition that affects between 10% and 20% of infected women in the third world. PID encompasses a range of inflammatory conditions of the upper reproductive tract and has several potential sequelae including infertility, ectopic pregnancy, among others (Hoyme, 1990; Tapsall, 2001).

The purulent exudates produced by infected men and the cervical secretions of women with gonorrhoeae contain bacteria attached to and within polymorphonuclear leukocytes (PMNs) (Apicella et al., 1996; Ovcinnikov and Delektorskij, 1971), which are the primary innate immune responders to bacterial and fungal infection and are capable of phagocytosing and killing a variety of microorganisms (Borregaard, 2010). Yet, in spite of the numerous PMNs at the site of gonorrheal infection, viable gonococci can be cultured from the exudates of Infected individuals suggesting that the PMNS driven innate immune response to *N. gonorrhoeae* are ineffective at clearing a gonorrheal infection (Johnson and Criss, 2011). Considering further that the humoral immune response against *N. gonorrhoeae* is extremely low in serum and in secretions of the human (male and female) during infection (Hedges et al., 1999; Hedges et al., 1998), the persistence of gonococcus can be explained by the presence of an ineffective immune response which facilitates the long-term colonization of hosts, creating enhanced opportunity for dissemination and transmission of gonorrhea.

The aim of this chapter is to review advances in our understanding of the immunity against *N. gonorrhoeae* and those mechanisms of evasion that seem to be responsible for the restricted immune response frequently observed.

2. Gonococcal membrane proteins and early steps of infection

Infection of genital epithelial cells by *N. gonorrhoeae* is a multi-step process, consisting of adherence, invasion, intracellular survival and exocytosis. These events are initiated and mediated by multiple interactions between gonococcal surface molecules and epithelial cells. These interactions activate signalling cascades in host cells and trigger the reorganization of the actin cytoskeleton, which is required for the entry of the bacteria into the cells. Pilus retraction from adherent gonococci on the epithelial cell surface activates calcium flux (Ayala et al., 2005), the PI3K/Akt pathway (Lee et al., 2005) and the MAP kinase ERK pathway (Howie et al., 2008). The interaction of opacity protein (Opa) with heparin sulfate proteoglycans (HSPG) activates phosphatidylcholine-specific phospholipase C (PLC) and the acid sphingomyelinase (Grassme et al., 1997). Opa also can trigger integrin-mediated protein kinase C (PKC) activation through binding to the serum-derived extracellular matrix proteins, fibronectin and vitronectin (Dehio et al., 1998a; Dehio et al., 1998b; Dehio et al., 1998c).

2.1 Type IV pili

Although there are many potential cell surface proteins of *N. gonorrhoeae* having a role in cell-host interaction, attention of most studies has focused on a few of them. This is the case of the gonococcal type IV pili which are composed of a major structural subunit, the pilin or PilE protein, assembled into helical pilus fibers (Parge et al., 1995). *In vitro* studies indicate that antigenic variation of this protein can affect pilus-mediated adherence to human cells (Jonsson et al., 1994; Long et al., 1998; Rudel et al., 1992). The binding of *N. gonorrhoeae* pili to host cells is thought to involve the complement regulatory protein CD46 (membrane cofactor receptor) (Kallstrom et al., 2001). In fact, the association of pili with CD46 in cervical carcinoma cells results in a cytoplasmic calcium flux derived from intracellular calcium stores (Kallstrom et al., 1998). However, not all studies support this role for CD46. Accordingly, no binding of piliated gonococci was observed on CD46-transfected cells and furthermore, specific down-regulation of CD46 expression in human epithelial cell lines did not alter the binding of piliated gonococci (Kirchner et al., 2005; Kirchner and Meyer, 2005; Tobiason and Seifert, 2001). Thus the topic remains controvertial. There are other potential receptors for pili attachment, i.e., integrins containing a domain known as I-domain. Edwards et al. demonstrated that pili bind to I-domain-containing integrins on primary cell cultures derived from cervical and male urethral epithelia (Edwards and Apicella, 2005; Edwards et al., 2002). In this regard, the complement receptor 3 (CR3; integrin αMβ2 or CD11b/CD18) serves as the key receptor mediating gonococcal adherence to human cervical epithelia, *in vivo*, as well as *ex vivo* (Figure 2) (Edwards et al., 2001).

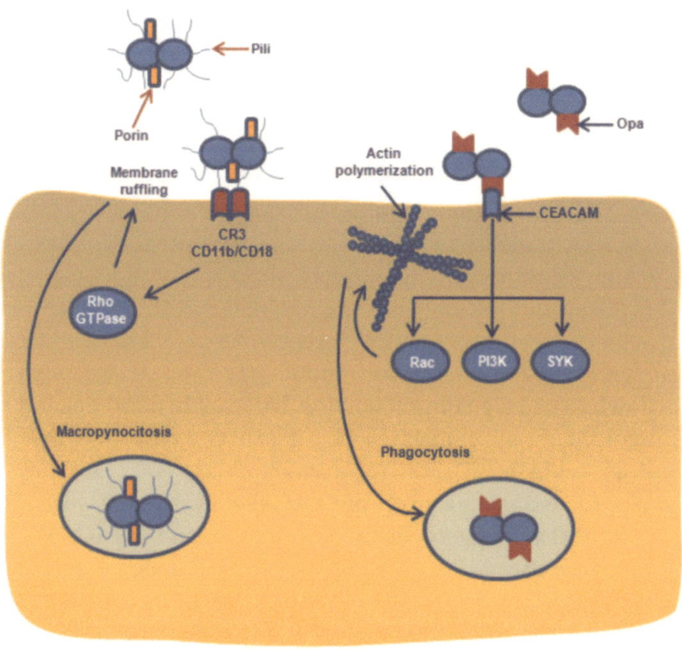

Fig. 2. Adhesion and internalization of N. gonorrhoeae in the host cell.

Pilus engagement has also been demonstrated to play a role in host cell cytoskeletal rearrangements (Edwards et al., 2000; Grassme et al., 1996; Griffiss et al., 1999; Merz et al., 1999; Merz and So, 1997). Membrane ruffles are induced in response to gonococci; epithelial cell invasion occur primarily in an actin-dependent manner, but it does not appear to require *de novo* protein synthesis by either the bacterium or the host cervical cell, eliciting substantial rearrangements of filamentous actin in the host cell cortex directly beneath sites of bacterial contact (Merz et al., 1999). Engagement of CR3 on primary cervical epithelial cells results in vinculin- and ezrin-enriched focal complex formation before membrane ruffle formation, bacteria reside within macropinosomes, and an accumulation of actin-associated protein occur in response to gonococcal infection (Edwards et al., 2000). Finally a signal transduction cascade that is dependent upon the activation of phosphatidylinositol 3-kinase or MAP kinases and Rho GTPases is activated (Edwards et al., 2001).

2.2 Opacity-associated (Opa) adhesin proteins

Opacity-associated adhesion proteins located in the gonococcal outer membrane facilitate the interaction of bacteria with a number of host cell types, including epithelial cells on mucosal surfaces and various immune cells, indicating a direct effect on the immune response. Receptor tropism of Opa proteins can be broadly divided into two categories, those that bind to members of the carcinoembryonic antigen cell adhesion molecule (CEACAM) family (Figure 2) and those that bind to HSPGs (Bos et al., 1997; Chen et al., 1995; Chen and Gotschlich, 1996; Chen et al., 1997; Gray-Owen et al., 1997a; Gray-Owen et al., 1997b; Popp et al., 1999; van Putten and Paul, 1995; Virji et al., 1999; Virji et al., 1996a; Virji et al., 1996b). These categories are represented by Opa50, i.e., Opa proteins that recognize HSPG, and Opa52, i.e., Opa proteins that recognize members of CEACAM familiy. Vitronectin and fibronectin function as required bridging molecules between the gonococcus and its target HSPG receptor(s) (Duensing and Putten, 1998; Duensing and van Putten, 1997; Gomez-Duarte et al., 1997; van Putten et al., 1998). Association with an integrin coreceptor (vß3 or vß5 for vitronectin-mediated adherence or vß1 for fibronectin-mediated adherence) triggers a signaling cascade within the target cell that is dependent upon the activation of PKC (Dehio et al., 1998c).

The binding sites of Opa proteins reside on the amino-terminal domains of the CEACAM family, which are largely conserved and therefore allow one or more Opa proteins to target distinct CEACAMs (Chen and Gotschlich, 1996; Muenzner et al., 2000; Virji et al., 1996b). As CEACAMs may contain immunoreceptor tyrosine-based inhibitory motifs (ITIMs) or immunoreceptor tyrosine-based activation motifs (ITAMs) (Hammarstrom, 1999), the consequences of downstream signaling following bacterial ligation depend on the receptor and target cell involved. From studies so far, it can be concluded that Opa–CEACAM interactions result in cellular invasion (Muenzner et al., 2000; Virji et al., 1999). The CEACAM receptor-mediated phagocytosis of Opa(52)-expressing *N. gonorrhoeae* results in a rapid activation of the acid sphingomyelinase. Furthermore, the CEACAM receptor-initiated stimulation activates a cascade via Src-like protein tyrosine kinases, Rac1 and PAK to Jun-N-terminal kinases (Hauck et al., 2000; Hauck et al., 1998).

The gonococcal opacity proteins are a well-studied example of phase-variable surface structures. Gonococcal strains express several antigenical distinct Opa proteins that are encoded by separate chromosomal alleles (Bhat et al., 1991; Connell et al., 1990; Dempsey et al., 1991). Each *opa* gene undergoes phase variation via frameshift mutations that cause changes in pentameric repeats in the *opa* structural gene (Murphy et al., 1989). Bacteria that express no Opa proteins, bacteria that express one Opa protein, and bacteria that express multiple Opa proteins simultaneously result from these reversible mutations. This is one of the earliest described mechanisms of immune evasion found in gonococcus.

2.3 Porin, the outer membrane protein channel

Porin, is membrane channel through which small molecules traverse the gonococcal outer membrane, is thought to play multiple roles in potentiating disease caused by *N. gonorrhoeae*. Porin molecules trigger different responses within host cells depending upon the particular porin and the host cell type. A feature of gonococcal porin is its ability to translocate into eukaryotic cell membranes (Lynch et al., 1984; Weel and van Putten, 1991), where it acts as voltage-gated channel that is modulated by host cell ATP and GTP (Rudel et al., 1996). It has also been demonstrated that *N. gonorrhoeae* infection of epithelial cells results in selective porin transport to the mitochondria (Muller et al., 2000; Muller et al., 2002). Within the cell mitochondrial membrane, porin initiates apoptosis by inducing a calcium influx and, consequently, calpain and caspase activity within these cells (Muller et al., 1999). In contrast to the porin-induced apoptosis observed in HeLa cells, gonococcal infection of primary human male urethral epithelial cells results in antiapoptotic events (Binnicker et al., 2003; Binnicker et al., 2004). Finally, porin also acts as an actin-nucleating protein in epithelial cells (Wen et al., 2000) facilitating the cytoskeletal rearrangements required for actin-mediated entry of the gonococcus into its target host cell.

2.4 Lipooligosaccharide (LOS)

Lipooligosaccharide is a major antigenic and immunogenic component of pathogenic *Neisseria* species. LOS produced by these bacteria consists of an oligosaccharide (OS) moiety and lipid A, and structural variation of the OS leads to LOS heterogeneity (Preston et al., 1996). Studies using primary male urethral epithelial cells demonstrated an association between the urethral epithelium and the gonococcus through the interaction of the asialoglycoprotein receptor (ASGP-R) and gonococcal LOS (Harvey et al., 2001). In primary cell culture, engagement of the ASGP-R by the gonococcus results in pedestal formation beneath the bacterium (Harvey et al., 1997). Pedestal formation is also observed in microscopic analysis of exudates collected from men with naturally acquired gonococcal urethritis (Apicella et al., 1996; Harvey et al., 1997). Evidence suggests that endocytosis occurs primarily by actin-dependent (Giardina et al., 1998) and clathrin-dependent processes (Harvey et al., 1997).

3. Immune response against *N. gonorrhoeae*

The immunity against bacterial infections is achieved by many levels of defense that are triggered depending on the type, number and virulence of the bacteria that enter to the body (Figure 3). If the infection is mild, the tissue phagocytes are able to kill the bacteria in the phagolysosomes by reactive oxygen and nitrogen intermediates and proteolytic enzymes. In addition, these cells are able to secrete pro-inflammatory cytokines such as interleukin (IL)-1, IL-6, IL-8 and Tumoral Necrosis Factor (TNF) which initiates inflammatory response. On the other hand, antigen processing and presentation, which is a crucial biological process for the initiation of adaptative immune response, might initiate antigen-specific immune response and a long lasting memory. Dendritic cells (DCs) are a subgroup of high-power antigen presenting cells (APC) with a unique ability to attract and interact with naive T cells to induce a primary immune response (Sabatos et al., 2008; Verhagen et al., 2008). Immature DCs (iDCs) reside in most peripheral tissues where they act as sentinels for incoming pathogens (Rowell and Wilson, 2009). After exposure to pro-inflammatory cytokines and microbial products, iDCs undergo a process termed maturation, which involve up-regulation of MHC molecules, co-stimulatory molecules, secretion of pro-inflammatory cytokines and migration to draining lymph node where mature DCs activate T cells (Xu et al., 2007). Following antigen stimulation by DCs, T cells begin an expansion process, as a result of extensive division. Under a control of DCs, helper T cells (Th) acquire the ability to respond to infection through the production of powerful cytokines like interferon gamma (IFN-γ), which is able to activate macrophages resisting infections by facultative and obligate intracellular microbes (Th1 cells) (Napolitani et al., 2005), or IL-17, which mobilize phagocytes at body surfaces to resist extracellular bacteria (Th17 cells) (LeibundGut-Landmann et al., 2007). Th17 cells represent a distinct lineage that originates mainly in the presence of TGF-β1 and IL-6 and need the presence of IL-23 for their expansion and/or maintenance (Annunziato et al., 2007). IL-23 is secreted by macrophages and DCs in response to microbial products and inflammatory cytokines (Langrish et al., 2004). Once differentiated, Th17 cells are able to secrete preferentially IL-17A, IL-17F and IL-22, a particular set of cytokines not secreted by the other Th cells (Ouyang et al., 2008). IL-17 plays a particularly significant role in regulating neutrophils (PMNn) recruitment and granulopoiesis via the production of IL-8 and MIP-2 (CXCL2) (Laan et al., 1999). In early stages of infections, interactions between *N. gonorrhoeae* and epithelial mucosa trigger immune response with release of IL-1, IL-6, IL-8 and TNF which serve to recruit and activate PMNn to the site of infection and promoting their bactericidal activity limiting bacterial penetration into submucosal tissues (Fisette et al., 2003; Maisey et al., 2003; McGee et al., 1999). In men, PMNs appear in urethral swabs and urine several days after infection and immediately prior to the onset of symptoms (Cohen and Cannon, 1999). In women with gonorrhea, the cervical secretions also contain PMNn (Evans, 1977) and bacteria are attached to and within PMNn (Johnson and Criss, 2011). In spite of the numerous PMNn at the site of gonorrheal infection, viable gonococci can be cultured from the exudates of infected individuals (Wiesner and Thompson, 1980). When bacteria crosses the layer of epithelial cells, obtaining access to submucosa, they have the first encounter with macrophages and DCs (Rarick et al., 2006). DCs interaction with *N. gonorrhoeae* surface factors like Pili and Opa is mediated by members of the CD66 family, CD46 and CR3. However, C-type lectins (macrophage galactose-type lectin -MLG- and DC-SIGN) constitute the main DCs expressed receptor for *N. gonorrhoeae* (Astier et al., 2010).

Most studies that have investigated antigonococcal immune responses have focused predominantly on humoral responses (Table 1). The hallmark of humoral immune response against *N. gonorrhoeae* is the extremely low levels of anti-gonococcal antibodies found in serum and secretions of the human (male and female) during infection (Hedges et al., 1999; Hedges et al., 1998), indicating that humoral immunity against gonococcus is highly limited (Hedges et al., 1999; Song et al., 2008). Antigenic heterogeneity is a major consideration for humoral immunity in gonococcal infection studies. Meanwhile Pili, protein I (PI), protein II

(PII), H.8, IgAl protease and LOS are quantitatively the most important antigens in generating antibody responses in gonococcal infection. It is clear that patients make antibodies against the pili of the infecting gonococcal strain. In women, pili appeared to be the predominant antigen in the immune response unlike men, that have higher levels of antibodies to other antigens than pili (Brooks and Lammel, 1989). Thus, antibodies generated are directed against other major membrane molecules, such as Opa proteins and Porin protein (Brooks and Lammel, 1989; Hedges et al., 1999; Hedges et al., 1998; Plummer et al., 1993; Plummer et al., 1994; Zheng, 1997). Although some of these have bactericidal activity, they are not protective and seem to be blocked by immunoglobulins against the outer membrane protein 3 (RmP). In fact, women with these antibodies were at increased risk to gonococcal infection (Plummer et al., 1993). The absence of induction of humoral response results on limited or no protection against re-infection with *N. gonorrhoeae* despite the generation of serum antibody responses against antigens produced by several prototype gonococcal vaccines (Boslego et al., 1991; McChesney et al., 1982; Tramont et al., 1981).

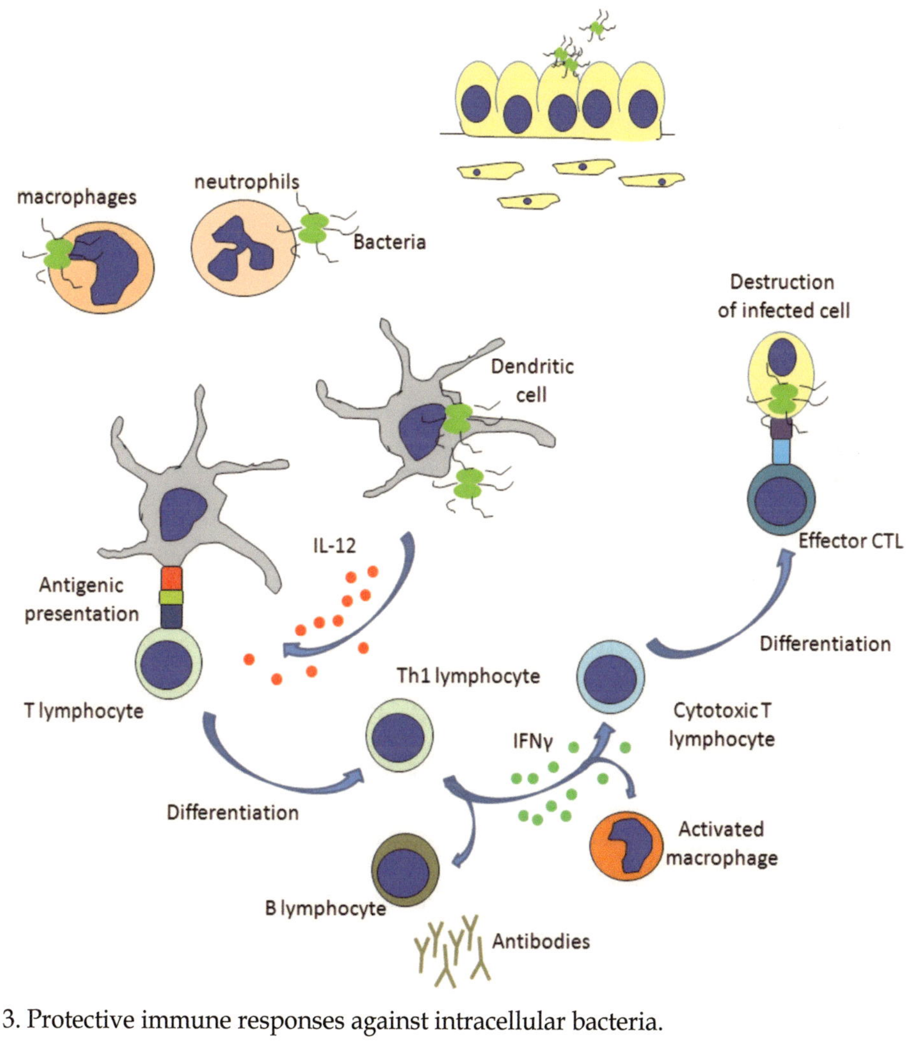

Fig. 3. Protective immune responses against intracellular bacteria.

Antigen	Effects on immune response	References
N. gonorrhoeae	IgG>IgM and sIgA>IgA	(Tapchaisri and Sirisinha, 1976)
Outer membrane protein I	IgA>IgG	(Jeurissen et al., 1987)
Outer membrane protein I	IgA>IgG	(Kohl et al., 1992)
Porin	Up-regulated B7-2 expression of B lymphocytes	(Wetzler et al., 1996)
Heat labile and fixed *N. gonorrhoeae*	IgG>IgA>IgM serum	(Cohen, 1967)
Pili and outer membrane protein II	IgG serum	(Lammel et al., 1985)
Outer membrane protein II	IgA serum	(Lammel et al., 1985)
Outer membrane protein I and II and pili	IgG and IgA vaginal fluid	(Lammel et al., 1985)
LPS	IgG>IgA in serum	(Ison et al., 1986)
Outer membrane protein III	IgG in serum	(Rice et al., 1986)
N. gonorrhoeae MS11	Slight increase of IgG and IgA in serum	(Hedges et al., 1999)
N. gonorrhoeae mice infection	Increased of neutrophils and macrophage in site of infection	(Song et al., 2008)
N. gonorrhoeae mice infection	IgG>IgA>IgM in vaginal fluid	(Song et al., 2008)
Whole-protein extractes of *N. gonorrhoeae* P9-17	Low titers of IgG in serum	(Imarai et al., 2008)
N. gonorrhoeae	Th17 profile immune response and increased IL-17	(Feinen et al., 2010)
IgA1 protease	Th1 pro-inflammatory profile with increased IFNγ and TNFα	(Tsirpouchtsidis et al., 2002)
IgA1 protease	IL-1β, IL-6, TNFα and IL-8	(Lorenzen et al., 1999)
Porin	Th2 pro-inflammatory profile with increased of IL-4	(Simpson et al., 1999)
Porin	B lymphocytes activation and up-regulation of CD40	(Snapper et al., 1997)
Pili	Activation and proliferation of $CD4^{+}$T Lymphocyte	(Plant and Jonsson, 2006)
Opa	Arrest of activation and proliferation of $CD4^{+}$ T lymphocytes binding CEACAM1	(Boulton and Gray-Owen, 2002)

Table 1. Anti-gonococcus immune responses.

Similarly, in the murine model of infection, no antibody induced response has been detected. In Balb/c mice, *N. gonorrhoeae* is able to reach the upper genital organs and to invade uterine tissue, as it occurs in humans (Imarai et al., 2008; Jerse, 1999). Interestingly, studies in this model revealed several features of infection that mimic a good spectrum of the characteristics of the human disease. Some of them seem highly valuable, (i) the bacteria introduced in the vagina not only invade and colonize the lower genital tract, but also spread to the upper organs (uterus and oviducts) (Inaba et al., 1992), (ii) infection occurs with no signs of the disease, just as it occurs in a high percentage of women during natural infection (Farley et al., 2003; Inaba et al., 1992) and (iii) the bacteria remains alive within the internal compartments of the infected cells, invading uterine tissues up to 22 days post inoculation (Imarai et al., 2008).

On the other hand, CD4+ T cell responses also occur with gonoccocal antigens. Antigenic stimulation with Porin induces an increase in the percentage of IL-4 producing CD4+ T cells, but no production of other cytokines such as IL-2, IL-10, IFN-γ, or TNF occurs, indicating that infected individuals produce a Th2 response against Porin (Simpson et al., 1999).

Moreover, gonococcal pili interaction with CD4+ T cells induces the activation and proliferation of lymphocytes and stimulates the secretion of IL-10 (Plant and Jonsson, 2006). In contrast, Opa proteins mediate binding to CEACAM-1 expressed by CD4+ T cells and suppress activation and proliferation of naive lymphocytes (Boulton and Gray-Owen, 2002; Lee et al., 2008). Rarick et al. showed a differential activation of peripheral blood mononuclear cells by *N. gonorrhoeae* that includes the early induction (96 hours) of IL-2, IL-12 and IFN-γ (Th1 cytokines), IL-4 (Th2 cytokine), IL-10 (immunosuppressive cytokine) and MCP-1, MCP-2 (chemotactic cytokines). The cytokine response observed in this study indicate that distinct gonococcal components produce antagonistic signaling and cytokines suggesting that *N. gonorrhoeae* infection cannot be initially categorized as Th1 or Th2 response (Rarick et al., 2006). Recent studies in the murine model of gonococcal genital tract infection showed that Th17 cells are involved in the immune response to *N. gonorrhoeae*. This response leads to IL-17 dependent secretion of IL-6, LIX and MIP2α and subsequent recruitment of PMNn, which is delayed in the presence of IL-17A blocking antibodies or deletion of IL-17RA prolonging infection (Feinen et al., 2010).

Overall, most known gonococcal antigens are able to induce humoral and cellular immune responses in the human, but a protective immune response has not been identified. Data suggest that the bacteria have mechanisms to evade destruction by PMNn, antibodies and T cells.

4. Mechanisms of immune evasion by *Neisseria gonorrhoeae*

Several studies suggest the promotion of direct inhibitory mechanisms by gonococcus to escape the immune response. Data indicate that bacteria induces transient reduction of CD4+ and CD8+T cells during acute gonococcal infection in HIV-1-positive woman, with increase in plasma HIV-1 RNA copy number and plasma concentration of IL-4, IL-6, IL-10 and TNF-α soluble receptor (Anzala et al., 2000). Gonococcal infection also correlates with suppression of activation and proliferation of CD4+ T lymphocytes (Boulton and Gray-Owen, 2002). In this respect, inhibitory effect is mediated by the ligation of gonococcus membrane component Opa52 present in blebs of outer membrane (OMV) to CEACAM1 (also known as CD66a or BGP) on lymphocyte (Lee et al., 2007). The interaction triggers the phosphorilation of the ITIM impeding the normal expression of early activation marker CD69 and the subsequent proliferation of T cells. This strategy represents an effective means by which to create a "zone of immunosuppression" surrounding the infected site (Lee et al., 2008). Opa-CEACAM1-induced immunosuppression might also control the development of a humoral response, decreasing the T cell help for B cell activation or targeting the CEACAM1-expressing B cells causing cell death (Pantelic et al., 2005) and subsequent inhibition of antibody production.

On the other hand, piliated gonococci enhances T-cell activation and proliferation, regardless of whether this is mediated by the pilus itself or is due to the act of binding to a pilus receptor such as CD46 or integrins. Upon pili-CD46 ligation, the IL-10-secreting type 1 regulatory T (Tr1) cells are elicited (Plant and Jonsson, 2006). Tr1 cells are able to suppress the activation of bystander T cells via induction of IL-10 (Jonuleit et al., 2001). In addition, IL-10 suppresses the production of pro-inflammatory cytokines thereby inhibiting the ability of APC to induce differentiation of Th1 cells, just the type of response associated to protection against intracellular pathogens such as gonococcus (McGuirk et al., 2002).

In regard to the role of regulatory T (Treg) cells, we showed that in Balb/c, the mouse model of gonococcus infections, *N. gonorrhoeae* induces transforming growth factor β1 (TGF-β1)+ $CD4^+$ T cells in the mucosal lymph nodes, including a subset of CD25+Foxp3+ Tregs, indicating that type of response may avoid the host mechanisms of protection (Imarai et al., 2008). Mature CD4+ CD25- T cells can be converted in Treg cells in peripheral tissues under immunosuppressive conditions, such as exposure to IL-10 or TGF-β1 made by antigen presenting cells (Sakaguchi, 2004). Treg cells inhibit the function of effectors T cells through the secretion of suppressive cytokines IL-10 and TGF-β1, or by a cell contact-dependent mechanism via CTLA4 or GITR molecules (Bending et al., 2009; O'Connor et al., 2008; Sakaguchi, 2004). Considering that, the source of TGF-β1 could be stromal and epithelial cells of reproductive organs (Nocera and Chu, 1995; Srivastava et al., 1996; Taylor et al., 2000), which are target of gonococcus infection, it is possible that the cytokine milieu found in reproductive tract subsidized the inductions of Tregs by *N.gonorrhoeae.* In fact, we must consider that the genital tract is an immune-privileged site with expression of regulatory cytokines which might induce a tolerogenic response against gonococcus (Nocera and Chu, 1995; Srivastava et al., 1996; Taylor et al., 2000). For instance, epithelia and stromal cells of the reproductive organs of the mouse and human, express high levels of TGF-β1 and other molecules involved in conditioning immune privilege sites (Chegini et al., 1994; Grant and Wira, 2003; Jin et al., 1992; Wada et al., 1996). Moreover, antigen presenting cells such as macrophages and DCs, regularly present in the reproductive tissues might also contribute to regulatory response, since they could promote T regulatory cells differentiation trough production of IL-10 and TGF-β1 after infection (Givan et al., 1997; Stagg et al., 1998).

The effects of interaction of different stable gonoccocal LOS phenotypes with human DCs were evaluated (van Vliet et al., 2009). Interestingly, this study revealed that LOS variants result in alterations of cytokine secretion profiles of DCs and in the induction of distinct adaptive CD4+ T helper responses. Gonococcus significantly increased IL-10 production, as well as pro-inflammatory cytokines, such as TNF-α, IL-6, IL-8 and IL-12. However, only IL-10 production was modulated by LOS variation. Supporting the anti-inflammatory or regulatory effects of gonococcus on APCs, recently we found that the bacterium was unable to induce significant up-regulation of cell surface co-stimulatory molecule CD86 in macrophages, as well in DCs (unpublished data). This suggests that, although *N. gonorrhoeae* is actually phagocytosed by macrophages and DCs, the bacteria can deteriorate antigen presenting function. Moreover, gonococcus was unable to induce up-regulation of MHC class II in macrophages, this molecule is involved in antigen processing and presentation, therefore this implies that macrophages do not have a proper antigen presenting function. In addition, gonococcus induced IL-10 and TGF-β1 in dendritic cells reaching an anti-inflammatory or regulatory response.

Altogether, studies so far show that *N. gonorrhoeae* might control immune response by inducing (1) suppression of activation and proliferation of CD4+ T lymphocytes, (2) secretion of tolerogenic-type cytokines, (3) inhibitory T cells (Tr1 and Tregs), and (4) by deteriorating antigen presenting function. This wide variety of immune evasion mechanism may explain the frequent appearance of persistent and asymptomatic infection (Figure 4).

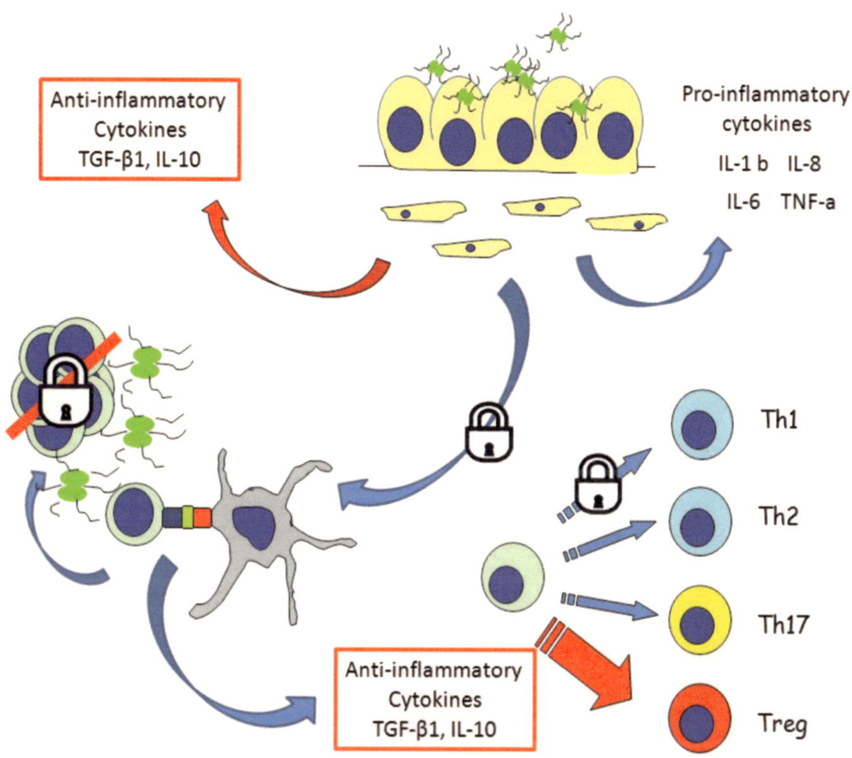

Fig. 4. *N. gonorrhoeae* interferes with immune responses.

5. Conclusion

Neisseria gonorrhoeae infects the reproductive tract of the human causing gonorrhea. Mechanisms of infection involved the early attachment of gonococcal membrane components, such as Pili, Opa, Porin and LOS, to cell host receptors. Frequently, the bacteria develop persistence and asymptomatic disease, which seem to be associated to the gonoccoccus ability to evade immune response. Several lines of research revealed that *N.*

gonorrhoeae is able to subvert polymorphonuclear cell phagocytic destruction, induces a weak humoral immune response, decreases antigen presenting properties of macrophages and dendritic cells, inhibits T cell proliferation and induces anti-inflammatory cytokines and T inhibitory cells. On the whole, this seems to be a complex network of immune evasion mechanisms responsible for the restricted immune response frequently observed during gonococcal infection.

6. Acknowledgment

We thanks the support of DICYT 021043IB, PBCT to CA and CONICYT Fellowship to KM and SR.

7. References

Annunziato F., Cosmi L., Santarlasci V., Maggi L., Liotta F., Mazzinghi B., Parente E., Fili L., Ferri S., Frosali F., Giudici F., Romagnani P., Parronchi P., Tonelli F., Maggi E. and Romagnani S., 2007. Phenotypic and functional features of human Th17 cells. J Exp Med 204, 1849-61.

Anzala A. O., Simonsen J. N., Kimani J., Ball T. B., Nagelkerke N. J., Rutherford J., Ngugi E. N., Bwayo J. J. and Plummer F. A., 2000. Acute sexually transmitted infections increase human immunodeficiency virus type 1 plasma viremia, increase plasma type 2 cytokines, and decrease CD4 cell counts. J Infect Dis 182, 459-66.

Apicella M. A., Ketterer M., Lee F. K., Zhou D., Rice P. A. and Blake M. S., 1996. The pathogenesis of gonococcal urethritis in men: confocal and immunoelectron microscopic analysis of urethral exudates from men infected with Neisseria gonorrhoeae. J Infect Dis 173, 636-46.

Astier A. L., Beriou G., Eisenhaure T. M., Anderton S. M., Hafler D. A. and Hacohen N., 2010. RNA interference screen in primary human T cells reveals FLT3 as a modulator of IL-10 levels. J Immunol 184, 685-93.

Ayala P., Wilbur J. S., Wetzler L. M., Tainer J. A., Snyder A. and So M., 2005. The pilus and porin of Neisseria gonorrhoeae cooperatively induce Ca(2+) transients in infected epithelial cells. Cell Microbiol 7, 1736-48.

Bending D., De La Pena H., Veldhoen M., Phillips J. M., Uyttenhove C., Stockinger B. and Cooke A., 2009. Highly purified Th17 cells from BDC2.5NOD mice convert into Th1-like cells in NOD/SCID recipient mice. J Clin Invest 119, 565-72.

Bhat K. S., Gibbs C. P., Barrera O., Morrison S. G., Jahnig F., Stern A., Kupsch E. M., Meyer T. F. and Swanson J., 1991. The opacity proteins of Neisseria gonorrhoeae strain MS11 are encoded by a family of 11 complete genes. Mol Microbiol 5, 1889-901.

Binnicker M. J., Williams R. D. and Apicella M. A., 2003. Infection of human urethral epithelium with Neisseria gonorrhoeae elicits an upregulation of host anti-apoptotic factors and protects cells from staurosporine-induced apoptosis. Cell Microbiol 5, 549-60.

Binnicker M. J., Williams R. D. and Apicella M. A., 2004. Gonococcal porin IB activates NF-kappaB in human urethral epithelium and increases the expression of host antiapoptotic factors. Infect Immun 72, 6408-17.

Borregaard N., 2010. Neutrophils, from marrow to microbes. Immunity 33, 657-70.

Bos M. P., Grunert F. and Belland R. J., 1997. Differential recognition of members of the carcinoembryonic antigen family by Opa variants of Neisseria gonorrhoeae. Infect Immun 65, 2353-61.

Boslego J. W., Tramont E. C., Chung R. C., McChesney D. G., Ciak J., Sadoff J. C., Piziak M. V., Brown J. D., Brinton C. C., Jr., Wood S. W. and et al., 1991. Efficacy trial of a parenteral gonococcal pilus vaccine in men. Vaccine 9, 154-62.

Boulton I. C. and Gray-Owen S. D., 2002. Neisserial binding to CEACAM1 arrests the activation and proliferation of CD4+ T lymphocytes. Nat Immunol 3, 229-36.

Brooks G. F. and Lammel C. J., 1989. Humoral immune response to gonococcal infections. Clin Microbiol Rev 2 Suppl, S5-10.

Cohen I. R., 1967. Natural and immune human antibodies reactive with antigens of virulent Neisseria gonorrhoeae: immunoglobulins G, M, And A. J Bacteriol 94, 141-8.

Cohen M. S. and Cannon J. G., 1999. Human experimentation with Neisseria gonorrhoeae: progress and goals. J Infect Dis 179 Suppl 2, S375-9.

Connell T. D., Shaffer D. and Cannon J. G., 1990. Characterization of the repertoire of hypervariable regions in the Protein II (opa) gene family of Neisseria gonorrhoeae. Mol Microbiol 4, 439-49.

Chegini N., Zhao Y., Williams R. S. and Flanders K. C., 1994. Human uterine tissue throughout the menstrual cycle expresses transforming growth factor-beta 1 (TGF beta 1), TGF beta 2, TGF beta 3, and TGF beta type II receptor messenger ribonucleic acid and protein and contains [125I]TGF beta 1-binding sites. Endocrinology 135, 439-49.

Chen T., Belland R. J., Wilson J. and Swanson J., 1995. Adherence of pilus- Opa+ gonococci to epithelial cells in vitro involves heparan sulfate. J Exp Med 182, 511-7.

Chen T. and Gotschlich E. C., 1996. CGM1a antigen of neutrophils, a receptor of gonococcal opacity proteins. Proc Natl Acad Sci U S A 93, 14851-6.

Chen T., Grunert F., Medina-Marino A. and Gotschlich E. C., 1997. Several carcinoembryonic antigens (CD66) serve as receptors for gonococcal opacity proteins. J Exp Med 185, 1557-64.

Dehio C., Freissler E., Lanz C., Gomez-Duarte O. G., David G. and Meyer T. F., 1998a. Ligation of cell surface heparan sulfate proteoglycans by antibody-coated beads stimulates phagocytic uptake into epithelial cells: a model for cellular invasion by Neisseria gonorrhoeae. Exp Cell Res 242, 528-39.

Dehio C., Gray-Owen S. D. and Meyer T. F., 1998b. The role of neisserial Opa proteins in interactions with host cells. Trends Microbiol 6, 489-95.

Dehio M., Gomez-Duarte O. G., Dehio C. and Meyer T. F., 1998c. Vitronectin-dependent invasion of epithelial cells by Neisseria gonorrhoeae involves alpha(v) integrin receptors. FEBS Lett 424, 84-8.

Dempsey J. A., Litaker W., Madhure A., Snodgrass T. L. and Cannon J. G., 1991. Physical map of the chromosome of Neisseria gonorrhoeae FA1090 with locations of genetic markers, including opa and pil genes. J Bacteriol 173, 5476-86.

Duensing T. D. and Putten J. P., 1998. Vitronectin binds to the gonococcal adhesin OpaA through a glycosaminoglycan molecular bridge. Biochem J 334 (Pt 1), 133-9.

Duensing T. D. and van Putten J. P., 1997. Vitronectin mediates internalization of Neisseria gonorrhoeae by Chinese hamster ovary cells. Infect Immun 65, 964-70.

Edwards J. L. and Apicella M. A., 2005. I-domain-containing integrins serve as pilus receptors for Neisseria gonorrhoeae adherence to human epithelial cells. Cell Microbiol 7, 1197-211.

Edwards J. L., Brown E. J., Ault K. A. and Apicella M. A., 2001. The role of complement receptor 3 (CR3) in Neisseria gonorrhoeae infection of human cervical epithelia. Cell Microbiol 3, 611-22.

Edwards J. L., Brown E. J., Uk-Nham S., Cannon J. G., Blake M. S. and Apicella M. A., 2002. A co-operative interaction between Neisseria gonorrhoeae and complement receptor 3 mediates infection of primary cervical epithelial cells. Cell Microbiol 4, 571-84.

Edwards J. L., Shao J. Q., Ault K. A. and Apicella M. A., 2000. Neisseria gonorrhoeae elicits membrane ruffling and cytoskeletal rearrangements upon infection of primary human endocervical and ectocervical cells. Infect Immun 68, 5354-63.

Evans B. A., 1977. Ultrastructural study of cervical gonorrhea. J Infect Dis 136, 248-55.

Farley T. A., Cohen D. A. and Elkins W., 2003. Asymptomatic sexually transmitted diseases: the case for screening. Prev Med 36, 502-9.

Feinen B., Jerse A. E., Gaffen S. L. and Russell M. W., 2010. Critical role of Th17 responses in a murine model of Neisseria gonorrhoeae genital infection. Mucosal Immunol 3, 312-21.

Fisette P. L., Ram S., Andersen J. M., Guo W. and Ingalls R. R., 2003. The Lip lipoprotein from Neisseria gonorrhoeae stimulates cytokine release and NF-kappaB activation in epithelial cells in a Toll-like receptor 2-dependent manner. J Biol Chem 278, 46252-60.

Giardina P. C., Williams R., Lubaroff D. and Apicella M. A., 1998. Neisseria gonorrhoeae induces focal polymerization of actin in primary human urethral epithelium. Infect Immun 66, 3416-9.

Givan A. L., White H. D., Stern J. E., Colby E., Gosselin E. J., Guyre P. M. and Wira C. R., 1997. Flow cytometric analysis of leukocytes in the human female reproductive tract: comparison of fallopian tube, uterus, cervix, and vagina. Am J Reprod Immunol 38, 350-9.

Gomez-Duarte O. G., Dehio M., Guzman C. A., Chhatwal G. S., Dehio C. and Meyer T. F., 1997. Binding of vitronectin to opa-expressing Neisseria gonorrhoeae mediates invasion of HeLa cells. Infect Immun 65, 3857-66.

Grant K. S. and Wira C. R., 2003. Effect of mouse uterine stromal cells on epithelial cell transepithelial resistance (TER) and TNFalpha and TGFbeta release in culture. Biol Reprod 69, 1091-8.

Grassme H., Gulbins E., Brenner B., Ferlinz K., Sandhoff K., Harzer K., Lang F. and Meyer T. F., 1997. Acidic sphingomyelinase mediates entry of N. gonorrhoeae into nonphagocytic cells. Cell 91, 605-15.

Grassme H. U., Ireland R. M. and van Putten J. P., 1996. Gonococcal opacity protein promotes bacterial entry-associated rearrangements of the epithelial cell actin cytoskeleton. Infect Immun 64, 1621-30.

Gray-Owen S. D., Dehio C., Haude A., Grunert F. and Meyer T. F., 1997a. CD66 carcinoembryonic antigens mediate interactions between Opa-expressing Neisseria gonorrhoeae and human polymorphonuclear phagocytes. EMBO J 16, 3435-45.

Gray-Owen S. D., Lorenzen D. R., Haude A., Meyer T. F. and Dehio C., 1997b. Differential Opa specificities for CD66 receptors influence tissue interactions and cellular response to Neisseria gonorrhoeae. Mol Microbiol 26, 971-80.

Griffiss J. M., Lammel C. J., Wang J., Dekker N. P. and Brooks G. F., 1999. Neisseria gonorrhoeae coordinately uses Pili and Opa to activate HEC-1-B cell microvilli, which causes engulfment of the gonococci. Infect Immun 67, 3469-80.

Hammarstrom S., 1999. The carcinoembryonic antigen (CEA) family: structures, suggested functions and expression in normal and malignant tissues. Semin Cancer Biol 9, 67-81.

Handsfield H. H., Lipman T. O., Harnisch J. P., Tronca E. and Holmes K. K., 1974. Asymptomatic gonorrhea in men. Diagnosis, natural course, prevalence and significance. N Engl J Med 290, 117-23.

Harvey H. A., Jennings M. P., Campbell C. A., Williams R. and Apicella M. A., 2001. Receptor-mediated endocytosis of Neisseria gonorrhoeae into primary human urethral epithelial cells: the role of the asialoglycoprotein receptor. Mol Microbiol 42, 659-72.

Harvey H. A., Ketterer M. R., Preston A., Lubaroff D., Williams R. and Apicella M. A., 1997. Ultrastructural analysis of primary human urethral epithelial cell cultures infected with Neisseria gonorrhoeae. Infect Immun 65, 2420-7.

Hauck C. R., Grassme H., Bock J., Jendrossek V., Ferlinz K., Meyer T. F. and Gulbins E., 2000. Acid sphingomyelinase is involved in CEACAM receptor-mediated phagocytosis of Neisseria gonorrhoeae. FEBS Lett 478, 260-6.

Hauck C. R., Meyer T. F., Lang F. and Gulbins E., 1998. CD66-mediated phagocytosis of Opa52 Neisseria gonorrhoeae requires a Src-like tyrosine kinase- and Rac1-dependent signalling pathway. EMBO J 17, 443-54.

Hedges S. R., Mayo M. S., Mestecky J., Hook E. W., 3rd and Russell M. W., 1999. Limited local and systemic antibody responses to Neisseria gonorrhoeae during uncomplicated genital infections. Infect Immun 67, 3937-46.

Hedges S. R., Sibley D. A., Mayo M. S., Hook E. W., 3rd and Russell M. W., 1998. Cytokine and antibody responses in women infected with Neisseria gonorrhoeae: effects of concomitant infections. J Infect Dis 178, 742-51.

Howie H. L., Shiflett S. L. and So M., 2008. Extracellular signal-regulated kinase activation by Neisseria gonorrhoeae downregulates epithelial cell proapoptotic proteins Bad and Bim. Infect Immun 76, 2715-21.

Hoyme U. B., 1990. Pelvic inflammatory disease and associated sexually transmitted diseases. Curr Opin Obstet Gynecol 2, 668-74.

Imarai M., Candia E., Rodriguez-Tirado C., Tognarelli J., Pardo M., Perez T., Valdes D., Reyes-Cerpa S., Nelson P., Acuna-Castillo C. and Maisey K., 2008. Regulatory T cells are locally induced during intravaginal infection of mice with Neisseria gonorrhoeae. Infect Immun 76, 5456-65.

Inaba K., Steinman R. M., Pack M. W., Aya H., Inaba M., Sudo T., Wolpe S. and Schuler G., 1992. Identification of proliferating dendritic cell precursors in mouse blood. J Exp Med 175, 1157-67.

Ison C. A., Hadfield S. G., Bellinger C. M., Dawson S. G. and Glynn A. A., 1986. The specificity of serum and local antibodies in female gonorrhoea. Clin Exp Immunol 65, 198-205.

Jerse A. E., 1999. Experimental gonococcal genital tract infection and opacity protein expression in estradiol-treated mice. Infect Immun 67, 5699-708.

Jeurissen S. H., Sminia T. and Beuvery E. C., 1987. Induction of mucosal immunoglobulin A immune response by preparations of Neisseria gonorrhoeae porin proteins. Infect Immun 55, 253-7.

Jin L. W., Inaba K. and Saitoh T., 1992. The involvement of protein kinase C in activation-induced cell death in T-cell hybridoma. Cell Immunol 144, 217-27.

John J. and Donald W. H., 1978. Asymptomatic urethral gonorrhoea in men. Br J Vener Dis 54, 322-3.

Johnson M. B. and Criss A. K., 2011. Resistance of Neisseria gonorrhoeae to neutrophils. Front Microbiol 2, 77.

Jonsson A. B., Ilver D., Falk P., Pepose J. and Normark S., 1994. Sequence changes in the pilus subunit lead to tropism variation of Neisseria gonorrhoeae to human tissue. Mol Microbiol 13, 403-16.

Jonuleit H., Schmitt E., Stassen M., Tuettenberg A., Knop J. and Enk A. H., 2001. Identification and functional characterization of human CD4(+)CD25(+) T cells with regulatory properties isolated from peripheral blood. J Exp Med 193, 1285-94.

Kallstrom H., Blackmer Gill D., Albiger B., Liszewski M. K., Atkinson J. P. and Jonsson A. B., 2001. Attachment of Neisseria gonorrhoeae to the cellular pilus receptor CD46: identification of domains important for bacterial adherence. Cell Microbiol 3, 133-43.

Kallstrom H., Islam M. S., Berggren P. O. and Jonsson A. B., 1998. Cell signaling by the type IV pili of pathogenic Neisseria. J Biol Chem 273, 21777-82.

Kirchner M., Heuer D. and Meyer T. F., 2005. CD46-independent binding of neisserial type IV pili and the major pilus adhesin, PilC, to human epithelial cells. Infect Immun 73, 3072-82.

Kirchner M. and Meyer T. F., 2005. The PilC adhesin of the Neisseria type IV pilus-binding specificities and new insights into the nature of the host cell receptor. Mol Microbiol 56, 945-57.

Kohl P. K., Kratofiel M., Gorner R., Kunze F., Senf-Blum A., Eggert-Kruse W., Gerhard I., Hoferer E. and Petzoldt D., 1992. [Local and systemic humoral immune response to protein I of Neisseria gonorrhoeae]. Hautarzt 43, 352-8.

Laan M., Cui Z. H., Hoshino H., Lotvall J., Sjostrand M., Gruenert D. C., Skoogh B. E. and Linden A., 1999. Neutrophil recruitment by human IL-17 via C-X-C chemokine release in the airways. J Immunol 162, 2347-52.

Lammel C. J., Sweet R. L., Rice P. A., Knapp J. S., Schoolnik G. K., Heilbron D. C. and Brooks G. F., 1985. Antibody-antigen specificity in the immune response to infection with Neisseria gonorrhoeae. J Infect Dis 152, 990-1001.

Langrish C. L., McKenzie B. S., Wilson N. J., de Waal Malefyt R., Kastelein R. A. and Cua D. J., 2004. IL-12 and IL-23: master regulators of innate and adaptive immunity. Immunol Rev 202, 96-105.

Lee H. S., Boulton I. C., Reddin K., Wong H., Halliwell D., Mandelboim O., Gorringe A. R. and Gray-Owen S. D., 2007. Neisserial outer membrane vesicles bind the coinhibitory receptor carcinoembryonic antigen-related cellular adhesion molecule 1 and suppress CD4+ T lymphocyte function. Infect Immun 75, 4449-55.

Lee H. S., Ostrowski M. A. and Gray-Owen S. D., 2008. CEACAM1 dynamics during neisseria gonorrhoeae suppression of CD4+ T lymphocyte activation. J Immunol 180, 6827-35.

Lee S. W., Higashi D. L., Snyder A., Merz A. J., Potter L. and So M., 2005. PilT is required for PI(3,4,5)P3-mediated crosstalk between Neisseria gonorrhoeae and epithelial cells. Cell Microbiol 7, 1271-84.

LeibundGut-Landmann S., Gross O., Robinson M. J., Osorio F., Slack E. C., Tsoni S. V., Schweighoffer E., Tybulewicz V., Brown G. D., Ruland J. and Reis e Sousa C., 2007. Syk- and CARD9-dependent coupling of innate immunity to the induction of T helper cells that produce interleukin 17. Nat Immunol 8, 630-8.

Long C. D., Madraswala R. N. and Seifert H. S., 1998. Comparisons between colony phase variation of Neisseria gonorrhoeae FA1090 and pilus, pilin, and S-pilin expression. Infect Immun 66, 1918-27.

Lorenzen D. R., Dux F., Wolk U., Tsirpouchtsidis A., Haas G. and Meyer T. F., 1999. Immunoglobulin A1 protease, an exoenzyme of pathogenic Neisseriae, is a potent inducer of proinflammatory cytokines. J Exp Med 190, 1049-58.

Lynch E. C., Blake M. S., Gotschlich E. C. and Mauro A., 1984. Studies of Porins: Spontaneously Transferred from Whole Cells and Reconstituted from Purified Proteins of Neisseria gonorrhoeae and Neisseria meningitidis. Biophys J 45, 104-7.

Maisey K., Nardocci G., Imarai M., Cardenas H., Rios M., Croxatto H. B., Heckels J. E., Christodoulides M. and Velasquez L. A., 2003. Expression of Proinflammatory Cytokines and Receptors by Human Fallopian Tubes in Organ Culture following Challenge with Neisseria gonorrhoeae. Infect. Immun. 71, 527-532.

McChesney D., Tramont E. C., Boslego J. W., Ciak J., Sadoff J. and Brinton C. C., 1982. Genital antibody response to a parenteral gonococcal pilus vaccine. Infect Immun 36, 1006-12.

McGee Z. A., Jensen R. L., Clemens C. M., Taylor-Robinson D., Johnson A. P. and Gregg C. R., 1999. Gonococcal infection of human fallopian tube mucosa in organ culture: relationship of mucosal tissue TNF-alpha concentration to sloughing of ciliated cells. Sex Transm Dis 26, 160-5.

McGuirk P., McCann C. and Mills K. H., 2002. Pathogen-specific T regulatory 1 cells induced in the respiratory tract by a bacterial molecule that stimulates interleukin 10 production by dendritic cells: a novel strategy for evasion of protective T helper type 1 responses by Bordetella pertussis. J Exp Med 195, 221-31.

Merz A. J., Enns C. A. and So M., 1999. Type IV pili of pathogenic Neisseriae elicit cortical plaque formation in epithelial cells. Mol Microbiol 32, 1316-32.

Merz A. J. and So M., 1997. Attachment of piliated, Opa- and Opc- gonococci and meningococci to epithelial cells elicits cortical actin rearrangements and clustering of tyrosine-phosphorylated proteins. Infect Immun 65, 4341-9.

Muenzner P., Dehio C., Fujiwara T., Achtman M., Meyer T. F. and Gray-Owen S. D., 2000. Carcinoembryonic antigen family receptor specificity of Neisseria meningitidis Opa variants influences adherence to and invasion of proinflammatory cytokine-activated endothelial cells. Infect Immun 68, 3601-7.

Muller A., Gunther D., Brinkmann V., Hurwitz R., Meyer T. F. and Rudel T., 2000. Targeting of the pro-apoptotic VDAC-like porin (PorB) of Neisseria gonorrhoeae to mitochondria of infected cells. EMBO J 19, 5332-43.

Muller A., Gunther D., Dux F., Naumann M., Meyer T. F. and Rudel T., 1999. Neisserial porin (PorB) causes rapid calcium influx in target cells and induces apoptosis by the activation of cysteine proteases. EMBO J 18, 339-52.

Muller A., Rassow J., Grimm J., Machuy N., Meyer T. F. and Rudel T., 2002. VDAC and the bacterial porin PorB of Neisseria gonorrhoeae share mitochondrial import pathways. EMBO J 21, 1916-29.

Murphy G. L., Connell T. D., Barritt D. S., Koomey M. and Cannon J. G., 1989. Phase variation of gonococcal protein II: regulation of gene expression by slipped-strand mispairing of a repetitive DNA sequence. Cell 56, 539-47.

Napolitani G., Rinaldi A., Bertoni F., Sallusto F. and Lanzavecchia A., 2005. Selected Toll-like receptor agonist combinations synergistically trigger a T helper type 1-polarizing program in dendritic cells. Nat Immunol 6, 769-76.

Nocera M. and Chu T. M., 1995. Characterization of latent transforming growth factor-beta from human seminal plasma. Am J Reprod Immunol 33, 282-91.

O'Connor R. A., Prendergast C. T., Sabatos C. A., Lau C. W., Leech M. D., Wraith D. C. and Anderton S. M., 2008. Cutting edge: Th1 cells facilitate the entry of Th17 cells to the central nervous system during experimental autoimmune encephalomyelitis. J Immunol 181, 3750-4.

Ouyang W., Kolls J. K. and Zheng Y., 2008. The biological functions of T helper 17 cell effector cytokines in inflammation. Immunity 28, 454-67.

Ovcinnikov N. M. and Delektorskij V. V., 1971. Electron microscope studies of gonococci in the urethral secretions of patients with gonorrhoea. Br J Vener Dis 47, 419-39.

Pantelic M., Kim Y. J., Bolland S., Chen I., Shively J. and Chen T., 2005. Neisseria gonorrhoeae kills carcinoembryonic antigen-related cellular adhesion molecule 1 (CD66a)-expressing human B cells and inhibits antibody production. Infect Immun 73, 4171-9.

Parge H. E., Forest K. T., Hickey M. J., Christensen D. A., Getzoff E. D. and Tainer J. A., 1995. Structure of the fibre-forming protein pilin at 2.6 A resolution. Nature 378, 32-8.

Plant L. J. and Jonsson A. B., 2006. Type IV pili of Neisseria gonorrhoeae influence the activation of human CD4+ T cells. Infect Immun 74, 442-8.

Plummer F. A., Chubb H., Simonsen J. N., Bosire M., Slaney L., Maclean I., Ndinya-Achola J. O., Waiyaki P. and Brunham R. C., 1993. Antibody to Rmp (outer membrane protein 3) increases susceptibility to gonococcal infection. J Clin Invest 91, 339-43.

Plummer F. A., Chubb H., Simonsen J. N., Bosire M., Slaney L., Nagelkerke N. J., Maclean I., Ndinya-Achola J. O., Waiyaki P. and Brunham R. C., 1994. Antibodies to opacity proteins (Opa) correlate with a reduced risk of gonococcal salpingitis. J Clin Invest 93, 1748-55.

Popp A., Dehio C., Grunert F., Meyer T. F. and Gray-Owen S. D., 1999. Molecular analysis of neisserial Opa protein interactions with the CEA family of receptors: identification of determinants contributing to the differential specificities of binding. Cell Microbiol 1, 169-81.

Preston A., Mandrell R. E., Gibson B. W. and Apicella M. A., 1996. The lipooligosaccharides of pathogenic gram-negative bacteria. Crit Rev Microbiol 22, 139-80.

Rarick M., McPheeters C., Bright S., Navis A., Skefos J., Sebastiani P. and Montano M., 2006. Evidence for cross-regulated cytokine response in human peripheral blood mononuclear cells exposed to whole gonococcal bacteria in vitro. Microb Pathog 40, 261-70.

Rice P. A., Vayo H. E., Tam M. R. and Blake M. S., 1986. Immunoglobulin G antibodies directed against protein III block killing of serum-resistant Neisseria gonorrhoeae by immune serum. J Exp Med 164, 1735-48.

Rowell E. and Wilson C. B., 2009. Programming perpetual T helper cell plasticity. Immunity 30, 7-9.

Rudel T., Schmid A., Benz R., Kolb H. A., Lang F. and Meyer T. F., 1996. Modulation of Neisseria porin (PorB) by cytosolic ATP/GTP of target cells: parallels between pathogen accommodation and mitochondrial endosymbiosis. Cell 85, 391-402.

Rudel T., van Putten J. P., Gibbs C. P., Haas R. and Meyer T. F., 1992. Interaction of two variable proteins (PilE and PilC) required for pilus-mediated adherence of Neisseria gonorrhoeae to human epithelial cells. Mol Microbiol 6, 3439-50.

Sabatos C. A., Doh J., Chakravarti S., Friedman R. S., Pandurangi P. G., Tooley A. J. and Krummel M. F., 2008. A synaptic basis for paracrine interleukin-2 signaling during homotypic T cell interaction. Immunity 29, 238-48.

Sakaguchi S., 2004. Naturally arising CD4+ regulatory T cells for immunologic self-tolerance and negative control of immune responses. Annu. Rev. Immunol. 22, 531-562.

Simpson S. D., Ho Y., Rice P. A. and Wetzler L. M., 1999. T lymphocyte response to Neisseria gonorrhoeae porin in individuals with mucosal gonococcal infections. J Infect Dis 180, 762-73.

Snapper C. M., Rosas F. R., Kehry M. R., Mond J. J. and Wetzler L. M., 1997. Neisserial porins may provide critical second signals to polysaccharide-activated murine B cells for induction of immunoglobulin secretion. Infect Immun 65, 3203-8.

Song W., Condron S., Mocca B. T., Veit S. J., Hill D., Abbas A. and Jerse A. E., 2008. Local and humoral immune responses against primary and repeat Neisseria gonorrhoeae genital tract infections of 17beta-estradiol-treated mice. Vaccine 26, 5741-51.

Srivastava M. D., Lippes J. and Srivastava B. I., 1996. Cytokines of the human reproductive tract. Am J Reprod Immunol 36, 157-66.

Stagg A. J., Tuffrey M., Woods C., Wunderink E. and Knight S. C., 1998. Protection against ascending infection of the genital tract by Chlamydia trachomatis is associated with recruitment of major histocompatibility complex class II antigen-presenting cells into uterine tissue. Infect Immun 66, 3535-44.

Tapchaisri P. and Sirisinha S., 1976. Serum and secretory antibody responses to Neisseria gonorrhoeae in patients with gonococcal infections. Br J Vener Dis 52, 374-80.

Tapsall J., 2001. Antimicrobial resistance in *Neisseria gonorrhoeae*. World Health Organization Department of Communicable Disease Surveillance and Response.

Taylor B. N., Saavedra M. and Fidel P. L., Jr., 2000. Local Th1/Th2 cytokine production during experimental vaginal candidiasis: potential importance of transforming growth factor-beta. Med Mycol 38, 419-31.

Tobiason D. M. and Seifert H. S., 2001. Inverse relationship between pilus-mediated gonococcal adherence and surface expression of the pilus receptor, CD46. Microbiology 147, 2333-40.

Tramont E. C., Sadoff J. C., Boslego J. W., Ciak J., McChesney D., Brinton C. C., Wood S. and Takafuji E., 1981. Gonococcal pilus vaccine. Studies of antigenicity and inhibition of attachment. J Clin Invest 68, 881-8.

Tsirpouchtsidis A., Hurwitz R., Brinkmann V., Meyer T. F. and Haas G., 2002. Neisserial immunoglobulin A1 protease induces specific T-cell responses in humans. Infect Immun 70, 335-44.
van Putten J. P., Duensing T. D. and Cole R. L., 1998. Entry of OpaA+ gonococci into HEp-2 cells requires concerted action of glycosaminoglycans, fibronectin and integrin receptors. Mol Microbiol 29, 369-79.
van Putten J. P. and Paul S. M., 1995. Binding of syndecan-like cell surface proteoglycan receptors is required for Neisseria gonorrhoeae entry into human mucosal cells. EMBO J 14, 2144-54.
van Vliet S. J., Steeghs L., Bruijns S. C., Vaezirad M. M., Snijders Blok C., Arenas Busto J. A., Deken M., van Putten J. P. and van Kooyk Y., 2009. Variation of Neisseria gonorrhoeae lipooligosaccharide directs dendritic cell-induced T helper responses. PLoS Pathog 5, e1000625.
Verhagen J., Sabatos C. A. and Wraith D. C., 2008. The role of CTLA-4 in immune regulation. Immunol Lett 115, 73-4.
Virji M., Evans D., Hadfield A., Grunert F., Teixeira A. M. and Watt S. M., 1999. Critical determinants of host receptor targeting by Neisseria meningitidis and Neisseria gonorrhoeae: identification of Opa adhesiotopes on the N-domain of CD66 molecules. Mol Microbiol 34, 538-51.
Virji M., Makepeace K., Ferguson D. J. and Watt S. M., 1996a. Carcinoembryonic antigens (CD66) on epithelial cells and neutrophils are receptors for Opa proteins of pathogenic neisseriae. Mol Microbiol 22, 941-50.
Virji M., Watt S. M., Barker S., Makepeace K. and Doyonnas R., 1996b. The N-domain of the human CD66a adhesion molecule is a target for Opa proteins of Neisseria meningitidis and Neisseria gonorrhoeae. Mol Microbiol 22, 929-39.
Wada K., Nomura S., Morii E., Kitamura Y., Nishizawa Y., Miyake A. and Terada N., 1996. Changes in levels of mRNAs of transforming growth factor (TGF)-beta1, -beta2, -beta3, TGF-beta type II receptor and sulfated glycoprotein-2 during apoptosis of mouse uterine epithelium. J Steroid Biochem Mol Biol 59, 367-75.
Weel J. F. and van Putten J. P., 1991. Fate of the major outer membrane protein P.IA in early and late events of gonococcal infection of epithelial cells. Res Microbiol 142, 985-93.
Wen K. K., Giardina P. C., Blake M. S., Edwards J., Apicella M. A. and Rubenstein P. A., 2000. Interaction of the gonococcal porin P.IB with G- and F-actin. Biochemistry 39, 8638-47.
Wetzler L. M., Ho Y. and Reiser H., 1996. Neisserial porins induce B lymphocytes to express costimulatory B7-2 molecules and to proliferate. J Exp Med 183, 1151-9.
WHO, 2011. Emergence of multi-drug resistant *Neisseria gonorrhoeae* - Threat of global rise in untreatable sexually transmitted infections.
Wiesner P. J. and Thompson S. E., 3rd, 1980. Gonococcal diseases. Dis Mon 26, 1-44.
Xu L., Kitani A., Fuss I. and Strober W., 2007. Cutting edge: regulatory T cells induce CD4+CD25-Foxp3- T cells or are self-induced to become Th17 cells in the absence of exogenous TGF-beta. J Immunol 178, 6725-9.
Zheng H., 1997. Analysis of the antigen-antibody specificity in the semen of patients with Neisseria gonorrhoeae. Chin Med Sci J 12, 47-9.

5

Syphilis

Roberto Saraiva et al.*
Santa Casa Hospital
Brazil

1. Introduction

Also known as lues venereum, syphilis is an infect-contagious chronic systemic disease, which is, in the majority of times, sexually transmitted. It is caused by the bacterium, *Treponema pallidum.* The illness is characterized by periods of activity between latency, becoming systemically worse throughout its different periods of virulence (1-5).

2. History

The name "syphilis" was first proposed by the physician and writer Girolamo Fracastoro who wrote about the disease in 1530, but it only became a medical term by the nineteenth century. He had published three epic books, in which he makes reference to a mythic Greek shepherd, *Syphilus,* whom *Apollo* had cursed with such an ailment (6).

The actual origin of this venereal condition is unknown. The first well described epidemic of the disease is dated from the fifteenth century. This European epidemic came about after the year of 1495, when the French, accompanied by the Spanish, invaded Italy. After the invasion, a strange and gruesome disease began to spread with sores, ulcers and skeletal pain, followed by physical incapacity and death. It then became known as the French disease. Of course, other names also followed, such as the Spanish disease, Italian, and so on (2-10).

It is not however, certain if this was syphilis' first appearance in the world; the pre-Colombian theory speculates that the bacterium was imported to Europe by sailors who went to America and many authors have observed bone deformity and treponemal lesions found in excavations and observations of the prehistoric period in different sites in America (9,10).

The Old World theory, states that Treponema has been around for thousands of years, but, like other living things, it suffered under nature's force and had to adapt through evolution. This theory is based on observations of diseases depicted throughout history and artefacts which seem to be in favour of different diseases caused by other species of spirochete bacterium. For example, it could have been misdiagnosed as leprosy for a long time. If this is true, its origin would mix with human history, far beyond a possible pinpoint in a timeline. Both theories remain inconclusive and are, as yet, not proven definitely one way or

*Augusto Daige, Joao Jazbik, Claudio Cesar, Marco Mello and Evandro Lopes

the other. What is true is that, even with such opposing theories, the *Renaissance* was a time of sexual freedom that helped the spread of sexual diseases (9,10). But, the new world theory or Columbia theory postulates that, since Columbus originated from continental Europe, where there was misleading evidence of syphilis, the origins could not be from Europe. Instead, his voyages contributed to the transmission, since his crew might have been infected on the voyages to the New World. Hence, the origin remains a mystery.

The discovery of the etiological factor of the disease - *Treponema Pallidum* - was of great importance. In 1905, in Hamburg, Germany, the zoologist Fritz Richard Schaudinn and the dermatologist Paul Erich Hoffmann presented the medical community with the discovery of the bacterium. Besides the natural controversies and disappointments of a new scientific discovery, it didn't take long for the world to recognize the new fact about the disease. From this point, research was made possible, helping the understanding of the pathology behind the bacterium (7-10). Another landmark for the classification of disease was the work developed by Wassermann in 1906, which led to serological test for syphilis. Treatment for the disease using arsenic-benzene was introduced by Paul Ehrlich in 1910, but it was only after the discovery of penicillin, and its introduction as treatment in 1943, that syphilis diminished its incidence and prevalence. A more recent discovery was the genomic sequence of the *Treponema pallidum* that can lead to a better understanding of the pathophysiology of the disease (10).

Another point in history that should be mentioned is the Tuskegee Syphilis Experiment. From 1932 until 1972 the US Public Health Services (PHS) left 399 black men untreated with diagnosed syphilis. Between those years, patients were given ineffective medicine (even aspirin) in order to keep track of the pathophysiology. Even with the cure for the disease accessible to all, these people were denied treatment with penicillin (11).

Many ethical issues have been exposed with this experiment, but the experiment took 30 years to finally end and many medical notes were revealed regarding the different phases of syphilis.

2.1 Epidemiology

It is a globally prevalent disease, most commonly found in cities. It does not have any predilection for race or sex, but it has been found to be more common among young people. From the 1960s there have been a growing number of syphilis cases because of sexual freedom, from use of birth control pills and higher rates of tourism and homosexuality (1,2,4).

There has been an expansion on the latent form of syphilis because of misdiagnoses and mistreatment of the disease. The fact that a person uses the antibiotics does not mean correct treatment, since the appropriate dosage must be applied. Hence many people go direct to the latent period of syphilis without the cure, with a high probability of recurrence (1,2,5,8).

With the advent of AIDS (Acquired Immunodeficiency Syndrome), atypical form of lues, with a more severe evolution of the disease, has been observed. Patients with other sexually transmitted diseases (STD) have been shown to have associated syphilis, for example, soft chancre (12-15%), donovanosis (45%), gonorrhoea (1-4%) and condyloma acuminatum (5%). This is the reason for the importance of screening patients with STDs for lues (1,2,8,12).

2.2 Pathophysiology

The causative agent of syphilis, *Treponema pallidum*, comes from a family of bacteria that are present in animals and insects without any harm to them, living in the digestive system of the animals. It is a gram-negative bacterium, spiral shaped (8 to 20 spirals), measuring from 4 to 10 μm in length to 0,25 μm in width. Except for its more irregular and delicate spirals, the bacterium is undistinguishable from others spirochetes. It is an obligate parasite of humans (1-8).

The initial multiplication of the parasite is intense, as there is an absence of antibodies and cellular immunity. They attach to cells of the mucosa by ligands on their surface, the adhesins, that facilitate bacterial adhesion to the host´s cells. The bacteria secrete hyaluronidase that will destroy the polysaccharide that holds animal cells together, making its penetration possible. It will need free iron and will bond to lactoferritin, lipoproteins, mucopolysaccharides, proteoglycans or glycosaminoglycans, that are necessary to its development and its protection and as they mix with these substances, the host will recognize the microorganism as itself (7).

There is no natural immunity against syphilis. The inoculation in healthy individuals will always cause the disease, by inducing a humoral and cellular response. The immune response to syphilis involves production of antibodies to a wide range of antigens, including non-specific antibodies and specific treponemal antibodies. The first demonstrable humoral response is the production of anti-treponemal IgM at the end of the second week, and IgG at approximately four weeks after the exposure. The cellular immunity will come after, exteriorized by disseminated infection (5-7).

With the development of the humoral and cellular immunity, the bacteria are gradually destroyed, living only in a few tissues. This is the latent phase of the disease, which can go for an undetermined period. They can remain inside the tissues or be eliminated through a biological cure. The microorganisms can be reactivated, when there is a decline in immunity efficiency, thus reinfecting the host (5-9).

T. pallidum cannot be cultured in the laboratory and therefore it is impossible to investigate it by using the conventional techniques. It does not live outside mammalian cells. It is researched through the inoculation of the bacteria inside rabbit or monkey cells.

It is contagious during the recent phase of the disease. Syphilis is transmitted primarily by sexual contact and the next most common is transfer across the placenta. Human contact, blood transfusion & accidental inoculation have also been reported as routes of transmission but are of minor importance. The bacterium penetrates the body through the mucosa or microabrasion on skin. Within a few hours of inoculation, it enters the lymphatics and blood, producing infection long before the appearance of the primary lesion. The concentration of *T. pallidum* in the blood of a person with the disease is around 10^7 per gram of tissue before the first lesions. The median incubation time is 21 days, ranging from 10 to 90 days. Studies in rabbits have shown that spirochetes can be found in the lymphatic system 30 minutes after primary inoculation (1-10,12-14). Congenital syphilis is contracted from an infected mother via transplacental transmission of T. pallidum at any time during pregnancy or at birth.

2.3 Primary syphilis

The primary lesion appears in the site of inoculation, persisting for 4 to 6 weeks, healing spontaneously. It is normally a single, painless papule, with a reddish halo around it, presenting a discrete serosity, that becomes indurated, which can erode (protosyphiloma). It measures from a few millimetres to 2 centimetres. The lesion can be painful if it is presented extragenital. It normally appears on the penis of heterosexual men. Lesions in homosexual men, are present in the anal canal, rectum or extragenital - perianal or perioral, for example. In women, the lesions are most commonly observed in the cervix and labia. Presence in the cervix can lead it to being undiagnosed. Extragenital lesions can appear on the lips, tongue, tonsil, nipple, fingers and anus. They usually heal within 4 to 6 weeks (ranging from 2 to 12 weeks); it does not leave any scar tissue. The lesion is highly contagious. If the protosyphiloma appears in a place that has been already inoculated with another pathogen, and presents a characteristic lesion, such as anal genital herpes or even anal fissures, the lesion can take the morphology of the first lesion. That is why every person with a genital ulcerated lesion should be tested for syphilis (1-6,8,15,16).

In relation to the primary lesion, other forms include:

Decapitated syphilis: syphilis that does not present with the primary lesion. Normally the infection occurs by transfusion or in patients that during the infection were using antibiotics that obscured the chancre, although the dosage was insufficient to eradicate the pathogen (1,17,18).

Chancre of Rollet: the association of a hard chancre (syphilitic) with a soft chancre, from *Haemophilus ducreyi* (chancroid) (1, 17,18).

Chancre Redux: Chancre redux is the presence of a gumma, reappearing at the site of the initial chancre, and "pseudochancre redux" is one solitary gumma on the penis (1,17,18)

A satellite bubo also appears 1 week after the primary lesion. Bubo is a lymphatic gland responsible in the drainage of the area containing the lesion. They become enlarged nonsuppurative and painless. From the affected gland, liquid can be aspirated for further diagnosis when the primary lesion does not have enough substance. When the lesion is anal or within the external genitalia, the nodes appear at the inguinal region. Rectal chancre usually cause perirectal lymphadenopathy, while lesions in the vagina or cervix result in iliac or perirectal adenopathy. This condition may persist for months, even after the primary lesion disappears (1-3,5, 6, 17,18).

Differential diagnosis: soft chancre and herpes are the basic pathologies that could be misdiagnosed, since both present with genital eruption.

2.4 Secondary syphilis

After 6 to 8 weeks of healing of the chancre, systemic manifestation and skin lesions begin to appear. Though, 15 to 25% of patients with secondary syphilis may still have the primary lesions, and up to 45% will have the lesion associated with AIDS. About 25% may not remember having a primary lesion. Some will take a few months for the disease to florid again, while others will never go through the secondary phase of syphilis (1-3,12, 18,19).

Symptoms include low-grade fever, nontender adenopathy, hyporexia, malaise and rash. Other symptoms that are less common are ophthalmia, arthralgia, iritis and other eye lesions, including pupillary abnormalities, optic neuritis, uveitis and retinitis pigmentosa. Acute meningitis may occur, but is rare; 30% of patients will only have proteins and cells present in the CSF, with only mild headache. Also gastrointestinal involvement, nephropathy and hepatosplenomegaly can occur (1-3,18).

The initial lesions are usually non-pruritic, with a wide aspect range, symmetric, and usually cover the entire body.

The skin lesions, *syphilides*, are very common. They consist of macular, papulosquamous, and sometimes pustular. Often, the different types of lesions may occur simultaneously (20). Initial lesions are bilateral, round macules measuring between 5 to 10mm in diameter, distributing on the trunk and proximal extremities. They are usually very discrete. After days or weeks, red papules also appear. These lesions will cover palms and soles, including face and scalp. After a few weeks, papular syphilides or papulosquamous (psoriform), and rarely pustulosis, appear. Biopsy shows numerous plasma cells with mononuclear infiltration and *endarteritis obliterans*. This endarteritis can lead to *papulosquamous syphilides* because of the isquemia and may finally lead to necrosis - *pustular syphilides*.

In black individuals, facial and anal lesions take on annular and circinated configurations ("elegant syphilids") (17,18).

Oral mucosa is also affected and the lesions are known as mucosal plaques. The plaques are multiple, erosive, asymptomatic, measuring about 1 centimeter, being usually of a round shape (17).

Follicular syphilides are the involvement of hair follicles that will lead to *alopecia areata*. On the head, there is usually loss of hair on the temporoparietal and occipital regions. It can affect the beard, eyebrows and eyelids. The alopecia is reversible and temporary; it ends after the control of the infection (1,18).

In intertriginous body areas, which are warm and moist, like the perineum and axillae, lesions will coalesce and erupt, becoming larger, moist, of pink colour or white, that is called *condyloma lata* or *flat condyloma*. These lesions have a high concentration of spirochetes and are the most infectious lesions in this phase. Laboratory techniques have shown a smaller concentration of the bacteria in the other lesions, suggesting that the rash is a direct consequence of the infection (17,20).

Differential diagnosis: skin lesions should be considered from drug usage and viruses. Mucous lesions have to be differentiated from candida, Lichen planus and leucoplasias. The condyloma from the genital and perianal area should be distinguished from the condyloma accuminatum.

The presentation of secondary syphilis is so wide that this disease can be thought as secondary diagnosis for any dermatitis that presents itself in an atypical manner.

2.5 Latent syphilis

Latent syphilis is diagnosed when serologic tests are positive, with normal CSF examination and absence of any clinical manifestation. It evolves from the secondary syphilis being untreated. It is suspected when there is a history of primary or secondary lesions, history of exposure, or a congenital case from a mother without a prior diagnosis. There is a possibility of headaches, different skin coloration and alopecia, because of mistreatment of secondary syphilis (1,2,5,8).

Early latent syphilis is the infection after primary or secondary phase have subsided, during the first year of infection, while late latent syphilis is diagnosed when the manifestations appears more than 1 year after infection. This period is variable; a patient can present at any moment presenting either secondary or tertiary syphilitic signs. There are still doubts as to what is the real outcome of the latent syphilis, since more than 50% may never present with another syphilitic lesion; although a spontaneous cure is controversial (1,2).

2.6 Late syphilis

Late or tertiary syphilis will appear in about one-third of untreated patients. Lesions will appear after 3 to 15 years of remission. The manifestations will appear as neurosyphilis, cardiovascular, cutaneous and others. And the most common manifestation of tertiary syphilis is aortitis (1,2,5,8,17).

2.7 Neurosyphilis

Symptoms begin after 1 year of infection for meningeal syphilis, between 5 to 10 years for meningovascular syphilis, 15 to 20 years for general paresis and 25 to 30 years for tabes dorsalis. The syndrome is nothing more than a chronic meningo-vasculitis, capable of producing vascular and parenchymal lesions on the brain and the spinal cord. It is not well known why some cases spontaneously resolve, evolve to asymptomatic neurosyphilis or to the symptomatic presentation. Nowadays, signs and symptoms are incomplete and mixed because of the antibiotic treatment (1,21).

Meningeal syphilis: 25% of patients will show the meningeal involvement as the first sign of syphilis. Clinical presentation alterations include headache, neck stiffness, nausea and vomiting. The main neurological alteration includes cranial nerve palsies, especially II, VI, VII e VIII, seizures and changes in mental status. Neurosensory deafness occurs in up to 20% of cases. Syphilitic hydrocephaly presents with intracranial hypertension, appearing from 3 to 7 months after the initial infection (1-3,21,22).

Meningovascular syphilis: involves practically any area of the central nervous system, being traditionally subdivided in cerebrovascular and spinal cord. The lesions are caused by ischemia, secondary to endarteritis, which is the result of vascular wall infiltration from lymphocytes and plasmocytes in small and medium arteries. Symptoms related to neurosyphilis are comparable to atherosclerotic disease. Manifestations may include hemiparesis, aphasia and seizures. The initial symptoms may be acute or may follow general symptoms, like headache, insomnia and humor changes. In older patients, these alterations may be mistaken for encephalic accident. In younger people, there is a mandatory screening for the disease (21,22).

Meningovascular syphilis is rare and involves a wide range of aspects, being associated with the cerebral disease. It clinically presents with alteration on sphincter function, legs paraparesia and weakness. Pain and paresthesia of the legs are common (1,21,22).

General paresis: is a rare, progressive and chronic meningoencephalitis, which will eventually evolve to dementia. The presentation is a consequence of multiple damage to the brain, which includes personality changes, affection disorders, hyperactive reflexes, Argyll Robertson pupils (small pupils that do not react to light, but reacts to accommodation), illusions, deliriums, hallucinations, alterations on recent memory, thinking capacity and speech. These signs may be confused with many psychiatric diseases with neurological signs. If not treated, the patient will become apathetic, hypotonic, demented and physically incapable, finally leading to death after 4 to 5 years of evolution. Treatment will stop the spread of the disease, but will not recover the damage already present (15,21-23).

Tabes dorsalis: Symptoms appear because of the demyelination of the posterior columns, dorsal ganglia and dorsal roots. Symptoms include ataxia, paresthesia, bladder disturbances, impotence, areflexia, Charcot's joints (trophic joint degeneration) loss of position, deep pain, alteration on temperature sensation, loss of pain sensation, that will finally result in perforation and ulceration of the feet, from the lack of sensation and optic atrophy. There is a history of terrible pain in this phase of the disease, although it is actually attributed to the heavy metals used for treatment in the past before the antibiotic treatment (21-23).

2.8 Cardiovascular syphilis

Among the lesions, the most common is the syphilitic aortitis. On the non-treated syphilis, aortitis can manifest after 10 to 40 years, after the initial sexual contact. The ascending aorta is the most targeted by the disease 50% of the cases, followed by the aortic arch, the descending aorta and the abdominal aorta, coronary ostia and aortic valve lesions (1,14, 24-29). Presently this entity is very rare.

The main cause of death, in about 80% of the cases, is sacular aneurism rupture, when it is not treated surgically (1,14, 24-29).

After infection, the *T. pallidum* can be observed on the aorta's wall, initially on the tunica adventitia and at the lymphatic vessels. This is one of the reasons for the spirochete's tropism for the ascending aorta, since the latter is rich in lymphatic vessels (1,15,17,18,24-29).

The vasa vasorum suffers an obliterative endarteritis process, media necrosis (mesoarteritis) and plasmocitary infiltrate. Consequently, the elastic tissue of the aorta is destroyed and substituted by scar tissue. The inflammatory process can go on for a long time and it can be found in the patient up to 25 years after the first contagion (1,15,17,18,24-29). The clinical features can be of angina pectoris, when there is coronary ostia obstruction, dyspnoea when there is aortic regurgitation. Although the most common clinical feature is thoracic pain, secondary to fast luetic aneurysm expansion. When the lesion is present only at the aorta, the patient may be asymptomatic (1,15,17,18,24-29). Differential diagnosis: hypertensive cardiomyopathy, rheumatic carditis, cardiac insufficiency, and coronary atherosclerosis.

2.9 Cutaneous syphilis

The cutaneous involvement of the secondary syphilis is rare and may appear as nodular syphilids and gumma. The nodules are firm, grouped, with tendency to a circinated disposition among them. With the progression, they tend to present with central cure and external progression. They are usually present on the face and back, although they can be present on any part of the body (1-7,15,16,18).

The gumma is the progression of the nodules that get larger and become necrotic and ulcerated, leading to adherent and caseous material. They are very destructive and painless. These can destroy the palate and uvula (15,17,18).

Differential diagnosis: pharmacodermias, tuberculosis, cancer, paracoccidiomicosis, *american tegumentary leishmaniasis, lupus and rosacea.*

2.10 Congenital syphilis

Without adequate treatment, pregnant women can infect the foetus, either transplacentary or during labour. Generally the more advanced the pregnancy, the chance of transmission decreases. Lesions usually occur after the fourth month of pregnancy, when the foetus begins to develop an immunologic system. This suggests that the disease depends on a response from the body rather than a direct effect from the *T. pallidum* (1,30,31).

The risk of congenital infection is 75 to 95% when syphilis is early and untreated in the mother. The risks drop to 35% when the maternal syphilis has more than 2 years of duration. The damage to the foetus can be prevented if treatment begins before the 16th week of pregnancy. Foetal loss can be as high as 40% when left untreated, another 30% may die shortly after birth; premature labour or congenital syphilis are other possible outcomes (31-35).

When the baby is born alive, only fulminant congenital syphilis is apparent at birth, and these babies have a very poor prognosis. Most babies are born apparently healthy (about two-thirds), from a serologic-positive mother. Live-born infants with congenital syphilis may be divided into early signs - appearing in the first 2 years of life - and late signs - appearing after 2 years, over the first two decades of life. Congenital syphilis can be clinically similar to other pathologies, such as toxoplasmosis, herpes simplex, cytomegalovirus and rubella, as well as sepsis, blood incompatibility and other neonatal disorders (1,31)

2.11 Early congenital syphilis

The manifestations of the early disease occur in the first two years of life. Most of symptomatic infants will have hepatomegaly, with normal liver function, but jaundice may be present, from hepatitis; usually associated with high hepatic enzymes. Splenomegaly may also be present in about 50% of cases. Liver disease may cure slowly or even worsen after treatment (1,13,34).

Mucocutaneous lesions are present in up to 70% of patients. They may be present at birth or appear within the first weeks of life. These lesions generally are compatible to the secondary syphilis, being more infiltrated. The typical lesions constitute a small red maculopapular lesion, affecting hands and feet more severely. Desquamation and crusts will be present after 1 to 3 weeks. Snuffles will appear because of the involvement of the nasal mucous membrane - syphilitic rhinitis, appearing in the first week of life. In syphilitic pemphigus, there is a discharge that can vary from blood tinged to purulent, when bacterial infection occurs. This secretion is rich in spirochetes; being highly infectious. Condyloma lata may be present, along with mucous patches. Fissures occur around the lips, nostrils and anus. Thrombocytopenia may cause petechiae (1,13,31,33,34). Bone involvement is present in 60 to 80% of these infants. The lesions are commonly symmetric and multiple. Periostitis and demineralization occur in long bones and osteochondritis affects the joints:

Parrot's pseudoparalysis: generally the bone lesions are very painful, leading the newborns to avoid movement with the affected area (36,37).

Wimberger sign: metaphyseal demineralization or destruction of the upper medial tibias are seen radiographically (36,38).

Usually within the first six months of life, the bone lesion will resolve spontaneously. Neurosyphilis is observed in 40 to 60% of babies in this phase.

2.12 Late congenital syphilis

Late syphilis occurs after 2 years of age with untreated syphilis, corresponding to the late acquired syphilis in the adult, because of the similarities of the lesions, as nodular syphilides, gumma and periostitis. In 60% of cases, the infection remains subclinical. Some lesions are characteristic of this phase (1,15,30,34):

Interstitial keratitis is the most common and serious lesion of this phase. Both eyes are normally affected; the patient presents with photophobia, pain and less visual acuity. Optic atrophy may also be present. Treatment will not affect the evolution of the manifestation (1,13,17,18).

Clutton's joints are painless synovitis, affecting knees. The radiologic finding is an increase in the articular space (1,3,13).

Bone involvements are periostitis of long bones, mainly tibia - that becomes bigger in size and presents an anterior curvature (Saber shins) (1,13,34).

Cranial nerve lesion is frequent , specially related to the VIII pair, which will gradually evolve to deafness (1,2,13).

Asymptomatic neurosyphilis is present in approximately 33% of the patients and 25% will display clinical neurosyphilis after the sixth year of age.

Characteristic stigmata presented in late congenital syphilis: Hutchinson's teeth: centrally notched, widely spaced, peg-shaped upper central incisors and "mulberry molars" - poorly developed teeth, present after the sixth year of life. The Hutchinson's triad includes the teeth lesion, interstitial keratitis and deafness. Facies is also abnormal and may include frontal bossing, saddle nose and curved maxillae. Linear scars at mouth and nose angles from secondary bacterial infection also appear (Rhagades) (1,2,13,34). Rarely, syphilis is found in children that that been sexually abused, thus it will behave as regular syphilis; going through each of the phases. Sexual transmission should be assumed unless another mechanism is identified. If precautious are not used, these children can transmit to healthcare providers that are unaware of the contagiousness.

2.13 Diagnosis

In the diagnosis of syphilis, apart from detailed clinical history and physical examination, microscopy and serologic tests are the most important aspects in diagnosis and monitoring treatment (15).

Dark field microscopic examination of the exudate present in lesions, such as chancre of primary syphilis and condyloma latum in secondary, is needed. If a single motile microorganism characteristic of syphilis is verified, it will be sufficient for diagnosis. Anal and oral lesions should not be evaluated through dark field since it is hard to differentiate the pathogen from other common bacteria present in these sites. A direct fluorescent antibody *T. pallidum* (DFA-TP) test is also available - it can be used for rectal/anal and oral and genital lesions. The most reliable method for detection is the rabbit infectivity testing (RIT), where the serum is inoculated into the animal and will provide definitive evidence of *T. pallidum*. However, the use of RIT for diagnostic procedure is impractical (1-3,13,39).

Serologic tests are divided between non-treponemal and treponemal tests. Non-treponemal tests are useful for screening, while treponemal tests are used as confirmatory tests.

Non-treponemal serologic tests: Detection of non-specific treponemal antibody. They detect and measure IgG and IgM against cardiolipine-lecithin-cholesterol antigen complex. They include Venereal Diseases Research Laboratory (VDRL) and rapid plasma reagin (RPR) tests. In these, the antibody is detected by microscopic or by macroscopic flocculation of antigen suspension. The limitation of the non-treponemal serologic tests is the lack of sensitivity in dark ground microscopic examination for positivity in primary and late syphilis (3,8,15).

The PRP and VDRL are both equally sensitive and may be used for initial screening or quantification of the antibody; the titter will reflect the disease's activity. A specific rise in the titter will be seen during the evolution of early syphilis. A persistent fall following treatment of early syphilis gives evidence of adequate response to therapy. PCR and VDRL are equal in sensitivity and may be used for the initial screening and quantitation of the serum antibody (3,815).

Treponemal: detects specific antibodies to cellular components of the bacterium. Treponema pallidum haemagglutination assay (TPHA), fluorescent treponemal antibody-absorbed test (FTA- ABS), enzyme immunoassay tests (EIA) and Polymerase Chain Reaction (PCR).

In TPHA, purified *T. pallidum* antigens are fixed into red cells to detect specific anti-treponemal antibodies from the patient's serum. If another particle from the patient's serum is attached, other than red blood cells, it is called Treponemal Pallidum Particle Agglutination (TPPA) test. FTA- ABS is an observer-dependent test that detects the presence on anti-treponemal antibodies microscopically, that were fixed with the treponema's antigen. Both agglutination assays and the FTA- ABS are very sensitive, although it may give false-positive results in up to 2% of the general population (15,39-41).

In the EIA chromogenic end products are measured from enzymatic reactions on antigen-antibody complex. These chromogenes are read in a spectrophotometric device. Other antigens can be used, like cardiolipin, purified treponemal antigen or recombinant treponemal antigen. In the case of cardiolipine usage, the test is known as non-treponemal test. Purified and recombinant treponemal antigen is the most available EIA tests. The EIA tests has the advantage of being more objective and automated, requiring less work. PCR is most useful where the treponema serologic tests are limited: in primary, early congenital syphilis and neurosyphilis (15,41-44).

The non-treponemal tests are non-reactive in approximately 15 to 25% of primary syphilis (RPR is positive in approximately 85% of primary syphilis and 98% in secondary, while VDRL is positive in 80% and 95%, respectively), hence the diagnosis should be confirmed by using either FTA- ABS or by repeating VDRL after 1 to 2 weeks of the initial negativity of the first test. In secondary syphilis, virtually all non-treponemal and treponemal tests are reactive; TPPA is positive in 75% and FTA- ABS in 85% in primary syphilis, while both are positive in 100% of the secondary syphilis. Non-reactivity virtually excludes the disease in the secondary phase, in a patient with the mucocutaneous lesions (1-3,5,15,39).

Titters of non-treponemal antibody reflect disease activity - a fourfold decrease suggests adequate therapy, whereas an equal increase indicates activity (treatment failure or reinfection). Within a year, the patient will show test negativity after adequate treatment of primary syphilis and within 2 years of secondary syphilis. Although a small percentage of patients that receives adequate therapy will remain positive, even with low titters (1-3).

About 1% of patients will have false-positive response in non-treponemal tests, although it will rarely exceed 1:8 titters. The antibody reacts with more than 200 non-*T. Pallidum* antigens. It can occur in some viral infections, such as varicella, measles and HIV; some systemic diseases - systemic lupus erythematosus, lymphoma, malaria, tuberculosis, hepatitis and endocarditis. A few patients will have high antibody quantity levels in serum, resulting in excess of free antibodies. This can be interpreted as false-negative - the prozone effect. It can be avoided by serial dilutions of the serum (1-3,15,39,45).

The diagnosis of neurosyphilis can be challenging, as about 25% of patients will present a non-reactive non-treponemal serologic test. Therefore, cerebrospinal fluid CSF examination is crucial for clinical evidence suggesting neurosyphilis. Cell count, protein analysis and VDRL titter are needed. With lymphocytosis, elevated CSF proteins are present. A reactive VDRL is diagnostic of neurosyphilis, but its negativity does not exclude the disease, since only 30% will have this test reactive in neurosyphilis. However, the treponemal test is highly sensitive; a non-reactive test almost always excludes neurosyphilis. Lumbar puncture should be performed in evaluation of late latent syphilis, syphilis of unknown duration, suspicion of neurosyphilis (neurologic signs and symptoms), in late complications other than symptomatic neurosyphilis or suspected treatment failure. In HIV patients, some authors believe that routine CSF examination should be done, since some patients coinfected have shown *T. pallidum* in the CSF even with completed standard treatment for syphilis (1-3, 21-23).

Studies have shown that sexually transmitted diseases (STD), such as syphilis, are associated with an increased risk for HIV acquisition. Initial serologic responses for early syphilis have shown to be equally present in HIV-positive and negative patients. Reports concerning false-positive and false-negative results in HIV-positive patients raise concern on serology. A biopsy to direct visualization and special staining should be considered. CSF evaluation should also be considered, but the magnitude of neurosyphilis presented in this population is unknown. It is difficult to diagnose neurosyphilis in HIV-positive patients, since there are similarities in CSF abnormalities in both syphilis and HIV. Hence clinical evaluation has great effect in appropriateness of this exam (1-3,15).

Early congenital syphilis is generally suspected on maternal serologic test, routinely done in the 3rd trimester and during delivery. Positive tests lead to a more thorough investigation; VDRL and PRP are used to titer the serum. Cord blood should not be used because of low specificity and sensitivity; instead dark field microscopy or fluorescent antibody tests are used to analyse the placenta and umbilical cord. Infants with positivity in serologic tests should also have the CSF analysed; long bone x-rays and liver function tests are indicated (31,32).

Diagnosis is confirmed through direct visualization of the spirochete. Serology in neonates can be false-positive because of transplacental IgG transfer. The positivity can be considered highly probable if neonatal titer is more than four times the maternal titer. Neonates with low titers should be considered with the illness if present with clinical manifestations, since acquired disease can be transmitted through the placenta before development of antibodies. Any positive non-treponemal test should always be confirmed with a specific treponemal test, but no delays on treatment should be considered if neonates are symptomatic or have a high risk for infection (31-33).

3. Treatment

Penicillin is considered the drug of choice for all stages of syphilis. Treatment is based on staging the disease; the longer the course of the disease, the longer the treatment, as *T. pallidum* has a slow bacterial replication.

Penicillin is the only drug used for neurosyphilis, congenital syphilis or during pregnancy. There is no evidence of bacterial resistance to penicillin, although there has been persistence of the disease after full treatment.

3.1 Recommendations with penicillin treatment

Primary or secondary syphilis – single dose of penicillin G benzathine 2.4 million units (IM).

In some countries will indicate 4.8 million units divided in two doses, with 1 week interval, for secondary syphilis is recommended.

Early latent syphilis – single dose of penicillin G benzathine 2.4 million units (IM) .

Late latent syphilis or latent syphilis of unknown duration - penicillin G benzathine 7.2 million units (IM) divided in 3 doses of 2.4 million units each at 1 week intervals.

Asymptomatic neurosyphilis (HIV negative) – penicillin G benzathine 7.2 million units (IM) divided in 3 of 2.4 million units each at 1 week intervals *plus* aqueous penicillin G or procaine penicillin G 9 million units (IM) in doses of 600,000 units/day for 15 days.

Symptomatic neurosyphilis or asymptomatic neurosyphilis (HIV positive) - aqueous penicillin G 2.4 million units (IV) every 4 hours for 10 to 14 days (some will consider adding oral penicillin to complement) *or* Procaine penicillin G 2.4 million (IM) plus probenecid 500 mg orally 4 times per day, both for 10 to 14 days.

Pregnancy - treatment appropriate to the stage of syphilis is recommended.

4. Congenital syphilis

For infants with confirmed or highly probable disease aqueous penicillin G 100,000 to 150,000 units/kg/day, administered a dose of 50,000 units /kg/dose (IV) every 12 hours during the first 7 days of life; every 8 hours thereafter for a total of 10 days *or* procaine penicillin G 50,000 units/kg/dose (IM) daily for 10 days.

Infants with normal physical examination and treponemal serologic titer, the same level or less than fourfold the maternal titer (with mother not treated, inadequately treated or with less than 4 weeks of treatment) aqueous penicillin G 100,000 to 150,000 units/kg/day administered 50,000 units /kg/dose (IV) every 12 hours during the first 7 days of life; every 8 hours thereafter for a total of 10 days *or* procaine penicillin G 50,000 units/kg/dose (IM) daily for 10 days *or* Penicillin G benzathine 50,000 units/kg-dose (IM) in single dose.

Infants with normal physical examination and treponemal serologic titer at the same level or less than fourfold the maternal titer (mother was treated *adequately* with no signs of reinfection or relapse) penicillin G benzathine 50,000 units/kg-dose (IM) in single dose.

Infants with normal physical examination and treponemal serologic titer at the same level or less than fourfold the maternal titer (with adequate mother treatment and mother's serological titer low and stable) NO treatment is required *or* penicillin G benzathine 50,000 units/kg-dose (IM) in single dose if follow-up is uncertain.

Children with syphilis aqueous penicillin G 200,000 to 300,000 units/kg/day administered 50,000 units/kg every 4 to 6 hours for 10 days (1,2,5,6,8, 14-18,29,31,34,35, 46).

5. Penicillin allergy

Penicillin is the drug of choice for neurosyphilis, congenital syphilis or in pregnant woman; HIV-positive patients should also be considered for this treatment. No other treatment has shown effectiveness as an alternative, consequently desensitization should be done (1,16,47).

5.1 Desensitization

Patients with positive skin tests for penicillin determinants can be desensitized. This procedure is safe and can be performed either IV or orally. The oral procedure is usually safer to perform. Patients should be in hospital for this procedure, since severe IgE mediated allergic reactions can occur. The entire desensitization is completed between 4 to 12 hours, after this period the first dose of penicillin is administered (1-3,16-18,47).

5.2 Alternatives to penicillin

Primary and secondary syphilis, non-pregnant penicillin allergic patients can be treated with alternative drugs.

Ceftriaxone, tetracycline, erythromycin, doxycycline and *azithromycin* have shown effectiveness against treponema in clinical trials, however the recommendation for their usage is restricted as an alternative to penicillin, since new studies have shown treatment failure with some drugs (1,2,5,6,8,14-18,29,31,34,35,46,48).

6. Jarisch-Herxheimer reaction

After treatment initiation, the dying bacteria release inflammatory molecules that can trigger a cytokine cascade, which can lead to this phenomenon. Symptoms include myalgia, fever, headache, tachycardia, increased respiratory rate, hypotension and increased circulating neutrophil count. Also exacerbation of current syphilitic lesions can occur, normally as rash and chancre. This reaction occurs in approximately 50% of patients with primary syphilis, 90% with secondary syphilis and 25% with early latent syphilis. It develops within 2 hours of treatment, with peak temperature at 7 hours and usually clears within 24 hours. The etiology is unclear, although studies have demonstrated induction of inflammatory mediators by treponemal lipoproteins. Management involves resting and aspirin. Patients should be informed of this possible aggravating side effect. Early labour and foetal distress have been reported as obstetric complications, although syphilis treatment should not be delayed. Obstetric care is mandatory if there is a decreased in foetal movement or uterine contractions are observed (1-3,17,18).

6.1 Surgery

Surgery is considered for cardiovascular lesions to treat aortic and coronary lesions (14,26-29,49,50).

6.2 Syphilis prevention

Sexually transmitted diseases are prevented through safe sex. Patient counselling should also advise not to share needles with others in the case of drug use, and only use clean needles.

Pre-natal care is important to prevent the spread of syphilis. At risk mothers should be screened. Screening is also advocated to city populations with high risks (1,2).

Although circumcision helps to prevent some sexually transmitted diseases, syphilis is not prevented (51).

7. References

[1] Braunwald E, Fauci A, Kasper D, Hauser S, Longo D, Jameson J. Harrison's Principle of Internal Medicine 16th Edition. McGraw-Hill. 2005.
[2] Medscape Reference. [Internet]. Syphilis. Updated: June 7, 2011. Available from: http://emedicine.medscape.com/article/229461-overview.
[3] Ho K. Review on Serologic Diagnosis of Syphilis. Hong Kong Dermatology & Venereology Bulletin. Mar 2002 ;(10)1:1-18.
[4] Passos M, Arze W, Maurici C, Barreto N, Varella R, Cavalcanti S, Giraldo P. Is There an Increasing Number of STD in Carnival? [Title Translated]. Rev Assoc Med Bras 2010; 56(4): 420-7.
[5] The Merk Manual. [Internet]. Syphilis. Cited on: July 11, 2011. Available from: http://www.merckmanuals.com/professional/sec15/ch205/ch205i.html
[6] Shmaefsky B : Syphilis. InfoBase Publishing; 2010 [Cited on July 11, 2011]. Available from: Google Books.
[7] Rodriguez-Martin C. Historical Background on Human Treponematoses. Rev Antrop Chile. Jul 2000;32 (2).
[8] Encyclopædia Britannica. [Internet]. Syphilis. [Cited on July 11, 2011]. Available from: http://www.britannica.com/EBchecked/topic/578770/syphilis.
[9] Souza E. A hundred years ago, the discovery of Treponema pallidum. An Bras Dermatol. 2005; 80(5): 547-8.
[10] Neto B, Soler Z, Braile D, Daher W. Syphilis in the 16th century: the impact of a new disease. Arq Ciênc Saúde. Jul-Sep2009; 16(3):127-9.
[11] Jones JH. *Bad Blood: The Tuskegee Syphilis Experiment* (new and expanded edition). New York: Free Press; 1993.
[12] Passoni L, Menezes J, Ribeiro S, Sampaio E. Lues maligna in an HIV-infected patient. Revista da Sociedade Brasileira de Medicina Tropical. Apr 2005; 38(2): 181-184.

[13] Wood C. Syphilis in Children: Congenital and Acquired. Semin Pediatr Infect Dis. 2005; 16:245-257.

[14] Saraiva RS, Albernaz C, Mello M. Syphilitic Aortitis: Diagnosis and Treatment. Case Report. *Rev Bras Cir Cardiovasc*, Sep 2010;(25)3: 415-418.

[15] Avellera J, Bottino G. Syphilis: diagnosis, treatment and control. *An Bras Dermatol. 2006; 81(2):111-26.*

[16] Fraser M, Norris J, Weinstock M, White O, Sutton G, Dodson R, Gwinn M, Hickey K, Clayton R, Ketchum A, Sodergren E, Hardham M, McLeod MP, Salzberg S, Peterson J, Khalak H, Richardson D, Howell JK, Chidambaram M, Utterback T, McDonald L, Artiach P, Bowman C, Cotton MD, Fujii C, Garland S, Hatch B, Horst K, Roberts K, Sandusky M, Weidman J, Smith HO, Venter JC. Complete Genome Sequence of *Treponema pallidum*, the Syphilis Spirochete. Science. July 1998; 281(5375):375-88.

[17] Wendel G, Stark B, Jamison R, Molina R, Sullivan T. Penicillin Allergy and Desensitization in Serious Infections during Pregnancy. N Engl J Med 1985; 312:1229-1232.

[18] Focaccia R. Tratado de Infectologia. São Paulo. Atheneu, 2009.

[19] Miranda M, Bittencourt M, Lopes I, Cumino S. Leucoderma syphiliticum - a rare expression of the secondary stage diagnosed by histopathology. *An Bras Dermatol. 2010; 85(4):* 512-5.

[20] Dylewski J, Duong M. The Rash of Secondary Syphilis. CMAJ. Jan 2007; 176(1): 33

[21] Medlink neurology. [Internet]. Cited in: July 2011. Available from: http://www.medlink.com.

[22] Barros A, Cunha A, Lisboa C, As M, Resende C. Neurossífilis *Revisão Clínica e Laboratorial.* ArquiMed, 2005;19(3): 121-129.

[23] Nadal L, Nadal S. Indications for Cerebrospinal Fluid Punction in Syphilis Patients. Rev bras Coloproct, 2006; 26(4): 459-462.

[24] Corso B, Kraychete N, Nardeli S, Moitinho R, Ourives C, Barbosa J, Pereira E. Aneurisma luético de arco aórtico roto, complicado pela oclusão de vasos braquiocefálicos e acidente vascular encefálico isquêmico: relato de caso tratado cirurgicamente. Rev Bras Cir Cardiovasc 2002; 17(2): 63-69.

[25] Mitsuru A, Hiroshi O Hanafusa Y, Kazuma H, Tanji M. Intramural hematoma and thoracic aortic aneurysm with syphilis. The Journal of Thoracic and Cardiovascular Surgery. 2006; (133) 4: 1085.

[26] Machado M, Trindade P, Miranda R, Maia L. Bilateral ostial coronary lesion in cardiovascular syphilis: case report. *Rev Bras Cir Cardiovasc 2008; 23(1): 129-131.*

[27] Pacini D, Mattioli S, Massimo P, Simone M, Ranocchi F, i Grillone G, Bartolomeo R, Pierangeli A. Syphilitic aortic aneurysm: A rare case of tracheomalacia. J Thorac Cardiovasc Surg 2003;126:900-2.

[28] Wang R, Blume G, Filho N, Moura L. Occlusion of the Left Coronary Trunk Secondary to Tertiary Syphilis. Arq Bras Cardiol 2009; 93(3) : 312-315.

[29] Oxford book of medicine [Internet]. Cardiovascular Syphilis. [Cited on July 11, 2011]. Available from: http://otm.oxfordmedicine.com.

[30] Alvares B, Mezzacappa M, Poterio C. *Congenital syphilis mimicking battered child syndrome – case report.* Radiol Bras 2002;35(4):251–254.

[31] Malcolm G. Congenital Syphilis. [Internet]. RPA Newborn Care Guidelines. Royal Prince Alfred Hospital. Protocol Book. [Cited on July 11, 2011]. Available from: http://www.sswahs.nsw.gov.au/rpa/neonatal/html/docs/syphilis.pdf.

[32] Ewing C, Roberts C, Davidson D, Arya O. Early Congenital Syphilis Still Occurs. Archives of Disease in Childhood, 1985; 60: 1128-1133.

[33] Barsanti C, Valderato F, Diniz E, Succi R. Diagnostic of congenital syphilis: a comparison between serological tests in mother and respective newborn. Revista da Sociedade Brasileira de Medicina Tropical. Nov 1999; 32(6):605-611.

[34] Centers for Disease Control and Prevention (CDC). Congenital syphilis - United States, 2003-2008. MMWR Morb Mortal Wkly Rep. Apr 2010; 59(14):413-417.

[35] Lorenzi D, Madi J. Congenital Syphilis as a Prenatal Care Marker. RBGO. 2001; (23)10: 647-652.

[36] Ghadouane M, Benjelloun S, Elharim-Roudies L, Jorio-Benkhraba M, el Malki-Tazi A. Skeletal lesions in early congenital syphilis (a review of 86 cases). Rev Rhum Engl Ed. Jun 1995;62(6):433-7.

[37] Rothner A, Klein N. Parrot's Pseudoparalysis, Revisited. Pediatrics 1975; (56)4: 604-605.

[38] Goraya S, Trehan A, Marwaha K. Wimberger's sign. Indian Pediatr. Dec 1997;34(12):1133-4.

[39] Egglestone S, Turner A. Serological diagnosis of syphilis. Commun Dis Public Health 2000; 3: 158-62 .

[40] Sato N, Melo C, Zerbini L, Silveira E, Fagundes L, Ueda M. Assessment of the Rapid Test Based on an Immunochromatography Technique For Detecting Anti-*Treponema pallidum* ANTIBODIES. Rev. Inst. Med. trop. S. Paulo .Dec 2003; 45(6):319-322.

[41] Moyer N, Hudson J, Hausler W. Evaluation of the hemagglutination treponemal test for syphilis. J Clin Microbiol. June 1984; 19(6): 849–852.

[42] Liu H, RODES B, CHEN C, STEINER B. New Tests for Syphilis: Rational Design of a PCR Method for Detection of *Treponema pallidum* in Clinical Specimens Using Unique Regions of the DNA Polymerase I Gene. J. Clin. Microbiol. May 2001; (39)5: 1941–1946.

[43] Grimpel E, Sanchez P, Wendel G, Burstain J, McCracken G, Radolf J, Nogard M. Use of Polymerase Chain Reaction and Rabbit Infectivity Testing To Detect Treponema pallidum in Amniotic Fluid, Fetal and Neonatal Sera, and Cerebrospinal Fluid. J. Clin. Microbiol. Aug 1991; (29)8: 1711-1718.

[44] Marangoni A, Sambri V, Storni E, D'Antuono A, Negosanti M, Cevenini R. *Treponema pallidum* Surface Immunofluorescence Assay for Serologic Diagnosis of Syphilis. Clin. Diagn. Lab. Immunol. May 2000; (7)3: 417–421.

[45] Butch A. Dilution Protocols for Detection of Hook Effects/Prozone Phenomenon. Clinical Chemistry 2000; (46): 10.

[46] All Sands [Internet]. The History of Syphilis and its Treatment. Cited on: July 11, 2011. Available from: http://www.allsands.com.

[47] Stoner B. Current Controversies in the Management of Adult Syphilis. Clinical Infectious Diseases 2007; 44: 130–46.

[48] Saraceni V, Leal M, Hartz Z. Evaluation of health campaigns with emphasis on congenital syphilis: a systematic review. Rev. Bras. Saúde Matern. Infant. Sep 2005; 5 (3): 263-273.

[49] Rocha M, Pedroso E. Fundamentos de Infectologia. Rio De janeiro. Rubio, 2009

[50] Kouchoukos N, Blackstone E, Doty D, Hanley F, Karp R. Cardiac Surgery. Salt lake City. Churchill Livingstone, 2005.

[51] Aaron A.R et al. Male Circumcision for the Prevention of HSV-2 and HPV Infections and Syphilis. N Engl J Med 2009; 360:1298-1309.

Part 3

Protozoal Infection

6

Human Trichomoniasis due to *Trichomonas vaginalis* – Current Perspectives

Nancy Malla
Department of Parasitology, Postgraduate Institute of Medical Education and Research, Chandigarh India

1. Introduction

Human trichomoniasis caused by protozoan parasite, *Trichomonas vaginalis* is one of the most prevalent non-viral sexually transmitted urogenital disease with more than 180 million cases annually worldwide. Annual incidence varies between 0-65 percent depending upon different geographical locations, age groups and population studied. In North America and Canada, more than 8 million new cases are reported annually, with an estimated rate of asymptomatic cases as high as 50 percent (Sobel, 2005). The number may be underestimated as symptomatic patients may be underdiagnosed because of insensitive wet mount procedure and most of the infected subjects remain asymptomatic, thus are not being reported (Petrin et al, 1998). Recent review on Global epidemiology in high risk populations and control of T.vaginalis has highlighed that the burden of infection is found in resource-limited settings and high risk groups in industrialized settings. The World Health Organization estimated global prevalence figures are based on a wet mount microscopy (sensitivity range of 60-80%), however recent data, using PCR suggests sensitivity may be lower (35-60%), thus underestimating global prevalence (Johnston and Mabey, 2008) In India, hospital based studies reveal 4-10 percent positivity in symptomatic women attending gynaecology clinics and almost similar percentage in asymptomatic women attending infertility, post-natal and family planning clinics (Sharma et al, 1988; Malla et al, 1989; Divekar et al, 2000; Vishwanath et al, 2000;Valadkhani et al, 2003; Chakraborty et al, 2005; Yadav et al, 2006). The significantly higher percentage has been observed amongst contraceptive users (7.31%), antenatal patients (7.59%) and women with gynaecological disorders (9.21%) compared to postnatal (3.62%) and infertile woman (2.83%) (Sharma et al, 1988). The association of infection with contraceptive practices indicates controversial figures. Lazer (1970) found an increase, McLellan et al (1982) found no such correlation while Krieger et al (1985) found prevalence to be less amongst women using oral contraceptive and Sharma et al (1988) found barrier contraceptive to be protective. This observation and the tendency for symptomatic disease to occur during menstrual periods, suggests a hormonal component to the susceptibility. In contrast, Demes et al (1988) reported fewer parasites in vaginas of infected women during menstruation, suggesting trichomonacidal effect of menstrual blood complement in-vivo and survival of parasites during menstrual bleeding has been explained by the existence of subpopulations of trichomonads that are resistant to complement lysis. The infection is low in women in higher socio-economic groups and high (55%) in the developing countries and in minority groups of industrialized populations (Tapsall et al, 1979). Based on family income, we have observed that 90% infected women belonged to middle and lower socio economic status, while only 10% were from upper socio-economic status, thereby indicating that socio-economic factors seem to play role in this infection (Kaur et al, 2008).

The infected men are usually asymptomatic, acting as carriers of infection. In men with non-gonococcal urethritis (NGU), although a median prevalence of 11 percent is suggested (Krieger, 1990), yet it varies from 10% to 21% in adolescents at high risk and 45% in those who have been in contact with infected women (Sobel, 2005). Report from India revealed that one (2.5%) out of 40 NGU male patients harboured *T.vaginalis* (Dawn et al, 1995). The rate of transmission from men to women appears to be higher (67-100%) than the other way round (14-80%) suggesting that in men, the disease is self limiting (Rein and Muller, 1990) and parasites are spontaneously cleared, possibly by the trichomonacidal action of prostatic secretions (Langley et al, 1987) or due to mechanical elimination of protozoa during micturition (Rein, 1990).

T.vaginalis and HIV infections are both sexually transmitted, yet there are controversial reports of the association of presence of T.vaginalis and HIV. No significant differences were observed between the presence of parasite and status of HIV infection from studies conducted in different geographical locations (Minkoff et al, 1999; Frankel and Monif, 2000; Susan et al, 2002; Klinger et al, 2006). It is concluded that HIV infection does not make a woman more likely to have prevalent, incident, persistent or recurrent trichomoniasis (Susan et al, 2002). No association of prevalence of *T.vaginalis* in HIV infected women and CD4+ cell count has been found (Sorvillo et al 1998). In support of this, in our study, none of the 100 HIV seropositive patients including 30% patients with <200/µl CD4+ cell count was found to harbour *T.vaginalis* (Kaur et al, 2008). The reason for absence of *T.vaginalis* in the study may be because most of the females (71%) were sexually inactive and 25% were using different contraceptive devices. In contrast, two cross-sectional studies in Africa (Ter Muelen et al, 1992; Ghys et al, 1995) and in Mexico (Bersoff-Matcha et al, 1998) have demonstrated an association between *T.vaginalis* and HIV infection in women. T.vaginalis was found in 18.6% HIV positive and 10.2% HIV negative pregnant women (Sutton et. al, 1999). *T.vaginalis* infected HIV women had 4.2 fold reduction in the quantity of cell-free HIV-I virus in vaginal secretions following metronidazole therapy (Wang et al, 2001). Study from Tanzania showed that treatment of trichomoniasis in HIV-infected women decreased vaginal HIV RNA levels. It is concluded that control of *T.vaginalis* infection may be single, most cost effective strategy for reducing the incidence of HIV transmission (Gosskurth et al,1995). It is postulated that although *T.vaginalis* infection may not be significantly high in HIV infected women, yet the Trichomonas infected subjects may be more susceptible and at higher risk of acquiring the HIV infection.

Although, sexual mode of transmission is the only documented route of acquisition of infection, yet, 2-17 percent female offspring of mothers infected with *T.vaginalis* acquired urinary tract trichomoniasis or vaginal infection (Rein and Muller, 1990) and 2 infants suffering from respiratory tract infection were delivered vaginally by infected mothers indicating respiratory route of infection (McLaren et al, 1983). The parasites have been reported from toilet seat towels and allied objects, but, so far, no case of fomite transmission has been documented (Heine and McGregor, 1993).

2. The parasite

Honigber and King (1964) have detailed out initially the morphological characteristics of this urogenital pathogen and further detailed morphological, parasitological, biochemical and clinical aspects of the parasite have been amply reviewed earlier (Petrin et al, 1998; Schwebke and Burgess, 2004). Recently with the cracking of the genome of the parasite, and identification of 26,000 confirmed genes, the new ways of diagnosing and treating the disease may come to light (Carlton et al, 2007). It is postulated that an additional 34,000 unconfirmed genes are on the way for identification.

3. Pathogenesis

The exact mechanism of pathogenesis is still under elucidation. Reports have revealed multifaceted interplay of parasite and host factors leading to different clinical spectrum. Initial events invariably have been focused on parasite factors revealing cell-to cell adhesion, haemolytic activity, pore-forming proteins, excretion of extracellular proteinases and cell detaching factors playing significant role in pathogenesis (Fiori et al, 1999). Host factors include role of Lactobacilii, local pH, hormonal components, humoral and cytokine responses and free radical generation (oxidative stress and No radicals).

3.1 Adherence and adhesions

Cytoadherence, one of the early steps in the infection process is essential for colonization. Initially, following cytoadherence, parasite changes its morphology from pear shape to amoeboid form with numerous cytoplasmic projections interdigetating with the microvilli of the host cell plasma membrane (Arroya et al, 1993) and allowing the formation of isolated intracelllular spaces (Gonzalez et al, 1995). The adherence is specifically mediated by four adhesion proteins (AP 65, 51, 33 and 23) which act in a specific receptor-ligand interaction and is time, temperature and pH dependent. The adhesions are concentrated on the side opposite the undulating membrane while laminin binding proteins are ubiquitous on the entire surface of the parasite (Costa et al, 1988). Parasite binds to numerous host macromolecules which may serve a nutritive purpose while few may protect the parasite by modifying their host defences, thereby helping in evasion of the host immunity (Honigberg, 1990). In Vitro studies have indicated time dependent significant difference in the percentage of vaginal epithelial cells (VEC) attached by trichomonads as well as number of parasites attached per VEC in *T.vaginalis* isolates from symptomatic and asymptomatic women. Significant difference in attachment of VEC's was observed only during first 15 minutes while maximum number of VEC's attached by parasite was significantly different at initial 20 to 25 minutes following incubation of VEC's and parasites (Valadkhani et al 2003). These observations suggest that adhesion proteins and / or other virulence markers may be playing significant role in the initial stages of attachment. Experimental studies revealed that sustained infection in mice could only be induced in presence of *Lactobacillus acidophilus* (McGrory and Garber, 1992). *L.acidophilus* may be playing role in sustaining trichomoniasis by providing low pH (4-4.5) in the environment. *In vitro* study demonstrated that in presence of *L.acidophilus* more number of VEC's were found attached by *T.vaginalis* as compared to controls and significant reduction was observed in presence of excretory secretory products of *L.acidophilus* (Valadkhani et al, 2003), thereby suggesting that adhesion of parasite to target cells is pH dependent.

T.vaginalis alpha-actinin is diffusely present throughout the parasite before interaction with target cell and gets localized in the peripheral regions of the amoeboid cell which is accompanied by an enhanced expression of the genes coding for some cytoskeletal components (Fiori et al, 1999). *T.vaginalis* cysteine proteinase 30 (CP30) has been found to bind to host cell surface and shown to play a role in cytoadherence (Menduza-Lopez et al, 2000). CP30 was detected in 40 fresh *T.vaginalis* isolates from both symptomatic and asymptomatic women, while intensity of CP30 band was significantly higher in isolates from symptomatic as compared to asymptomatic women. In long term culture maintained isolates, the band was detected in all the 20 (100%) isolates from symptomatic women and only in 14 (70%) isolates from asymptomatic women, thereby suggesting that CP30 expression of isolates leading to symptomatic infection appears to be more stable characteristic (Yadav et al, 2007). Further, CP30 was detected in serum and vaginal washes of 100% *T.vaginalis* infected women and in 65% serum and 80% vaginal wash samples from 15 asymptomatic infected women. Antibody to CP30 was detected in 100% serum samples of both symptomatic and asymptomatic women, in 54.5% vaginal washes of symptomatic and 35% asymptomatic women and also in 3/20 (15%) serum samples from uninfected women, thereby suggesting that besides CP30, other factors may also be playing role in leading to symptomatic infection (Yadav et al, 2007a).

3.2 Haemolysis

T.vaginalis is capable of producing haemolysis and utilizing haemoglobin as a source of iron. Experimental studies have indicated that virulence of parasite is reduced under iron depleted conditions (Ryu et al, 2001). The parasite possibly causes lysis of red blood cells both by contact dependent (Krieger et al, 1985; Fiori et al, 1999; Valadkhani et al, 2003) and contact independent mechanisms (Pindak et al, 1993). The contact of parasite with RBC's is thought to derive lipids and iron. This is suggested mechanism to exacerbate the symptoms during and following menstruation. The temperature and Ca^{2+} dependent mechanisms of haemolysis suggest the role of pore-forming proteins, which are able to insert themselves in the lipid bilayer of the target cell, forming transmembrane channels that lead to cell death, by osmotic lysis. The size of the pores formed on the target cell membrane is between 1.14 and 1.34 nm and alteration of membrane permeability eventually leads to cell lysis and loss of haemoglobin. The pore-forming proteins are active at pH lower than 6.5 and at 37°C. Electron microscopic studies have revealed that following parasite and target cell interaction, the change in shape of the target cell is due to loss of spectrin, the predominant protein of the RBC cytoskeleton and acid intact, metabolically active parasites can disrupt the target cell spectrin which is contact dependent (Fiori et al, 1999). The parasite has a haemolytic Phospholipase A (pore forming proteins) which is rich in membranes, hydrogenosomes, vesicles and vacuoles. The three pathogenic isolates showed maximum hemolytic activity at pH 6.0 and 8.0, indicating that the parasite have both acidic and alkaline hemolysins and activity was also related to type of RBC's from different sources, rat and human (Vargas - Villarreal et al, 2003).

3.3 Free radical generation

It is apparent that free radicals play a critical role in a variety of normal regulatory pathways and oxidant-antioxidant balance is important for immune cell function. Trichomonads are equipped with several oxygen scavenging systems localized in both cytoplasm and hydrogenosomes. The main systems operating in the cytoplasm consists of NADH and NADPH oxidases, (Linstead & Bradley, 1988) which reduce O_2 to H_2O and H_2O_2 respectively. Polymorphs recruited at the site of infection and when activated, initiate oxidative stress by releasing toxic oxidants such as superoxide anion and H_2O_2, which lead to cell damage surrounding VEC's. Shaio et al (1991) observed that neutrophil could kill *T.vaginalis* only in presence of normal human serum, indicating that trichomonicidal activity is complement dependent. However, low concentration of C' in vagina may explain survival of the parasite in presence of significant number of PMN's. Davis and Lushbaugh (1993) observed inter-strain heterogenity in the oxidative stress response of *T.vaginalis*. The parasite has developed mechanisms to deal with oxidative stress and upon exposure to H_2O_2, it upregulates the production of various heat shock proteins (Bozner,1997). Experimental study showed that vaginal tissue (VT) of mice infected with isolates from symptomatic women generated significantly higher superoxide radicals (SOD) while vaginal washes (VW) and blood samples generated less SOD as compared to mice infected with isolates from asymptomatic women(Valadkhani et al, 2006). It is suggested that different responses by VT, VW and blood may be due to functional differences in different tissue and circulating PMN's.

Nitric oxide appears to play an important function as a cytotoxic effector molecule for several parasites. Significant increase in reactive nitrogen intermediates (RNI) levels in mice infected with *T.vaginalis* isolates from infected women as compared to uninfected controls has been reported (Malla et al, 2004). The inducible nitric oxide synthase (iNOS) protein and RNI was detected in leucocytes (stimulated with *T.vaginalis* in vitro) and VW of all the *T.vaginalis* infected 22 symptomatic and 20 asymptomatic women studied. The mean iNOS protein band intensity was significantly higher in leucocytes of asymptomatic as compared to symptomatic women, while no significant difference was observed in VW between symptomatic and asymptomatic women. The study suggested that reactive nitrogen radicals may be playing role in limiting *T.vaginalis* infection (Yadav et al, 2006).

3.4 Other mechanisms

Host humoral immune responses to the parasite seem to be important determinants of virulence. High concentrations of IgG, IgM and IgA antibody to trichomonads have been observed in serum from experimental infected animals and infected subjects. Specific IgG and IgA are present in vaginal washes from women with trichomoniasis and significantly higher IgA levels have been found in vaginal secretions in asymptomatic than symptomatic women suggesting its role in preventing the establishment of infection (Ackers et al, 1975; Sharma et al, 1991). Significant increase in specific IgG and particularly IgG_1 was observed in experimental study (Yadav et al, 2005) and in infected human subjects (Kaur et al 2008). It is suggested that the IgG and IgM may be playing significant role in establishing symptomatic infection. *T.vaginalis* can coat itself with host plasma proteins, thus hosts immune system does not recognize the parasite as foreign (Peterson and Alderete, 1982) and continuous release of antigens may neutralize antibody or cytotoxic T lymphocytes, thus short-circulating specific anti-*T.vaginalis* defense mechanisms (Alderete and Garza, 1984). Numerous CP's secreted by the parasite degrade IgG, IgM and IgA, allowing the parasite to survive the antibody response (Provenzano and Alderete, 1995). It is proposed that the balance between different IgG subclasses influences the clinical outcome of infection in various parasitic diseases.

Cytokines and chemokines provide a mechanism for initiation, amplification or containment of inflammation during disease status. Experimental studies have revealed that the Th-I cytokine (IL2 and IFN-γ) responses might play a role in the elimination of *T.vaginalis* (Paintlia et al, 2002; Malla et al, 2007) and thus might be maintaining low levels of infection in asymptomatic infected subjects.

It is observed that the parasite induces cell death in host cells via apoptosis. The study indicated that p38 MAPK signaling cascade is requisite to apoptosis of *T.vaginalis* infected macrophage, and apoptotic process occurs via the phosphorylation of p38 MAPK, which is located downstream of mitochondria-dependent caspase activation, conferring insight into the plausible molecular mechanism of *T.vaginalis*- immune evasion from macrophage attack (Chang et al, 2006).

Recently, the influence of *T.vaginalis* lysate and excretory-secretory products (ESP) on the fate of neutrophils has been reported. The study revealed that *T.vaginalis* lysate inhibits apoptosis of human neutrophils. It is suggested that an intrinsic mitochondrial pathway of apoptosis was involved in *T.vaginalis* lysate-induced delayed neutrophil apoptosis and this phenomenon may contribute to local inflammation in trichomoniasis (Song et al, 2010).

3.5 Molecular mechanisms

Molecular analysis of the membrane molecules and virulence factors have begun. The recent sequencing of the T.vaginalis genome has allowed comprehensive computational analysis of the general transcription machinery and the identification of novel eukaryotic DNA involved in directing gene expression in this parasite. Identification of Genes, particularly, required for synthesis of an unusual nucleotide sugar found in *T.vaginalis* lipophosphoglycan, the monosaccharide rhamnose, which is absent in the human host, may make it a potential drug target. Genes involved in sialic acid biosynthesis consistent with the reported presence of this sugar on the parasite surface were identified. It is suggested that the discovery of previously unknown metabolic pathways, the elucidation of pathogenic mechanisms, and the identification of candidate surface proteins likely involved in facilitating invasion of human mucosal surfaces may provide potential leads for the development of new therapies and novel methods for diagnosis (Carlton et al, 2007).

Control of gene expression is essential to the survival of an organism and with the available genome data, additional analyses have been made possible. The wealth of data present in the *T.vaginalis* genome has been utilized to identify aspects of an array of biological processes, including small nuclear RNAs involved in splicing of introns, components of transcriptional complexes and the presence of discrete DNA elements that direct basal transcription. It is suggested that both evolutionarily conserved and novel features of T.vaginalis serve to inspire further questions specifically concerning this parasite, as well as the molecular mechanisms shared with other eukaryotic groups (Smith and Johnson, 2011).

4. Clinical spectrum

The clinical spectrum in women ranges from asymptomatic carrier state in approximately 50 percent infected women while symptomatic patients may complain of vaginal discharge in 50-75 percent, with pruritus in 25-50 percent and dysuria in 30-50 pertcent and dyspareunia in 10-50 percent (Heine and McGregor, 1993; Valadkhani et al, 2003; Kaul et al, 2004). Infection during pregnancy may be associated with premature rupture of membranes, preterm delivery, low birth weight babies and also respiratory infection in infants. The disease may be associated with endometritis and cervical erosion with predisposition to malignant transformation. There are contrasting reports of association of cervical carcinoma and presence of *T.vaginalis*. Kharsany et al (1993) in the study conducted in Durban have found no association while reports from other areas (Boyle et al, 1989; Zhang & Begg, 1994; Zhang et al, 1995; Vikki et al, 2000) indicated significant association. *T.vaginalis* could not be isolated in any of the 100 cervical cancer patients in our earlier study (Kaur et al, 2008).

In infected females, perspeculum examination usually reveals copious loose discharge that pools in the posterior vaginal formix and bubbles may be seen in about 10 to 33 percent. The vaginal epithelium is inflamed in 15 percent with small punctate haemnorrhagic spots on vaginal and cervical mucosa in 2 percent (Rein, 1990).

In men, the clinical spectrum varies from asymptomatic carrier state to acute state characterized by profuse purulent urethritis and mild symptomatic infection including scanty clear to mucopurulent discharge, dysuria and mild pruritus or burning sensation immediately after sexual intercourse (Krieger, 1990; Schwebke and Burgess, 2004).

5. Laboratory diagnosis

Laboratory diagnosis is established by examination of wet mount preparation of vaginal discharge and / or urine specimen. This method is least cost-effective but has low sensitivity (38% - 82%) (Petrin et al, 1998). Best results are obtained, if wet smear preparation is examined in bed side laboratory, within half an hour, as parasites thereafter loose motility. Low sensitivity is attributed to the loss of motility after the parasite has been removed from body temperature. The broth culture method is the gold standard, has been found most sensitive for routine diagnosis and requires 300 to 500 trichomonads/ml of inoculum (Sharma et al, 1991a; Petrin et al, 1998). "In Pouch™ culture has been found with added advantages and can be conveniently transported from the site of collection to the laboratory (Sood and Kapil,2008).The main limitation for its routine use is the high cost involved. Cell culture technique is reported superior to broth culture, since it is able to detect *T.vaginalis* at a concentration as low as 3 parasites/ml (Garber et al, 1987). However, it is not routinely performed because it is expensive and not convenient for rapid diagnosis (Petrin et al, 1998). Although, antigen in vaginal secretions and specific circulating and local antibody response have been demonstrated in infected subjects (Ackers et al, 1975; Alderete, 1984; Sharma et al, 1991), yet it has limited value in diagnosis due to lower sensitivity than culture technique. Anti-trichomonad, IgA antibodies decreased significantly post treatment and appear to be specific to the presence of parasite in the urogenital tract (Sharma et al, 1991). Review of reports indicates that DNA detection in clinical samples by PCR yielded higher sensitivity than wet mount and culture (Schwebke and Burgess, 2004). It requires expertise and availability. Further research is required to develop cheap, point of care diagnostic tests which will allow a greater understanding of *T.vaginalis* epidemiology (Johnston and Mabey, 2008).

6. Strain variation

The reasons for different clinical spectrum ranging from asymptomatic to acute and chronic symptomatic state and complications are still unclear, although, data supports that in addition to host factors, differences in parasite intrinsic virulence play role in such phenomenon. The differences in virulence in different strains by In-Vivo (Honigberg et al, 1966) and In-Vitro (Honigberg, 1990) assays have been reported. The In-Vivo virulence assays in experimental mouse model have shown that intraperitoneal infection of trichomonads produces visceral (pancreatic and hepatic) necrosis and extent of necrosis is proportional to the level of virulence of the inoculated strain, which can result in death. The effect of two strains, one highly virulent and other very mild strain on chick embryo fibroblast cultures was quite different. The pathogenic changes caused by the virulent parasites appeared much sooner and were far more extensive than those observed with mild-strain. A correlation between the length of time *In Vitro* of *T.vaginalis* strains and the attenuation of their virulence for cell cultures was observed. Although, the extrapolation of data from In Vitro experiments and In-Vivo animal models to human situation needs to be interpreted with caution, few recent molecular studies support these earlier observations. Antigenic heterogenicity (Krieger et al, 1985a) has differentiated *T.vaginalis* isolates and has been correlated with pathogenicity (Mason and Gwanzura, 1988). Isoenzyme analysis (Soliman et al, 1982;Vohra et al, 1991) and restriction digestion patterns (Sapru et al, 1994) could not differentiate clinical isolates from symptomatic and asymptomatic women. Phenotypic (Alderete et al, 1986, 1987) and genotypic variation by RAPD analysis (Vanacova et al, 1997) have demonstrated the presence of different strains, We have reported that dendogram based on RAPD data obtained from fresh 30 (15 each from symptomatic and asymptomatic women) *T.vaginalis* isolates showed upper branch representing 7 out of 15 isolates, from symptomatic women and other eight isolates constituted another cluster, whereas all the isolates from 15 asymptomatic women were represented in lower branch of the tree. The study indicated that the RAPD traits can be of utmost importance in differentiating isolates from symptomatic and asymptomatic women (Kaul et al, 2004).

Further, the same 30 isolates were maintained in culture for long term (6 months to 2 yrs) and were subjected to RAPD analysis. Following long term cultivation changes in RAPD patterns were observed. The phylogenetic tree of same 30 long term (up to 2 years) culture maintained isolates divided the isolates into two distinct branches. The upper half of tree represented all 15 isolates from symptomatic women, while the lower half of the tree represented all 15 isolates from asymptomatic women (Fig. 1.) (Kaul 2004a).

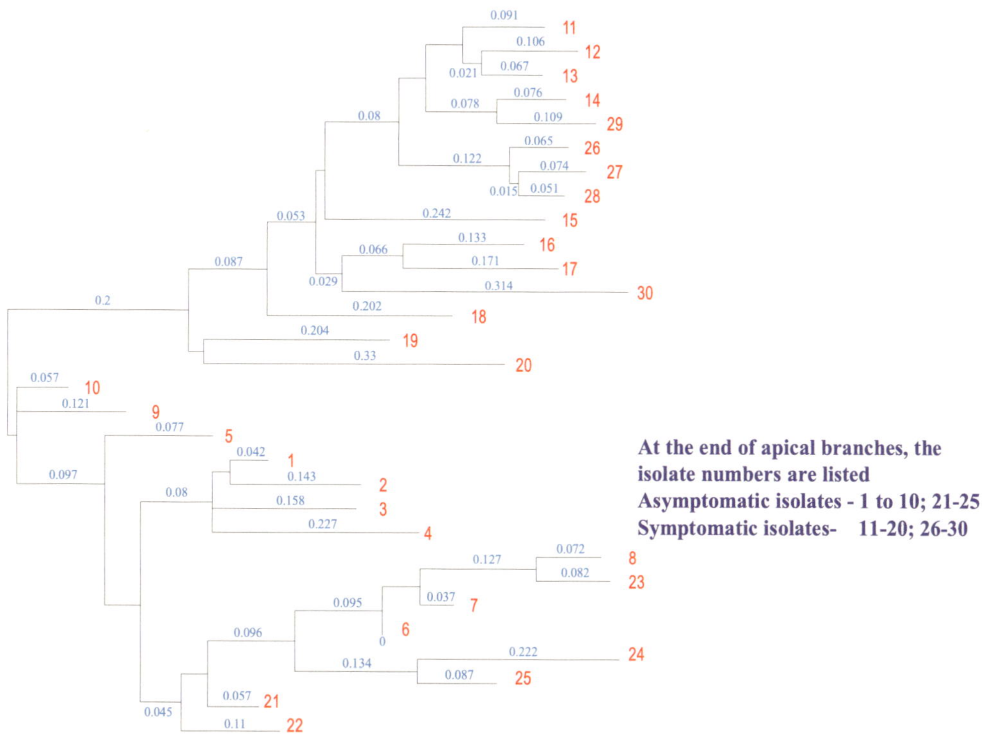

Fig. 1. Dendrogram constructed by RAPDistance programme for 30 long term culture isolates of *T.vaginalis*. The integers represent branch lengths, which reflect the genetic distance between the isolates.

7. Trichomonas Vaginalis Virus (TVV)

Double stranded RNA virus has been identified in *T.vaginalis* (Wang and Wang, 1985) and was found in about 50% clinical isolates. It was thought that most probably this virus is transferred from parent to progeny. Presence of TVV correlated with 270 kDa surface protein (P270) positive isolates and on long term culture loss of TVV was associated with absence of P270 (Wang et al, 1987). The loss of viral dsRNA and concomitant absence of the surface disposition of specific immunogens strengthens the likelihood of involvement of virus in the sequestration of immunogens into trichomonal membranes. All virus harbouring trichomonads contained at least three dsRNA segments (5.5, 4.8 to 4.3 kb) and the study suggested segmented nature of the TVV (Khoshnan and Alderete, 1993). Different studies from different geographical locations indicated different sizes of the segments of TVV (Tai et al, 1993; Shaio et al, 1993). It is suggested that *T.vaginalis* may be reservoir for several different dsRNA viruses simultaneously (Benchmol et al, 2002). Older women patients, infected with *T.vaginalis* were found with virus positive isolates as compared to younger patients and men. We analysed presence of dsRNA virus in *T.vaginalis* same 30 Indian isolates (15 each from symptomatic and asymptomatic women) in whom RAPD analysis was carried earlier (Kaul et al, 2004) and presence of three bands (5.5, 2.5 and 1.5 kb) were observed in all the 30 fresh isolates, while following long term cultivation (up to 2 years) TVV was observed only in 7 isolates, (3 from symptomatic and 4 asymptomatic women isolates) (Malla et al, 2011). The study suggests that genetic changes might be taking place during *in vitro* cultivation of parasites and this might be related to phenotypic variation and loss of dsRNA virus. No significant association was found between isolates from symptomatic and asymptomatic women and presence of TVV ($P > 0.05$), which is in agreement with an earlier report (Wendel et. al, 2002). The same fresh isolates were also subjected to *in vitro* metronidazole drug resistance assay. The study suggests that the presence of TVV alone may not be a virulence marker and loss of TVV on long term cultivation of *T.vaginalis* isolates appear to be related to drug resistance. Correlation of absence of TVV and drug resistance ($p<0.05$) in our study supports the earlier studies (Wang and Wang, 1985; Snipes et al, 2000). However, on retrospective analysis of presence of TVV and drug sensitivity with RAPD analysis of isolates, no significant correlation was found, which is in agreement to the earlier report (Stiles et al, 2000), whereby no significant correlation between metronidazole resistance and RFLP subtypes was reported. In contrast, Vanacova et al. (1997) have reported that all the 5 isolates refractory to metronidazole constituted single branch of tree by RAPD analysis. Out of these 5 isolates, 4 were metronidazole resistant while fifth was susceptible to metronidazole by *in vitro* assay. Metronidazole resistance existing in a closely related group of isolates indicated that only one or few mutations have occurred which resulted in resistance. It is suggested that some genealogical line of *T.vaginalis* may be genetically predisposed for the development of metronidazole resistance and same may be true for the capability of strains to cause disease in patients. The contrasting correlations in different reports from different geographical locations may be due to phenotypic and genotypic variations.

8. Treatment and drug resistance

Nitromidazole derivatives are drugs of choice for the treatment of trichomoniasis. The standard treatment is metronidazole 250 mg thrice a day given orally for 7 days or in a single 2 gm dose. The infected patient and sexual partner, both should be treated irrespective of symptomatology, to prevent reinfection. The drug does cross placental barrier, therefore is not prescribed during first trimester of pregnancy (Lossick and Kent, 1991).

Drug resistant cases have been reported (Sobel, 1999). It can be due to several mutational changes and can affect both aerobic and anaerobic mechanisms of metabolism (Upcroft and Upcroft, 2001). In the parasites resistant by aerobic mechanisms, the transcription of ferridoxin (Fd) gene is reduced, thereby decreasing the ability of cell to activate the drug. However, gene knock out mice were not found resistant to the drug under aerobic or anaerobic conditions and it is postulated that Fd gene product eliminated in knock out cells is neither necessary for hydrogen production nor metronidazole production (Land et al, 2004). Metronidazole has to be first reduced by certain mechanism(s) in *T.vaginalis* at the relatively low redox potential, before it exerts the antitrichomonad action (Muller et al, 1983). It is suggested that reductase(s) responsible for reducing metronidazole or its precursor, could be transitional product of dsRNA in *T.vaginalis*. The studies suggest that it might be possible to identify a marker for resistance that could lead to improved treatment strategies.

Many alternative drugs and treatments have been tested in vivo in cases of refractory trichomoniasis, as well as in vitro with some successes including the broad spectrum anti-parasitic drug nitazoxanide. Drug resistance incidence of *T.vaginalis* appears to be on the increase and improved surveillance of treatment failures is urged (Dunne et al, 2003).

9. Prevention and control

The main focus to prevent and control the disease should be on the identification of infected women and treatment of both the sexual partners. High rates of asymptomatic infection in male partners of infected females and subsequent re-infection have significant implications for control programmes. HIV-infected women are at increased risk of trichomoniasis and local HIV prevention strategies should target such women for intervention efforts. In addition, the effect of treatment on outcome of pregnancy and HIV acquisition requires further study. This will, in turn, facilitate operational studies evaluating optimal control strategies and their impact on the complications of *T.vaginalis* (Johnston and Mabey, 2008).

Vaccine

The Solco Trichovac Vaccine prepared from inactive Lactobacilli was thought to induce protection, however, further reports indicated its inconclusive efficacy. Experimental studies revealed that the mice which were inoculated whole, live trichomonads with adjuvant/s subcutaneously and then infected intravaginally, had significantly less intravaginal infection than control groups (Abraham et al, 1996). High levels of proteolytic activity found in T.vaginalis and involvement of some of these proteases in the colonization of the host suggest that proteases may have protective role. Intranasal immunization of T.vaginalis 62 kDa protease in a murine model induced significant IgG and IgA response against this antigen in the vaginal washes and suggests that the 62kDa protease is a potential vaccine candidate against trichomoniasis (Hernandez et al, 2006). The reports provides hope for the goal of vaccine development in future.

10. References

Abraham, M.C., Desjardins, M., Fillon, L.G. And Garber, G.E. (1996). Inducible immunity to *Trichomonas vaginalis* in a mouse model of vaginal infection. Infect Immun. 64, 3571-3575.

Ackers, J.P., Lumsden, W.H.R., Catterall, R.D., Coyle, R. (1975). Antitrichomonal antibodies in the vaginal secretions of women infected with *T.vaginalis*. Br. J. Vener. Dis. 51, 319-23.

Alderete, J.F. (1984). Enzyme linked immunosorbent assay for detecting antibody to *T.vaginalis*. Br. J. Vener. Dis. 60, 164-70.

Alderete, J.F. and Garza, G.E.(1984). Soluble *Trichomonas vaginalis* antigens in cell-free culture supernatants. Mol. Biochem. Parasitol. 13, 147-158.

Alderete, J.F., Kasmala, L., Metcalfe, E., Garza, G.E. (1986). Phenotypic variation and diversity among *Trichomonas vaginalis* isolates and correlation of phenotype with trichomonal virulence determinants. Infect. Immun. 53, 285-293.

Alderete, J.F., Demes, P., Gombosova, A., Valent, M., Yanoska, A., Fabusova, H., Kasmala, L., Garza, G.E., Metcalfe, E.C. (1987). Phenotypes and protein epitope phenotypic variation among fresh isolates of *Trichomonas vaginalis*. Infect. Immun. 55(5), 1037-1041.

Arroya R., Gonzalez-Robles, A., Martinex Palomo, A., Alderete, J.F. (1993). Signaling of *Trichomonas vaginalis* for amoeboid transformation and adhesion synthesis followed cyto-adherence. Mol. Microbiol. 7,299-309.

Benchmol, M., Chang, T.H., Alderete, J.F. (2002). *Trichomonas vaginalis* observation of coexistence of multiple viruses in the same isolate. FEMS Microbiol. Let. 215,197-201.

Bersoff-Matcha, S.J., Horgan, M.M., Fraser, V.J., Mundy, L.M., Stoner, B.P. (1998). Sexually transmitted disease acquisition among women infected with human immunodeficiency virus type 1. Journal of Infectious Diseases,178, 174-7.

Boyle, C.A., Lowell, D.M., Kelsey, J.L., Livolsi, V.A., Boyle, K.E. (1989). Cervical intraepithelial neoplasia among women with *Papillomavirus* infection compared to women with *T.vaginalis* infection. Cancer. 64, 168-72.

Bozner, P. (1997). Immunological detection and subcellular localization of Hsp70 and Hsp60 homologs in *Trichomonas vaginali.* J. Parasitol. 83, 224-229.

Carlton, J.M., Hirt, R.P., Silva, J.C., Delcher, A.L., Schatz, M., Zhao, Q., Wortman, J.R., et al. (2007). Draft genome sequence of the sexually transmitted pathogen *Trichomonas vaginalis*. Sci. 315, 207-211.

Chakraborty, T., Mulla, S.A., Kosambiya, J.K., Desai, V.K. (2005). Prevalence of *T.vaginalis* infection in and around Surat. Ind. J. Pathol. Microbiol. 48, 542-45.

Costa e Silva Filko, F., Souza W de and Lopex, J.D. (1988). Presence of Laminibinding proteins in Trichomonads and their role in adhesion. Proc. Natl. Acad. Sci.85, 8042-8046.

Chang, J.H., Kim, S.K., Choi, I.H., Leed, S.K., Morio (2006). Apoptosis of macrophages induced by *Trichomonas vaginalis* through the phosphorylation of p38 mitogen activate protein kinase that locates at downstream of mitochondria-dependent caspase activation. Int. J. Biochem. Cell Biol. 38, 638-647.

Davis, S. and Lushbaugh, W.B. (1993). Oxidative stress and *Trichomonas vaginalis*: The effect of hydrogen peroxide in vitro. Am. J. Trop. Med. Hyg. 48(4), 480-7.

Dawn, G., Sharma, M., Kumar, B., Malla, N. (1995). Prevalence of microorganisms in patients with non-gonococcal urethritis from North India. Ind. J. Sex. Trans. Dis. 16, 9-14.

Demes, P., Gombosova, A., Valent, M., Fabusova, H., Janoska, A. (1988). Fewer *Trichomonas vaginalis* organisms in vaginas of infected women during menstruation. Gen. Med. 64, 22-24.

Divekar, A.A., Gotate, A.S., Shivkar, L.K., Gotate, S., Badhwar, V.R. (2000). Disease prevalence in women attending STD clinic in Mumbai, India. Int. J. STD & AIDS 11, 45-48.

Fiori, P.L., Paola, R., Maria, F.A., 1999. The flagellated parasite *Trichomonas vaginalis*: new insights into cytopathogenicity mechanisms. Micro. Inf. 2,149-156.

Frankel, T.L., Monif, G.R. (2000). *T.vaginalis* and bacterial vaginosis: coexistence in vaginal wet mount preparations from pregnant women. J. Rep. Med. 45, 131-4.

Garber, G.E., Sibou, L., Ma, R., Proctor, E.M., Shaw, C.E., Bowis, W.R. (1987). Cell culture compared with broth for detection of *Trichomonas vaginalis*. J. Clin. Microbiol. 25,1275-1279.

Ghys, P.D., Diallo, M.O., Ettiegne-Traore, V., Yeboue, K.M., Gnaore, E., Lorougnon, F. et al. (1995). Genital ulcers associated with HIV related immunosupression in female sex workers in Abidjan, Ivary Coast. J. Infect. Dis. 172, 1371-4.

Gosskurth, H., Mosha, F., Todd, J. (1995). Impact of improved treatment of STDs on HIV infection in rural Tanzania: demised controlled trail. Lancet 346, 530-6.

Gonzalez-Robles, A., Lazaro-Haller, A., Espinosa-Castellano, M., Anaya-velazques, F., Martinez-alomo, A. (1995). *Trichomonas vaginalis*: Ultrastructural basis of the cytopathic effect. J. Euk. Microbil. 42, 641-51.

Heine, P. and McGregor, J.A. (1993). *Trichomonas vaginalis*: a reemerging pathogen. Clin. Obst. Gyncol. 36, 137-144.

Hernandez, H., Figueredo, M., Garrido, N., Sariego, I., Sarracent, J. (2006). Protective effect of a protease against *Trichomonas vaginalis* infection of the murine gential tract. Biotecnologia Aplicada, 23(3). 248-250.

Honigberg, B.M. and King, V.M. (1964). Structure of *Trichomonas vaginalis* (Donne). J. Parasitol. 50, 345-364.

Honigberg, B.M., Livingston, M.C., Frost, J.K. (1966). Pathogenecity of fresh isolates of *Trichomonas vaginalis*: "The moust assay" versus clinical and pathologic findings. Acta Cytol. 10, 353-361.

Honigberg, B.M. (1990). Host cell trichomonad interactions and virulence assays using in vitro systems. In: Trichomonads parasitic in humans. Springer-Verlag, New York, pp 155-212.

Johnston, V.J. and David, CM. (2008). Global epidemiology and control of *Trichomonas vaginalis*. Current Opinion in Infectious Diseases, 21, 56-64.

Kaul, P., Gupta, I., Sehgal, R., Malla, N. (2004). *Trichomonas vaginalis*: random amplified polymorphic DNA analysis of isolates from symptomatic and asymptomatic women in India. Parasitol. Int. 53,255-262.

Kaul, P. (2004a). Molecular and biochemical characterization of *Trichomonas vaginalis* isolated from symptomatic and asymptomatic women. Ph.D. Theses submitted to Postgraduate Institute of Medical Education & Research, Chandigarh, India.

Kaur, S., Khurana, S., Bagga, R., Wanchu, A., Malla, N. (2008). Trichomoniasis among women in North India: A hospital based study. Ind.Jl. Of Sexually Transm. Dis., 29, 76-81.

Kaur, S., Khurana, S., Bagga, R., Wanchu, A. and Malla, N. (2008). Kinetics of immunoglobulins G, M, A and IgG subclass responses in human intravaginal trichomoniasis. Parasit. Res., 103 (2), 305-312.

Kharsany, A.B.M., Hoosen, A.A., Moodley, J., Bagaratee, J., Gouws, E. (1993). The association between sexually transmitted pathogens and cervical intra epithelial neoplasia in a developing community. Gen. Med. 69, 357-360.

Khoshnan, A. and Alderete, J.F. (1993). Multiple double stranded RNA segments are associated with virus particles infecting *Trichomonas vaginalis*. J. Viro. 67(12), 6950-6955.

Klinger, E.V., Kapiquasn, Sam, N.E., Aboud, S., Chen, C.Y., Ballard, R.C. et al. (2006). A community based study of risk factors of *T.vaginalis* infection among women and their male partners in Moshi Urban Districts, North Tanzania. STD 33, 712-18.

Krieger, J.N., Ravdin, J.I., Rein, M.F. (1985). Contact-dependent cytopathogenic mechanisms of *Trichomonas vaginalis*. 50, 778-786.

Krieger, J.N., Holmes, K.K., Spence, M.R., Rein, M.F., McCormack, W.M. and Tam, M.R. (1985a). Geographic variation among isolates of *Trichomonas vaginalis*. Demonstration of antigenic heterogeneity by using monoclonal antibodies and the indirect immunofluorescence techniques. J. Inf. Dis. 152, 979-984.

Krieger, J.N. (1990). Epidemiology and clinical manifestations of urogenital trichomoniasis in men. In: BM Honigberg Ed, *Trichomonads parasitic in humans*, Springer-Verlag, New York, N.Y.

Land, K.M., Delgadillo-correa, M.G., Tachezy, J., Vanacova, S., Hsieh, C.L., Sutak, R., Johnson, P.J. (2004). Targeted gene replacement of a ferredoxin gene in *Trichomonas vaginalis* does not lead to metronidazole resistance. Mol. Microbiol. 51(1), 115-122.

Langly, J.G., Goldsmith, J.M., Davies, N. (1987). Venereal trichomoniasis: Role of men. Genito. Med.63, 264-267.

Lazar, A. (1970). *Trichomonas vaginalis* infection: Incidence with use of various contraceptive methods. J. Med. Soc. 67,225-227.

Linstead, D.J. And Bradley, S. (1988). The purification and properties of two soluble reduced nicotinamide: acceptor oxidoreductases from *Trichomonas vaginalis*. Mol. Biotech. Parasit. 27, 125-133.

Lossick, J.G. and Kent, H.L. (1991). Trichomoniasis: trends in diagnosis and management. Am. J. Obst. Gynae. 165, 1217-1222.

Malla, N., Wattal, C., Khan, I.A., Kaul, R., Raina, V. (1989). Study of trichomoniasis in Kashmir (North India). Ind. J. Med. Microbiol. 7,121-126.

Malla, N., Valadkhani, A., Harjai, K., Sharma, S., Gupta, I. (2004). Reactive nitrogen intermediates in experimental trichomoniasis induced with isolates from symptomatic and asymptomatic women. Parasitol. Res. 94, 101-105.

Malla, N., Yadav, M., Gupta, I. (2007). Kinetics of serum and local cytokine profile in experimental intravaginal trichomoniasis induced with *Trichomonas vaginalis* isolated from symptomatic and asymptomatic women. Parasit. Immunol. 29, 101-105.

Malla, N., Kaul, P., Sehgal, R and Gupta, I. (2011). The presence of DsRNA virus in *Trichomonas vaginalis* isolates from symptomatic and asymptomatic Indian women and its correlation with *in vitro* metronidazole sensitivity. Ind. Jl. Of Med. Microbiology, 29(2), 152-157.

Mason, P.R. and Gwanzura, L. (1988). Mouse spleen cell responses to trichomonal antigens in experimental *Trichomonas vaginalis* infection. J. Parasitol. 74(1), 93-97.

McGrory, T. and Garber, G.E. (1992). Mouse intravaginal infection with *Trichomonas vaginalis* and role of *Lactobacillus acidophilus* in sustaining infection. Infect. Immun. 60, 2375-2379.

Mc Laren, L.C., Davis, L.E., Healy, G.R., James, C.G. (1983). Isolation of *Trichomonas vaginalis* from the respiratory tract of infants with respiratory disease. Paediatr. 71, 888-90.

McLellan, R., Spence, M.R., Brockman, M., Raffel, L., Smith, J.L. (1982). The clinical diagnosis of trichomoniasis. Obst. Gynae. 60, 30-34.

Menduza-Lopez, M.R., Garcia, C.B., Fattel-Facenda, L.V., Avila-Gonzales, L., Ruiz-Tachiquin, M., Oriego Lopez, J., Aproyo, R. (2000). CP30-a cysteinase involved in *Trichomonas vaginalis* cytoadherence. Infect. Immun. 4907-12.

Minkoff, H.L., Eisenberger-Matityahu, D., Feldman, J., Burk, R., Clarke, L. (1999). Prevalence and incidence of gynaecological disorders among women infected with HIV. Am. J. Obst. Gynae. 180, 824-36.

Muller, M. (1983). *Trichomonas vaginalis* and other sexually transmitted protozoan infections. In: International perspectives of neglected STDs. Holmes, K.K. And Mardh, P. Eds. Hemisphere Publishing Corporation, New York, pp 113-124.

Paintlia, M.K., Kaur, S., Gupta, I., Ganguly, N.K., Mahajan, R.C., Malla, N. (2002). Specific IgA response, T-cell subtype and cytokine profile in experimental intravaginal trichomoniasis. Parasit. Res. 88, 338-343.

Peterson, K.M. and Alderete, J.F., 1982. Host plasma proteins on the surface of pathogenic *Trichomonas vaginalis*. Infect. Immun. 37, 755-762.

Petrin, D., Delgaty, K., Bhatt, R., Garber, G. (1998). Clinical and Microbiological aspects of *Trichomonas vaginalis*. Clin. Microbiol. Rev. 11(2), 300-317.

Pindak, F.F., Mora de Pindak, M., W.A Gardner, Jr. (1993). Contact- independent cytotoxity of *Trichomonas vaginalis*. Genito. Med. 69, 35-40.

Provenzano, D. and Alderete, J.F. (1995). Analysis of human immunoglobulin degrading cysteine proteinases of *Trichomonas vaginalis*. Infect. Immun. 63, 3388-3395.

Rein, M.F. (1990). Clinical manifestations of urogenital trichomoniasis in women. In: Trichomonads parasitic in humans. Honigberg BM Ed. Springer-Verlag, New York, pp225-234.

Rein, M.F. and Muller, M. (1990). *Trichomonas vaginalis* and trichomoniasis. In: Sexually transmitted diseases. 2nd ed. Holmes, K.K., Mardh, P.A., Sparling, P.F., Wiesner, P.J., Cates, W. Jr., Lemon, S.M. and Stamm, W.E. Eds. McGraw-Hill, New York.

Ryu, J.S., Choi, H.K., Min, D.Y., Ha, S.E., Ahn, M.H. (2001). Effect of iron on the virulence of Trichomonas vaginalis. J. Parasit. 87(2), 457-60.

Sapru, P., Mohan, K., Gupta, I., Ganguly, N.K., Mahajan, R.C., Malla, N. (1994). DNA banding patterns of *Trichomonas vaginalis* strains isolated from symptomatic and asymptomatic subjects. J. Protozo. Res. 4, 40-47.

Shaio, M.F., Chang, F.Y., Hou, S.C., Lee, C.S., Lin, P.R. (1991). The role of immunoglobulin and complement in enhancing the respiratory burst of neutrophils against *Trichomonas vaginalis*. Parasit. Immun. 13, 241-50.

Shaio, M.F., Lin, P.R., Lee, C.S. (1993). Killing of *Trichomonas vaginalis* by complement mediated lysis is not associated with the presence of *Trichomonas vaginalis* virus. Intern. J. Parasitol. 23, 675-680.

Sharma, P., Malla, N., Gupta, I., Ganguly, N.K., Mahajan, R.C. (1988). Prevalence of trichomoniasis in symptomatic and asymptomatic subjects using different contraceptive devices. Ind. J. Med. Microbiol. 6,315-322.

Sharma, P., Malla, N., Ganguly, N.K., Mahajan, R.C. (1991). Anti-trichomonad IgA antibodies in Trichomoniasis before and after treatment. Folia Microbiol. 36(3),302-304.

Sharma, P., Malla, N., Gupta, I., Ganguly, N.K., Mahajan, R.C. (1991a). A comparison of wet mount, culture and enzyme linked immunosorbent assay for the diagnosis of Trichomoniasis in women. Trop. Geog. Med. 43, 257-260.

Schwebke, J.R. and Burgess, D. (2004). Trichomoniasis. Clin. Microbiol. Rev. Oct, 794-803.

Smith, A., Johnson, P. (2011). Gene expression in the unicellular eukaryote *Trichomonas vaginalis*. Research in Microbiology, 162, 646-654.

Sobel, J.D. (1999). Metronidazole resistance vaginal trichomoniasis - an emerging problem. N. Eng. J. Med. July, 292.

Sobel, J.D. (2005). What's new in bacterial vaginosis and trichomoniasis? Infect. Dis. Clin. N. Am. 19, 387-406.

Soliman, M.A., Ackers, J.P., Catterall, R.D. (1982). Isoenzyme characterization of *Trichomonas vaginalis*. Bri. J. Venerol. Dis. 58,250-253.

Song, Hyun-Ouk, Young-Su Lim, Sun-Joo Moon, Myoung-Hee Ahn and Jae-Sook Ryu. (2010). Delayed human neutrophil apoptosis by *Trichomonas vaginalis* lysate. Korean Parasitol., 48 (1), 1-7.

Sood, S., Kapil, A. (2008). An update on *Trichomonas vaginalis*. Indian J. Sex Transm. Dis., 29(1), 7-14.

Sorvillo, F., Kovacs, A., Kerndet, P., Stek, A., Muderspach, L., Sanchez-Keeland, L. (1998). Risk factors for trichomoniasis among women with human immunodeficiency virus (HIV) infection at a public clinic in Los Angeles county, California implications for HIV prevention. Am. J. Trop. Med. Hyg. 58(4), 495-500.

Snipes, L.J., Gamard, P.M., Narcisi, E.M., Beard, C.B., Lehmann, T., Secor, W.E.(2000). Molecular epidemiology of Metronidazole resistance in a population of *Trichomonas vaginalis* clinical isolates. J. Clin. Microbiol. 38, 3004-3009.

Stiles, J.K., Shah, P.H., Xue, L., Meake, J.c., Lushbaugh, W.B., Cleary, J.D., Finely, W. (2000). Molecular typing of *Trichomonas vaginalis* isolates by HSP70 and restriction fragment length polymorphism. Am. J. Trop. Med. Hyg. 62(4), 441-445.

Susan, C.U., Hyejin, K., Denise, J.J., Joseph, W.H., Paula, S., Jean, A. et al. (2002). Prevalence, incidence and persistence or recurrence of trichomoniasis among Human Immunodeficiency Virus (HIV) - positive women and among HIV negative women at high risk for HIV infection. Clin. Infect. Dis. 34, 1406-11.

Sutton, M.Y., Stenberg, M., Nsuami, M., Behets, F., Nelson, A.M., St Louis, M.E. (1999). Trichomoniasis in pregnant HIV infected and HIV uninfected Congolese women: prevalence, risk factors and association with low birth weight. Am. J. Obstet. Gynae. 181, 656-62.

Tai, J.H., Su, H.M., Tsai, J., Shaio, M.F., Wang, C.C. (1993). The divergence of *Trichomonas vaginalis* virus RNAs among various isolates of *Trichomonas vaginalis*. Exp. Parasitol. 76, 278-286.

Tapsall, J.W., Puglisi, J., Smith, D.D. (1979). *Trichomonas vaginalis* infections in Sydney: Laboratory diagnosis and prevalence. Med. J. Aus. 1, 193-4.

Ter Muelen, J., Mgaya, H.N., Chang-Claude, J., Luande, J., Mtiro, H., Mhina, M. et al., 1992. Risk factors for HIV infection in gynaecological inpatients in Dar Es Salaam, Tanzania, 1988-90. East Afr. Med. J. 69, 688-92.

Upcroft, J.A. and Upcroft, P. (2001). Drug susceptibility testing of anaerobic protozoa. Antimicrob Ag. Chemother. June 45, 1810-1814.

Valadkhani, Z., Sharma, S., Harjai, K., Gupta, I., Malla, N. (2003). In vitro comparative kinetics of adhesive and haemolytic potential of *T.vaginalis* isolates from symptomatic and asymptomatic females. Ind. J. Pathol. Microbiol. 46(4), 693-699.

Valadkhani, Z., Sharma, S., Harjai, K., Gupta, I., Malla, N. (2004). Evaluation of *Trichomonas vaginalis* isolates from symptomatic and asymptomatic patients in mouse model. Ira. J. Pub. Hlth. 33,60-66.

Valadkhani, Z., Sharma, S., Harjai, K., Gupta, I., Malla, N. (2006). Superoxide radical formation in isolated PMN from experimental vaginal trichomoniasis. Ira. J. Pub. Hlth. 35,76-82.

Vanacova, S., Tachezy, J., Kulda, J., Flegr, J. (1997). Characterization of trichomonad species and strains by PCR Fingerprinting. J. Euk. Microbiol. 44(6), 545-52.

Vargas - Villarreal, J., Mata-Cardenas, B.D., Gonzalez-Salazar, F., Lozano-Garz, H.G., Cortes-Gutierrez, E.I., Palacios-Corona, R., Martinez-Rodriguez, H.G., Ramirez-Bun, E., Said Fernandez, S. (2003). *Trichomonas vaginalis*: identification of a phospholipase A dependent haemolytic activity in a vesicular subcellular fraction. J. Parasitol. 89(1), 105-112.

Vikki, M., Pukkala, E., Nieminen, P., Hakama, M. (2000). Gynaecological infections as risk determinants of subsequent cervical neoplasia. Acta Oncol. 39, 71-5.

Vishwanath, S., Talwar, V., Prasad, R., Coyaji, K., Elias, C.J., De Zoysa, I. (2000). Syndromic management of vaginal discharge among women in reproductive health clinic in India. Sex. Trans. Infect. 76, 303-306.

Vohra, H., Sharma, P., Sofi, B.A., Gupta, I., Ganguly, N.K., Mahajan, R.C., Malla, N. (1991). Correlation of zymodeme patterns, virulence and drug sensitivity of *Trichomonas vaginalis* isolates from women. Ind. J. Med. Res. 93, 37-39.

Wang, A.L. and Wang, C.C. (1985). A linear double stranded RNA in *Trichomonas vaginalis*. J. Biol. Chem. 260, 3697-702.

Wang, A., Wang, C.C. and Alderete, J.F. (1987). *Trichomonas vaginalis* phenotypic variation occurs only among trichomonads with the double stranded RNA virus. J. Exp. Med. 166, 142–150.

Wang, C., McClelland, S., Reilly, M., Overbaugh, J., Emery, S.L., Mandaliya, K. et al. (2001). The effect of treatment of vaginal infections on shedding of HIV-type 1. J. Infect. Dis. 183, 1017-22.

Wendel, K.A., Rampalo, A.M., Erbelding, E.J., Chang, T.H., Alderete, J.F. (2002). Double stranded RNA viral infection of *T.vaginalis* infected patients attending a STD clinic. J. Infect. Dis. 186, 558-61.

Yadav, M., Gupta, I., Malla, N. (2005). Kinetics of immunoglobulin G, M, A and IgG subclass responses in experimental intravaginal trichomoniasis: prominence of IgG_1 response. Parasit. Immunol. 27,461-467.

Yadav, M., Dubey, M.L., Gupta, I., Malla, N. (2006). Nitric oxide radicals in leucocytes and vaginal washes of *Trichomonas vaginalis* - infected symptomatic and asymptomatic women. Parasitol. 132,339-43.

Yadav, M., Dubey, M.L., Gupta, I., Bhatti, G., Malla, N. (2007). Cysteine proteinase 30 in clinical isolates of *T.vaginalis* from symptomatic and asymptomatic infected women. Exp. Parasitol. 116(4), 399-406.

Yadav, M., Dubey, M.L., Gupta, I., Malla, N. (2007a). Cysteine proteinase 30 (CP30) and antibody response to CP30 in serum and vaginal washes of symptomatic and asymptomatic *Trichomonas vaginalis* infected women. Parasit. Immunol. 29, 359-365.

Zhang, Z.F. and Begg, C.B. (1994). Is *T.vaginalis* a cause of cervical neoplasia? Results from combined analysis of 24 studies. Internat. J. Epidemiol. 23, 682-90.

Zhang, Z.F., Graham, S., Yu, S.Z., Marshall, J., Zielezny, M., Chen, Y.X. et al. (1995). *Trichomonas vaginalis* and cervical cancer. A prospective study in China. Ann. Epidemiol. 5, 325-32.

Part 4

Human Papilloma Virus Infection

7

Human Papillomavirus Infection in Croatian Men: Prevalence and HPV Type Distribution

Blaženka Grahovac[1], Anka Dorić[2], Željka Hruškar[2], Ita Hadžisejdić[1] and Maja Grahovac[2]
[1]*Department of Pathology, School of Medicine, University of Rijeka, Rijeka*
[2]*Polyclinic of Dermatovenerology, Infectious Diseases and Cytology Virogena Plus, Zagreb*
Croatia

1. Introduction

Human papillomavirus (HPV) infection has been identified as a major risk factor for cervical intraepithelial neoplasia (CIN) and invasive cervical cancer (zur Hausen, 2002; Bosch et al., 2002; Munoz et al., 2003). HPV infection is one of the most common sexually transmitted infections, generally asymptomatic, with the worldwide prevalence in women with normal cytology of 11.4% (11.3-11.5%; 95%CI) (WHO/ICO Information Centre on HPV and Cervical Cancer. Summary report 2010). Epidemiological studies in the USA have reported that 75% of the 15-50 year-old population is infected with genital HPV during their lifetime. Among those, 60% are with transient infection, 10% with persistent infection (confirmed by detection of HPV-DNA in genital samples), 4% with mild cytological signs, and 1% with clinical lesions (WHO/ICO Information Centre on HPV and Cervical Cancer. Papillomavirus and Related Cancers in United States of America. Summary Report 2010). To date, more than 100 genotypes of HPV have been identified, with more than 40 anogenital types, at least 15 of which are oncogenic (Munoz et al. 2003; Clifford et al., 2005). Anogenital HPV types have been further classified into low-risk types (lrHPV, e.g., 6 and 11), which are associated with anogenital warts and mild dysplasia, and high-risk types (hrHPV, e.g., 16, 18, 31, and 33), which are associated with high-grade dysplasia and anogenital cancers, such as cervical and anal carcinoma. (Bosch et al., 2002; Smith et al., 2007). In Croatia, HPV testing is widely used as a secondary test to triage borderline cytology and as a follow-up after treatment of severe cervical lesions, in addition to conventional cytological screening (Grce et al., 2007). Grahovac et al. (2007) investigated the HPV prevalence and type distribution among 361 women regularly attending gynecological examinations, and showed 67.9% overall prevalence of hrHPV in women with abnormal PAP smears compared to 35.6% in women with normal cytology. Study done by Hadžisejdić et al., (2006) on prevalence of HPV genotypes in cervical cancer also revealed high prevalence of HPV-DNA in cervical lesions; 93% in CIN III, 92.6% in squamous cell carcinoma (SCC) and 92.5% in adenocarcinoma (ADC).

While much is known about the epidemiology and pathogenesis of genital HPV infections in women, relatively little is known about the natural history of anogenital HPV infection and diseases in men. Available data suggest that, as with women, most genital HPV infections in men are asymptomatic and unapparent (Baldwin et al., 2003; Partridge & Koutsky, 2006; Dunne et al., 2006; Bleeker et al., 2008; Colon-Lopez et al., 2010). Each year in the U.S. there are about 400 men who get HPV-related penile cancer and 1,500 men who get HPV-related anal cancer (US Center for Disease Control and Prevention, STD Facts-HPV and Men, 2009).

According to the Croatian National Cancer Registry (Croatian National Cancer Registry, 2010), the average incidence of cervical cancer in 2008 was 15.6 new cases per 100,000 women, and incidence of penile and anal cancer were 1.3 and 0.4 new cases per 100,000 men, respectively.

Compared with cervical cancer, penile and anal cancers are rare diseases in the general population. However, its incidence is increasing in the general population with age. Majority of cervical, penile and anal cancers are caused by HPV-16 and HPV-18, together accounting for about 70% cases globally. The importance of different hrHPV varies between countries and regions, but type 16 has the greatest contribution to the genital cancer in all regions (WHO/ICO, Summary Report, 2010.).

Anal HPV infection and disease also remain poorly understood. Although HPV is transmitted sexually and infects the genitals of both sexes, the cervix remains biologically more vulnerable to malignant transformation than does the penis or anus in men. An understanding of male HPV infection is therefore important in terms of reducing transmission of HPV to women and improving women's health (Palefsky, 2007, 2010; Monsonego, 2011; Giuliano et al., 2011.). Improved sampling techniques of the male genitalia and cohort studies in progress should provide important information on the natural history of anogenital HPV infection and disease in men, including risk factors for HPV acquisition and transmission (Bleeker et al. 2002, 2005; Weaver et al. 2004.; Lajous et al., 2005; Nielson et al., 2007; Dunne et al., 2006; Giuliano et al., 2007.). The understanding of HPV infection and associated diseases in men has increasing importance due to advent of highly efficacious HPV prophylactic vaccines and possibility that the same vaccines may be also useful in preventing HPV infection in men. (Palefsky, 2010., Elbasha & Dasbach, 2010). Also, the impact of HPV vaccination in women, on male anogenital HPV infection needs to be assessed as well.

To date, there are no relevant studies investigating genital HPV prevalence and type distribution among men in Croatia. The aim of our investigation is to assess the prevalence and type distribution of HPV among patients visiting outpatient sexually transmitted diseases (STD) clinic, urologic and dermatovenerologic clinics in Zagreb and Rijeka, Croatia, in period between 2006 and 2008 and to compare obtained results with available epidemiologic literature data. To date there is no consensus regarding methods and recommendations for sampling or optimal male anatomic sites for HPV DNA detection. We have adapted the analytical approach by using scraped materials from external genitals and brushed exfoliated cells from distal urethral canal for HPV DNA detection and genotyping. We used consensus and type-specific primers directed polymerase chain reaction (PCR) focusing on the most prevalent lrHPV (6,11) and hrHPV (16, 18, 31, 33) accounting together for more than 80% of HPV related genital lesions globally (WHO/ICO Information Centre on HPV and Cervical Cancer. Summary Report 2010.).

2. Materials and methods

The retrospective cross-sectional study was performed among men attending STD, urology and dermatovenerology outpatient clinics in Zagreb and Rijeka between 2006 and 2008. During this period 581 men participated in the study. All men who were included in the study signed informed consent previously approved by The Ethical Committee. Saline-wetted cotton swabs were taken from urethral canal (up to 1 cm into urethral meatus) with scrapes from the penile surface including glans, coronal sulcus and penile shaft and placed into a specimen transportation medium (Digene Corp., Gaithersburg, MD). The samples containing exfoliated epithelial cells were kept at 4°C until analyses were performed. DNA was isolated by Nucleospin Tissue isolation kit (Macherey-Nagel GmbH, Duren, Germany) according to manufacturer's instruction. HPV DNA detection and genotyping was performed by consensus and type-specific primers directed PCR (Gravitt et al., 2000, Walboomers et al., 1999, Shimada et al. 1990, Fujinaga et al., 1991). The samples for HPV DNA analyses were collected by experienced physicians.

2.1 PCR analysis

To assess the quality of extracted DNA, β-globin PCRs were performed using primer combinations spanning 250 and 408 bp (Takara Biomedicals, Japan). Poor or no β-globin amplification indicated a lack of sufficient cellular material for PCR or the presence of PCR inhibitors. Primers targeting highly conserved regions within the L1 and E6/E7 open reading frame (ORF) were used to detect HPV DNA. These included the MY9/MY11 (Gravitt et al. 2000) primers of the L1 ORF and primers from Human Papillomavirus Typing Set (Takara Biomedicals, Japan), which amplify sequences within E6 and E7 ORF (Fujinaga et al. 1991). The HPV types in positive samples were further characterized by restriction enzyme digestion and type specific PCR amplifying sequences of HPV-16, 18, 31 and 33 within E6 and E7 ORF (Human Papillomavirus Detection Set, Takara Biomedicals, Japan - Shimada et al., 1990) and primers recommended by Walboomers et al., 1999.

2.2 Statistical analysis

HPV prevalence was expressed as percentage of HPV positive samples against all HPV tested cases. When determining the prevalence of hrHPV and lrHPV types, men were counted more than once if they harboured multiple infections. The prevalence of individual HPV types was determined as they appeared as either single or multiple infections. Multiple HPV infection was defined as two or more HPV types. The two times two contingency tables and Fisher's exact test were used to assess statistical significance of differences in the prevalence and distribution of hrHPV and lrHPV, and to examine the relationship between HPV types within different anatomical sampling sites. Statistical significance was established at the $p<0.05$ level.

3. Results

During study period 581 men were enrolled in the cross-sectional study, mean age was 34.6±8.3 years (range 18-54 years). They were mostly asymptomatic, self-referring to the clinics either for primary screening for STDs or having symptoms suggestive of an STD, unspecific urogenital problems, having partners with diagnosed STD or high-risk sexual behaviour in the last several months (weeks). The patient's specimens were collected from the external genitals (scrapes from penile surface including glans, coronal sulcus and penile shaft) and exfoliated cells from the urethral canal. From the total of 581 men enrolled in the study we were able to collect 392 samples from the external genitals. In this group of 392 patients, 295 men also gave permission for urethral sampling in addition to the external genital swab (59 patients refused to give permission for urethral sampling). From 38 urethral samples β-globin PCRs were negative and subsequently considered as inadequate for HPV DNA testing. Additionally, in another group of 189 samples, swabs were taken from both anatomical sites, external genitals and urethra, and combined into one specimen. They were used in calculation of total HPV DNA prevalence as external swab specimens. By using several combinations of consensus and type specific primers, we were able to successfully amplify all specimens from external genitals and 86.8% urethral samples. The overall prevalence of HPV DNA in men was 27.4% (159/581) as shown on Table 1. and Fig. 1.

	HPV positive (%)	Low-risk HPV (%)	High-risk HPV (%)	HPV indeterm. types (%)	Multiple HPV infection (%)
Whole tested group N=581	159 (27.4%)	80 (13.8%)	82 (14.1%)	24 (4.1%)	25 (4.3%)

Table 1. Prevalence of HPV DNA in men and distribution of lrHPV, hrHPV, HPV of indeterminate type and multiple HPV infection in study group; values are number of HPV DNA positive samples and their percentage are indicated in parentheses. HPV positive = all samples with positive HPV DNA test result.

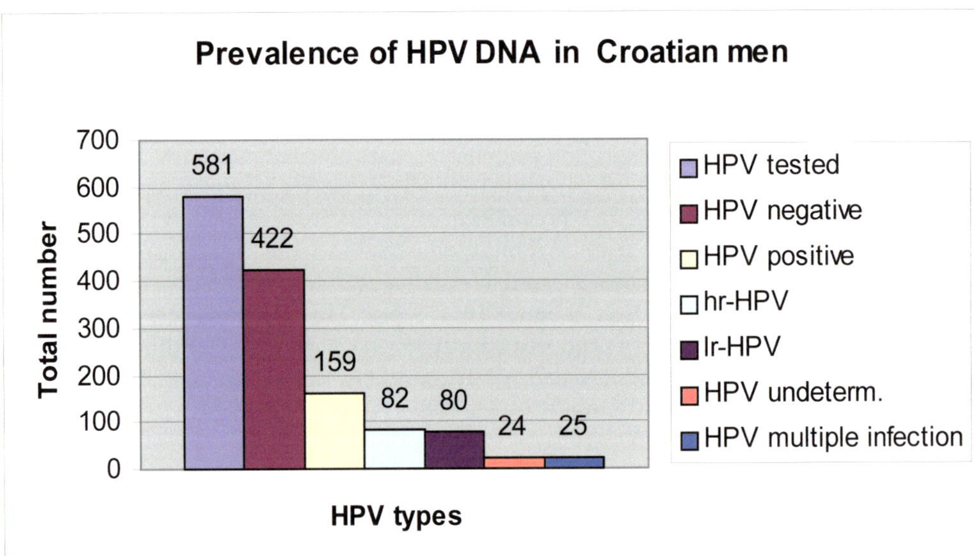

Fig. 1. Overall prevalence of HPV-DNA in study group of 581 Croatian men, presented as number of cases.

HrHPV DNA was detected in 82/581 (14.1%) and lrHPV DNA in 80/581 (13.8%) cases. Unclassified HPV type was detected in 24/581 (4.1%) and infection with multiple HPV types was detected in 25/581 (4.3%) cases (Table1.). LrHPVs and hrHPV types were detected as part of mixed HPV infections or as single infection as shown on Fig. 2.

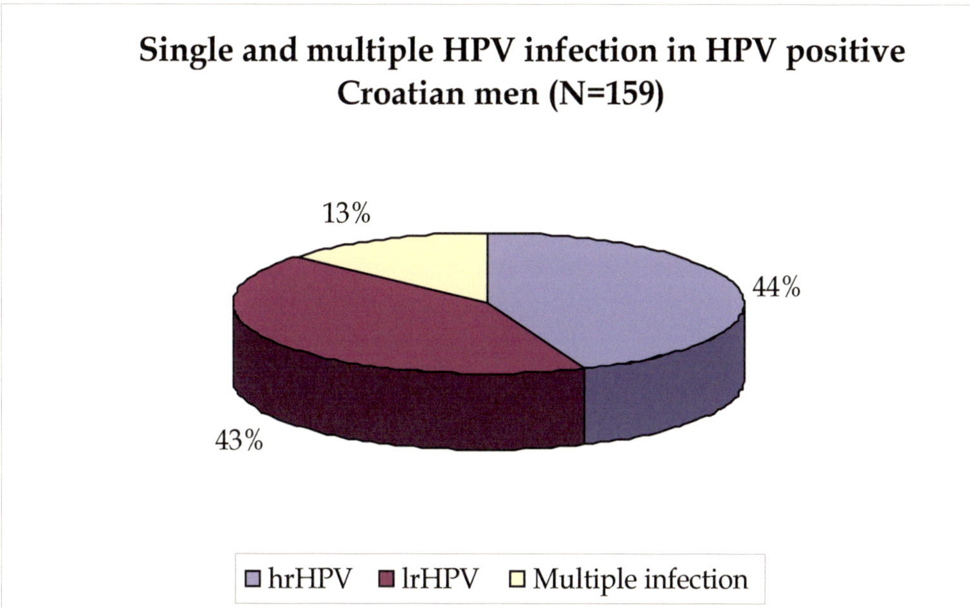

Fig. 2. Single hrHPV , lrHPV and multiple HPV infection in HPV positive Croatian men.

As single infection the most prevalent hrHPV type was HPV 16 detected in 32/82 (39%) cases followed by HPV 18 (10/82; 12.2%), HPV 31 (8/82; 9.8%) and HPV 33 (8/82; 9.8%). (Fig. 3.)

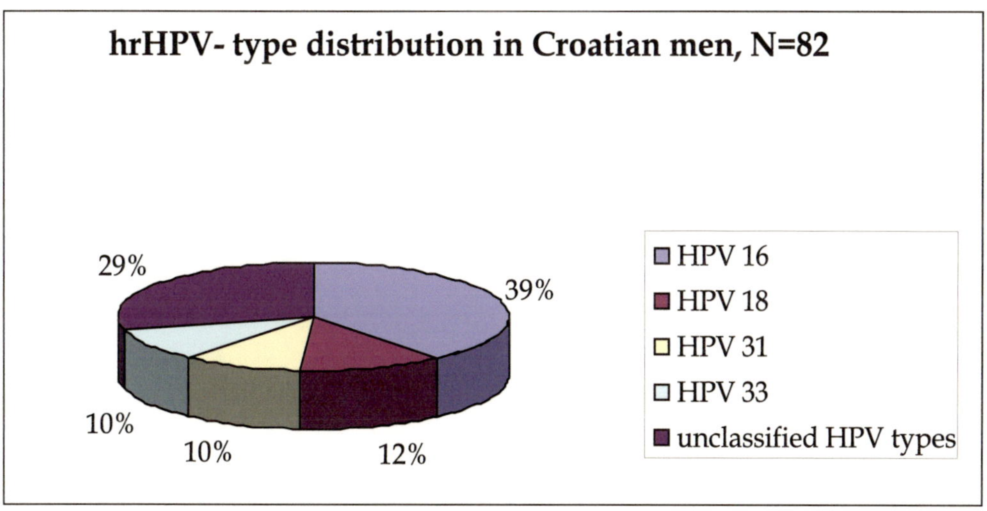

Fig. 3. Distribution of hrHPV types in HPV DNA positive cases.

Our findings indicate that in asymptomatic male the prevalence of major hrHPV, HPV 16 and HPV 18 exceeded 51.2% (42/82). Statistical evaluation revealed that the prevalence of HPV16/18 is significantly different ($p<0.0001$) compared to the prevalence of HPV31/33 (Table 3.). To determine the optimal genital anatomic site for the assessment of HPV DNA prevalence in men, we have analyzed the samples from two genital sites: penile surface and urethral canal (Fig. 4). The difference in overall HPV DNA prevalence between the penile surface including glans/coronal sulcus and penile shaft and the urethra was statistically significant ($p<0.0001$) with 25.3% (99/392), compared to 9.8% (29/295) respectively. The prevalence of lrHPV (17.1%) and hrHPV (15.1%) at external genitals was significantly different compared to the prevalence in urethral canal with 9.8% hrHPV and 7.1% lrHPV, ($p= 0.0051$ and 0.0016, respectively). Prevalence and distribution of HPV-DNA types in samples collected from external genitals (glans, coronal sulcus and penile shaft) and urethral meatus demonstrate that the external genitals are more likely to be HPV positive, harboring the risk of transmission of HPV infection between sexual partners (Fig.5).

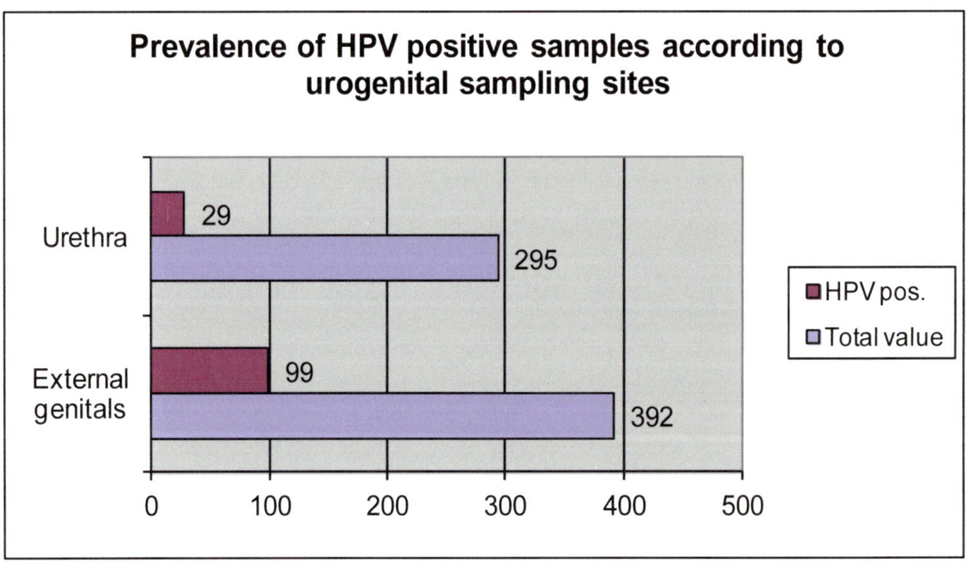

HPV pos - all samples with positive HPV DNA test result.

Fig. 4. Prevalence of HPV DNA positive samples related to different sampling site.

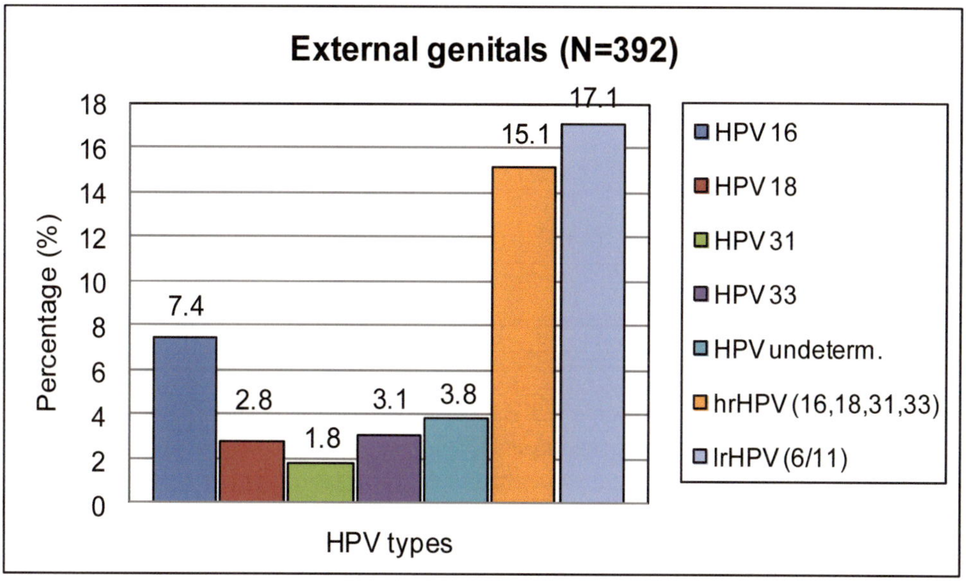

A

hrHPV-high risk HPV types; lrHPV-low risk HPV types; HPV undeterm.-unclassified HPV types.

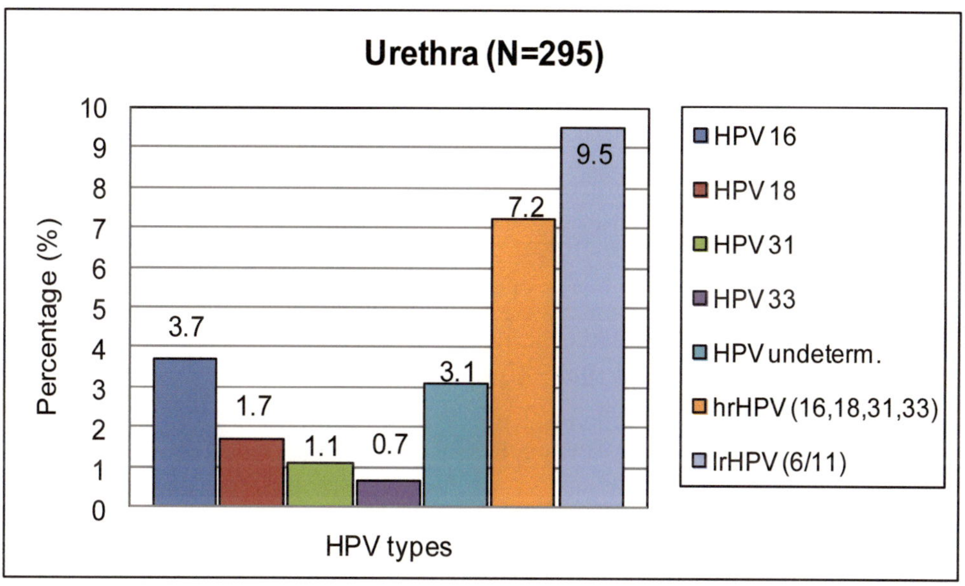

B

hrHPV-high risk HPV types; lrHPV-low risk HPV types; HPV undeterm.-unclassified HPV types.

Fig. 5. Prevalence and distribution of HPV-DNA types in samples collected A) from external genitals (glans, coronal sulcus and penile shaft) and B) urethral meatus.

Anatomical sites	HPV positive	HPV 6/11	HPV 16	HPV 18	HPV 31	HPV 33	HPV indeterm.	Multiple HPV infection
External genitals (N=392)	99 (25.3%)	67 (17.1%)	29 (7.4%)	11 (2.8%)	7 (1.8%)	12 (3.1%)	15 (3.8%)	18 (4.6%)
Urethra (N=295)	29 (9.8%)	28 (9.5%)	11 (3.7%)	5 (1.7%)	3 (1.1%)	2 (0.7%)	9 (3.1%)	7 (2.4%)

Table 2. Prevalence and distribution of HPV types in HPV DNA positive samples taken from external genitals and urethra. Multiple HPV infections made impact on overall HPV prevalence while they were counted more than once; values are number of HPV DNA positive samples and their percentage is indicated in parentheses. HPV positive = all samples with positive HPV DNA test result.

Category	hrHPV positives cases	HPV 16/18	HPV 31/33	External genitals N=392	Urethra N=295	p Fisher's exact test
	82	42	16			<0.0001
HPV positive cases per sampling sites				99 (25.3%)	29 (9.8%)	<0.0001
lrHPV types *per* sampling sites				67 (17.1%)	28 (9.5%)	0.0051
hrHPV types *per* sampling sites				59 (15.1%)	21 (7.1%)	0.0016

hrHPV-high risk HPV; lrHPV-low risk HPV

Table 3. Statistical evaluation of differences in prevalence of hrHPV- HPV16/18 compared to HPV31/33 and prevalence of lrHPV and hrHPV in relation to genital sampling sites.

4. Discussion

Many questions exist regarding clinical utility of HPV testing in men. Screening for HPV infection is not recommended for men for many reasons: infection is very common, no FDA-approved test is available and finding HPV infection does not indicate an increased risk of disease or cancer in men or their sexual partners. In addition, there is no specific treatment for HPV per se (Palefsky, 2007; 2010). The evaluation and treatment of male sexual partners of women with clinical or subclinical infection (genital warts or abnormal Pap smear results) is also not known to have a clinical benefit (Bleeker et al., 2002; 2005.)

Until the last few years relatively little was known about the epidemiology of penile HPV infection, in part due to the lack of standardization of penile cell sampling techniques for HPV DNA detection. Several techniques have been published and have been used to better define the prevalence, incidence, and clearance of penile HPV infection (Giuliano, 2007; 2011; Nielson, 2007). However, the epidemiology of penile disease, its relationship to HPV infection, and the role of penile disease in transmission of HPV between partners remains poorly understood (Palefsky, 2010). Global data on prevalence of HPV infection in men are essential for future efforts to prevent HPV-related diseases.

Recent literature data demonstrate a wide range of HPV DNA prevalence among men, depending on the study population and the type and number of anatomic sites evaluated.

In populations of similar age, the prevalence of specific HPV types is usually lower in men than in women (Partridge & Koutsky, 2006). Whether this observation could be related to natural history of HPV infection in men with lower incidence or shorter duration of infection has to be determined. Differences in sexual behaviour may also be important predictors of genital HPV infection (Partridge & Koutsky, 2006).

We have obtained similar results in the pilot study conducted in Zagreb from 2003 to 2004. The prevalence of HPV DNA was investigated by consensus and type specific PCR methods in the group of 340 patients attending the outpatient STD clinic (205 female and 135 male patients). The results demonstrated that overall HPV and hrHPV prevalence (HPV 16, 18, 31 and 33) in women was 43.4% and 22.4%, respectively, and in men 25.2% and 11.9%, respectively. The lrHPV prevalence (HPV 6 and 11) in women and men was almost the same (11.2% and 11.1%, respectively) (Grahovac, 2004, unpublished data).

To our knowledge, this was the first study to examine HPV prevalence among men in Croatia. The current retrospective cross-sectional study performed among men attending STD, urology and dermatovenerology outpatient clinics in Zagreb and Rijeka between 2006 and 2008 is the first large study performed in Croatia. During this period 581 men participated in the study. The overall prevalence of HPV DNA among men in current Croatian study group was 27.4% (159/581), which is almost identical result to our previous study. For comparison, the overall HPV prevalence in men in HPV Study group from Brazil, Mexico and USA (HIM Study) was between 40% to 72.3% in Brazil, between 42% to 44.6% in Mexico and between 28.2% to 45.5% in USA. In our study hrHPV was detected in 14.1% (82/581) and lrHPV in 13.8% (80/581) cases. Unclassified HPV type was identified in 4.1% (24/581) cases and HPV infection with multiple HPV types occurred in 4.3% (25/581) cases. In HIM Study prevalence of oncogenic HPV types (type 16 and 18) was detected in 8.2% cases while non-oncogenic types (6 and 11) were identified in 8.1% of participants.

Approximately 15% of men (10-20%) in HIM Study were positive for unclassified HPV types while in our study group it accounted only for 4.1% cases. The differences should be interpreted with caution since method of genotyping in HIM Study was based on hybridization, using Linear Array HPV genotyping test (Roche Diagnostics), while we were using type specific PCR method directed to recognize the main lrHPV and hrHPV types, relevant for prophylactic vaccination. Out of hrHPV positive specimens, HPV 16 was the predominant type found in 39 % cases, followed by HPV 18 (12.2%), HPV 31 (9.7%) and HPV 33 (9.7%). Our findings indicate that in asymptomatic male, prevalence of major hrHPV, HPV 16 and HPV 18 exceeded 51.2% (42/82). Statistical evaluation revealed that the prevalence of HPV16/18 is significantly different ($p<0.001$) compared to the prevalence of HPV31/33. HPV DNA detection was higher at the penile surface including glans/coronal sulcus and penile shaft with frequency of 25.3% (99/392), compared to 9.8% (29/295) in the urethra.

In HIM Study the prevalence of anogenital HPV infection, identified on the penis, scrotum, and perianal area, was remarkably constant as a function of age. The prevalence of anogenital HPV infection in these men was high, approximately 60%, a prevalence that is also remarkably similar to recent report of the age-related prevalence of HPV infection in men (Smith et al., 2011). In this global review, the data demonstrate that genital HPV infection in men varies widely, from 2 to 93%, both between and within high and low-risk men groups and by geographic region.

Giuliano et. al., 2011, presented recently in The Lancet a prospective study on the incidence and clearance of HPV infection in men. The results revealed important new information demonstrating considerable differences between the natural history of male and female HPV infection. Although the prevalence of HPV infection in men is higher or similar to that in women, the HPV-related disease rate in men is lower. Penile intraepithelial neoplasia (PIN) is 10-20 times less frequent than CIN and HPV-induced cancers of the penis, which are extremely rare (Monsonego, 2011).

HPV prevalence in men was between 1.3%-72.9% in studies in which multiple anatomic sites or specimens were evaluated; HPV prevalence varied on the basis of sampling and processing methods. The best anatomic sites for sampling in men—taking into consideration convenience of sampling, adequacy of the sample, and detection of HPV DNA—appear to be the glans, corona, prepuce, and shaft of the penis. It is possible that combined samples from these sites may be optimal. Scrotum samples are often adequate, but, in most studies, they were less likely to yield HPV DNA. The prepuce, when present, is possibly the best single site for HPV DNA detection. Specimens that are less useful include urine, semen, and urethral swabs. Semen and urethral specimens often have adequate β-globin and HPV DNA but are difficult and sometimes uncomfortable to collect. β-globin and HPV DNA detection is often poor from urine specimens, although these specimens could be the easiest to obtain (Bleeker et al. 2002, 2005; Weaver et al. 2004.; Lajous et al., 2005; Nielson et al., 2007; Dunne et al., 2006; Giuliano et al., 2007; D`Hauwers & Tjalma, 2009).

Persistent infection with hrHPV is the main risk factor for developing cervical, penile and anal cancer. Large and worldwide epidemiological studies will enable better understanding of natural history of HPV infection in men. They will also support the future decision making whether HPV infected men should be treated as HPV reservoir and transmitters of HPV disease and consequently screened for HPV.

5. Conclusion

Our study revealed that the overall prevalence of HPV DNA in Croatian men study group was 27.4% (159/581). HrHPV was detected in 14.1% (82/581) and lrHPV in 13.8% (80/581) cases, respectively. Out of hrHPV positive specimens, HPV 16 was the predominant type found in 39 % cases, followed by HPV 18 (12.2%), HPV 31 (9.7%) and HPV 33 (9.7%). Our findings indicate that in asymptomatic male carriers prevalence of oncogenic types, HPV 16 and 18 exceeded 51.2% (42/82). HPV DNA was detected more frequently at the penile surface, including glans/coronal sulcus and penile shaft, with 25.3% (99/392) positive samples, in comparison to 9.8% (29/295) positive sample in the urethra. The external genitals are more likely to be HPV positive, harbouring the higher risk of oncogenic HPV type transmission between sexual partners. Our study demonstrated that the optimal anatomic sites for sampling in men considering convenience of sampling, adequacy of the sample, and detection of HPV DNA—appear to be combined sample of scrapes from glans/coronal sulcus and penile shaft.

6. References

Baldwin, S.B., Wallace, D.R., Papenfuss, M.R., Abrahamsen, M., Vaught, L.C Kornegay, J.R., Hallum, J.A., Redmond, S.A. & Giuliano, A.R. (2003) Human Papillomavirus infection in men attending a sexually transmitted disease clinic, J Infect Dis, 187:1064–70.

Bleeker, M.C., Hogewoning, C.J., van den Brule, A.J., Voorhorst, F.J., Van Andel, R.E., Risse, E.K., Starink, T.M. & Meijer, C.J. (2002) Penile lesions and human papillomavirus in male sexual partners of women with cervical intraepithelial neoplasia. J Am Acad Dermatol. Vol.47, No.(3):351-357.

Bleeker, M.C., Hogewoning, C.J., Berkhof,J., Voorhorst, F.J., Hesselink, A.T., van Diemen, P.M., van den Brule, A.J. & Snijders, P.J. (2005). Concordance of specific human papillomavirus types in sex partners is more prevalent than would be expected by chance and is associated with increased viral loads. Clin Infect Dis, Vol.41, No.(5), pp.612-620.

Bleeker, M.C., Heideman, D.A., Snijders, P.J., Horenblas, S., Dillner,J. & Meijer C.J. (2008). Penile cancer: epidemiology, pathogenesis and prevention. World J Urol, Vol.27,No.(2), pp.141-150.

Bosch, F.X., Lorincz, A., Muñoz, N., Meije,r C.J. & Shah, K.V.(2002) The causal relation between human papillomavirus and cervical cancer. J Clin Patho, Vol.55, pp. 244-265.

Clifford, G.M., Gallus, S., Herrero, R., Muñoz, N., Snijders, PJ., Vaccarella, S., Anh,P.T., Ferreccio, C., Hieu, N.T., Matos, E., Molano, M., Rajkumar, R., Ronco, G., de Sanjose, S., Shin, H.R., Sukvirach, S., Thomas, J.O., Tunsakul, S., Meijer, C.J. & Franceschi, S. IARC HPV Prevalence Surveys Study Group. (2005). Worldwide distribution of human papillomavirus types in cytologically normal women in the International Agency for Research on Cancer. HPV prevalence surveys: a pooled analysis. Lancet, Vol.366, No.(9490), pp. 991-998.

Colon-Lopez, V., Ortiz, A.P. & Palefsky, J.M.(2010). Burden of Human Papillomavirus Infection and Related Comorbidities in Men. Implication for Research, Disease Prevention ana Health Promotion among Hispanic Men. P R Health Sci J, Vol.29, No.(3), pp. 232-240.

Croatian National Cancer Registry, Cancer Incidence in Croatia, Bulletin No. 33 Croatian National Institute of Public Health, Zagreb, 2008.

Dunne, E.F., Nielson, C.M., Stone, K.M., Markowitz, L.E. & Giuliano, A.R.(2006) Prevalence of HPV Infection among Men:A Systematic Review of the Literature.J Infect Dis, Vol.194, pp. 1044-1057.

zur Hausen, H. (2002). Papillomaviruses and cancer: from basic studies to clinical application. Nat Rev Cancer. Vol.2, pp. 342-350.

D`Hauwers, K.W. & Tjalma W.A. (2009). Screening for human papillomavirus: Is urine useful?.Indian J Cancer, Vol.46, pp. 190-193.

Elbasha, E.H. & Dasbach, E.J. (2010). Impact of vaccinating boys and men against HPV in the United States. Vaccine, Vol. 28, pp. 6858-6867.

Fujinaga, Y., Shimada, M., Okazawa,K., Fukushima, M., Kato, I. & Fujinaga, K. (1991). Simultaneous detection and typing of genital human papillomavirus DNA using the polymerase chain reaction. J Gen Virol, Vol. 72, pp. 1039-1044.

Garland, S.M. (2010). Prevention strategies against human papillomavirus in males. Gynecologic Oncology, Vol.117, pp. 520-525.

Giuliano, A.R., Nielson C.M., Flores, R., Dunne E.F., Abrahamsen, M., Papenfuss, M.R., Markowitz, L.E., Smith, D. & Harris, R.B. (2007). The optimal anatomic sites for sampling heterosexual men for human papillomavirus (HPV) detection: the HPV detection in men study. J Infect Dis, Vol.196, pp. 1146-1152.

Giuliano, A.R., Lee, J.H., Fulp, W., Villa, L.L., Lazcano, E., Papenfuss, M.R., Abrahamsen, M., Salmeron, J., Anic,G.M., Rollison, D.E. & Smith,D. (2011). Incidence and clearance of genital human papillomavirus infection in men (HIM): a cohort study. Lancet, Vol.377, No.(9769), pp. 932-940.

Grahovac, M., Račić, I., Hadžisejdić, I., Dorić, A. & Grahovac, B.(2007) Prevalence of Human Papillomavirus among Croatian Women Attending Regular Gynecological Visit. Coll Antropol, Vol.31, Suppl. (2), pp. 73-77.

Gravitt, P.E., Peyton, C.L.,Alessi, T.Q., Wheeler, C.M., Coutlee, F., Hildesheim, A., Schiffman, M.H., Scott, D.R. & Apple, R.J. (2000) Improved Amplification of Genital Human Papillomaviruses. J Clin Microbiol,Vol. 38, No.1, pp. 357-361.

Grce,M., Grahovac,B., Rukavina,T., Vrdoljak-Mozetič,D., Glavaš-Obrovac, Lj., Kaliterna, V. & Žele-Starčević, L. (2007) HPV Testing for Cervical Cancer Screening in Croatia. Coll Antropol, Vol. 31, Suppl.(2), pp. 67-71.

Hadžisejdić, I., Šimat, M., Bosak, A., Krašević, M. & Grahovac, B. (2007) Prevalence of Human Papillomavirus Genotypes in Cervical Cancer and Precursor Lesions. Coll Antropol, Vol.30, No.(4), pp. 315-319.

HPV and men-fact sheet.Centers for Disease Control and Prevention Web site. http://www.cdc.gov/std/hpv/STDFACT-HPV-and-men.htm. Accessed August 20, 2011.

HPV Study group in men from Brazil, USA and Mexico.(2008) Human Papillomavirus infection in men residing in Brazil, Mexico and the USA. Salud publica de Mexico, Vol.50, No. (5), pp. 408-418.

Lajous, M., Mueller, N., Cruz-Valdez, A., Aguilar, L.V., Franceschi, S., Hernandez-Avila, M. & Lazcano-Ponce, E. (2005) Determinants of prevalence, acquisition, and persistence of human papillomavirus in healthy Mexican military men. Cancer Epidemiol Biomarkers Prev Vol.14, No.(7), pp. 1710-1716.

Monsonego, J. (2011) Genital infection with HPV in men: research into practice. Lancet, Vol. 377, pp. 881-883.

Muñoz, N., Bosch, F.X., de Sanjosé, S., Herrero, R., Castellsagué, X., Shah, K.V., Snijders, P.J.F. & Meijer, C.J.L.M. (2003) International Agency for Research on Cancer Multicenter Cervical Cancer Study Group. Epidemiologic classification of human papillomavirus types associated with cervical cancer. N Engl J Med, Vol.348, pp. 518-527.

Nielson, C.M., Flores,R.,Harris R.B., Abrahamsen, M., Papenfuss, M.R., Dunne, E.F., Markowitz, L.E. & Giuliano, A.R.(2007) Human Papillomavirus Prevalence and Type Distribution in Male Anogenital Sites and Semen. Cancer Epidemiol Biomarkers Prev, Vol.16, No.(6), pp. 1107-1114.

Palefsky, J.M. (2007). HPV infection in men. Disease Markers, Vol.23, No.(4), pp. 261-272.

Palefsky, J.M. (2010). Human Papillomavirus-Related Disease in Man: Not Just a Women's Issue. J Adolesc Health , Vol.46, Suppl.(4), pp.S12-S19.

Partridge, J.M., Hughes, J.P., Feng, Q., Winer, R.L., Weaver, B.A., Xi, L.F., Stern, M.E., Lee, S.K., O'Reilly, S.F., Hawes, S.E., Kiviat, N.B. & Koutsky, L.A. (2007). Genital human papillomavirus infection in men: incidence and risk factors in a cohort of university students. J Infect Dis, Vol.196, No.(8), pp. 1128-1136.

Partridge, J.M. & Koutsky, L.A. (2006). Genital human papillomavirus infection in men. Lancet Infect Dis, Vol.6, pp. 21-31.

Shimada, M., Fukushima, M., Mukai, H., Kato, I., Nishikawa, A. & Fujinaga, K.(1990) Jpn J Cancer Res, Vol. 81, pp. 1-5.

Smith, J.S., Gilbert, P.A., Melendy, A., Rana, R.K. & Pimenta, J.M.(2011). Age-Specific Prevalence of Human Papillomavirus Infection in Males: A Global Review. J Adolest Health, Vol.48, No. (6), pp.540-552.

Stanley, M. (2007). Prophylactic HPV vaccines: prospects for eliminating ano-genital cancer. British Journal of Cancer, Vol.96, pp. 1320-1323.

Vardas, E., Giuliano, A.R., Goldstone, S., Palefsky, J.M., Moreira, E.D Jr., Penny, M.E., Aranda, C., Jessen, H., Moi, H., Ferris, D.G., Liaw, K-L., Marshall, B., Vuocolo, S., Barr, E., Haupt, R.M., Garner, E.I.O. & Guris, D. (2011). External genital human papillomavirus prevalence and associated factors among heterosexual men on 5 continents.J Infect Dis, Vol.203, No.(1), pp. 58-65.

Walboomers, J.M.M., Jacobs, M.M.V., Manos, M.M., Bosch, F.X., Kummer, J.A., Shah, K.V., Snijders, P.J.F., Peto, J., Meijer, C.J.L.M. & Munoz, N. (1999) Human papillomavirus is necessary cause of invasive cervical cancer worldwide. J Pathol, Vol.189, pp. 12-19.

WHO/ICO Information Centre on HPV and Cervical Cancer. Summary Report 2010. Web site. http://www.who.int/vaccine research/diseases/viral cancer. Accessed July 20, 2011.

Weaver, B.A., Feng, Q., Holmes, K.K.,Kiviat, N., Lee, S-K., & Meyer, C. (2004). Evaluation of genital sites and sampling technique for detection of human papillomavirus DNA in men. J Infect Dis, Vol.189, pp. 677-685.

8

Human Papilloma Virus and Anal Cancer

João Batista de Sousa and Leonardo de Castro Durães
University of Brasilia
Brazil

1. Introduction

Anal cancer is a rare tumor, whose incidence has increased in recent years. Its incidence is approximately 1.5 / 100,000 in the general population (Jemal et al, 2009, Siegel et al, 2011). Historically anal cancer is more common in women, however the incidence in men has been increasing, especially among those who practice anal sex with men (MSM).

Among the risk factors are human papillomavirus (HPV), smoking, immunosuppression and anal sex (Uronis et al, 2007)

The most common anal cancer is the squamous cell carcinoma. It may be keratinized or non-keratinized. Adenocarcinoma may occur, however, it resembles the lower rectal cancer and should follow its principles of treatment. (Nivatvongs, 2006) According to the World Health Organization (WHO), approximately 80% of tumors of the anal canal are squamous cell type and these are divided in squamous cell carcinoma tumors, basaloid (cloacogenic) and mucoepidermoid. In this classification of tumors of the anal region, WHO considers the anal verge, anal canal, the anal transition zone and the rectal type mucosae of the anal canal. Therefore, other histological types of tumors can arise in the anal canal. Adenocarcinomas may originate in the rectal type mucosae in the anal canal and in the path of a long evolution anal fistula or in the epithelium of the anal glands. Other tumors may be lymphoma, melanoma, Kaposi's sarcoma, Bowen's disease and Paget's disease. (Table 1)

HISTOLOGICAL TYPE	ORIGIN
SQUAMOUS CELL CARCINOMA	SKIN AND ANAL VERGE
ADENOCARCINOMA	RECTAL TYPE MUCOSAE ANAL GLANDS FISTULA'S PATH
LYMPHOMAS	ANAL CANAL
MELANOMA	ANAL CANAL ANAL VERGE
KAPOSI	ANAL CANAL ANAL VERGE
BOWEN	ANAL VERGE
PAGET	ANAL VERGE

Table 1. Histological types of malignant tumors of the anal canal and its origin in the anorectal region.

The human papilloma virus (HPV) belongs to Papillomavirus genus of the family Papillomaviridae. It causes the lesion called condyloma acuminata (from the greek "Kondilus", that means rounded tumor, and the latin "acuminare" meaning make sharp). Infection by HPV is a sexually transmitted viral disease most common in sexually active population. According to the Centers for Disease Control and Prevention (CDC) between 1966 and 1981 there was a 500% increase in the incidence of condyloma acuminata. In 1996 it was estimated that the incidence per year was 500 thousand to 1 million new cases and 25% of the population was infected. Therefore, the Human Papilloma Virus (HPV) is the most common sexually transmitted disease. Its association with cervical cancer is well established. However, their role in anal cancer as the primary cause, not just as a cofactor, is being increasingly accepted. There are several serotypes of HPV, with different risks of inducing cancer.

2. Anatomy of the anal canal

The anal canal is a small area that extends from the anal verge to the rectal mucosa, bypassing the dentate line. It is a complex area that has different histological features. The diversity of cells in this region is wide for being the junction of embryonic layers. According to World Health Organization (WHO), the anal canal is defined as the terminal part of the large intestine, beginning at the upper surface of the anorectal ring and passing through the pelvic floor at the anus. The lower part extends from the dentate line and downwards to the anal verge. This was therefore the surgical anal canal. The lateral limit is 5 to 6 cm from anal verge. (Nivatvongs, 2006). The skin of the anal margin consists of a keratinized squamous epithelium and eccrine and apocrine glands and other appendages such as hair follicles and may thus be compromised for any condition that affects the skin itself and its structures such as malignant tumors.

Lymphatic drainage above the dentate line is for the lymphatic chain of the lower mesenteric vessels passing trough the lymphatic chain of the superior rectal vessels. Lymphatic drainage below the dentate line runs to the inguinal lymph nodes.

The anal canal represents the end of the squamous mucosa and the beginning of a transition zone for non-squamous mucosa. There is a transition from squamous epithelium to an immature epithelium, in which a squamous epithelium overlaps a columnar epithelium, to a squamous metaplastic area of tissue that occurs above the dentate line, which has a columnar epithelium.

Therefore tumors of this region may be keratinized or non-keratinized, but with similar biology and prognosis.

3. Human Papilloma Virus (HPV)

HPV is a sexually transmitted disease of high incidence. HPV is a DNA Papilloma virus with an 8-kilobase genome. Systematic reviews of the literature showed a prevalence of genital HPV infection ranging from 1.3% to 72.9%. These variations are due to different study populations and different diagnostic methods. (Dietz et al. 2011, Uronis et al. 2007, Bean et al. 2009, Chin Hong et al. 2004, Darragh et al. 2011, Fox 2006, Giuliano et al. 2010)

In most patients, the virus is rapidly recognized by the immune system, with only 1% of patients developing clinical symptoms of infection (anal warts). The estimated prevalence of subclinical infection varies between 10 and 46% (Welton et al. 2004)

Transmission of the virus is not entirely preventable by using condoms and sexual abstinence is the only way to effective prevention. The virus can remain in the secretion at the base of the penis and scrotum, making the condoms ineffective.

Chronic infection occurs in a minority of patients who are exposed to HPV. For this to occur the virus must gain access to the basal and parabasal cells of the anorectal transition zone through erosion or disruption of normal mucosal barrier, which can occur in anal sex, anorectal trauma from other causes, or concomitant presence of infections of other sexually transmitted diseases. There are more than 80 different subtypes of HPV. Among them, at least 23 have potential for infection of the anogenital mucosa. Each subtype has a different potential to induce malignancy. HPV 6 and 11 serotypes are most associated with genital warts and have less oncogenic potential. Already serotypes 16,18,31, 33, 35, 39, 45, 50, 51, 53, 56, 58, 59 and 68 are most commonly identified in high-grade dysplasia or carcinoma (Uronis et al, 2007). The serotype can be evidenced by specific test for DNA. Serotype 16 is the most prevalent and associated with 70% of cases of anal cancer.

Anal warts are a benign condition not associated with mortality. However, it is a disease that causes psychosocial stress, shame and embarrassment. The incubation period is 3 weeks to 8 months; most of them develop 2-3 months after infection with HPV. Over 90% of warts are caused by serotypes 6 and 11, however approximately one third achieve co-infection with oncogenic serotypes.

Several cancers are attributed to HPV infection. These include cancers of the cervix, vagina, vulva, penis, oral cavity, head and neck and anal canal. The two most common HPV-associated cancers are anal cancer and cervical cancer. Both occur in the mucous epithelium, while anal cancer also occurs in the perianal keratinized epithelium.

Several epidemiological studies have assessed the association between HPV and anal CA. In a recent study, DURAES and SOUSA showed a strong correlation between CA and anal HPV in Brazil. (Duraes & Sousa, 2010)

Anal sex is the major risk factor for HPV infection, but heterosexual men who did not have sex with men may present with HPV infection.

The prevalence of HPV infection in men who have sex with men (MSM) HIV negative reaches 57% (Chin-Hong et al, 2004)

4. Anal cancer

Anal cancer accounts for approximately 2.6% of carcinomas of the large intestine. Its incidence is increasing in the United States, Europe and South America. The American incidence has been increasing over the past 40 years. In 2003, there was an estimated 4,000 new cases in the United States. In 2007, about 4650 new cases, and in 2009 the number was estimated to be 5,290 new cases (2100 men and 3190 women). In 2011 the figure was 5820 new cases (2140 men and 3680 women) (Siegel et al, 2011).

The incidence rate is higher in women in all age groups, however the incidence in men has increased. The incidence rates are 1.4 per 100,000 in men and 1.7 per 100,000 in women.

Anal cancer was initially associated with chronic inflammatory conditions such as Crohn's disease. Then viral genital infections were associated. HPV infection, with or without immune compromise was seen as the main risk factor for the development of anal dysplasia, which is the precursor lesion of anal cancer.

Other associated risk factors are anal sex, number of sexual partners, smoking and history of anal warts. For women the history of vulvar intraepithelial neoplasia and high-grade cervical or vulvar cancer are considered risk factors. Imunossupressed post-transplant patients are also considered high risk.

The populations most at risk for anal cancer are men who have sex with men (MSM), regardless of HIV infection. Other risk groups are imunossupressed individuals and HIV positive.

Although it is a rare cancer, the incidence in men who have sex with men (MSM) HIV-positive has been increasing, especially in those using antiretroviral therapies. The incidence of anal cancer in HIV-negative MSM is approximately 35 per 100000. In the HIV-positive MSM the incidence range from 42 to 137 per 100,000 per year.

Symptoms include rectal bleeding (in half of patients), pain, and rectal mass sensation. 20% of patients have no symptoms. Cancer of the anal canal extends to the rectum or perianal skin in half of the cases.

Anal cancer can give metastases via the lymphatic system, and less frequently, can be hematogenous. Anal cancer below the dentate line is at risk of metastasis to the inguinal and femoral nodes. Above the dentate line the risk of metastasis is to the perirectal lymph nodes.

The diagnosis in early stage is possible by clinical evaluation by detecting the presence of a papular nodule or tumor in the anal canal, of varying size and hardness, which may be fixed or not the muscle planes. You can often see a fissure at the anal inspection, presenting itself as an ulcerated lesion with raised borders and irregular, hard, lumpy, very painful that easily bleeds when touched. Proctological examination for evaluation and biopsy is often only possible with the anesthetized patient. In advanced disease, vegetative ulcers lesions are often observed, advancing extensively to the perineum, vulva, vagina and sacrococigeal region. These advanced lesions can cause pain to urinate, evacuate or even walk. The not diagnosed, untreated disease evolves compromising the anal sphincter apparatus and leads to progressive stenosis of the anal canal and can result in fecal incontinence and production of foul-smelling discharge. The differential diagnosis should be done with various anorectal diseases, and the anal fissure disease that requires further attention. The typical pain of the fissure that occurs after the evacuation can also occur in early carcinoma, but with the progression of the disease the pain becomes continuous, persistent and almost unbearable. The atypical location, outside the median line and above the dentate line is important data to rule out idiopathic anal fissure.

5. Anal cancer staging

The staging for anal cancer is done through the TNM system (tumor, node, metastasis). The TNM is based on the anatomical extent, where T refers to the primary tumor, N refers to lymph node metastases, and M refers to the presence or absence of distant metastases.

As for the T rating:

Tis or carcinoma in situ.

T1: Tumor measures 2 cm or less.

T2: Tumor is between 2 and 5 cm.

T3: Tumor is larger than 5 cm.

T4: Tumor of any size invading adjacent structures such as the urethra, vagina or bladder.

Regarding the classification N:

N0: No lymph node metastases

N1: Metastasis in perirectal lymph nodes

N2: Unilateral metastasis in inguinal lymph nodes or unilateral internal iliac nodes

N3: Bilateral metastasis in inguinal lymph nodes or bilateral internal iliac

As for the M rating:

M0: No distant metastases.

M1: Distant metastases.

6. Staging

The staging of anal carcinoma requires a digital rectal exam, a CT scan of chest, abdomen and pelvis. In any suspicion of affected lymph nodes, fine needle aspiration biopsy should be performed. The use of PET CT is not well established.

Stage	T	N	M
Stage 0	Tis	N0	M0
Stage I	T1	N0	M0
Stage II	T2	N0	M0
Stage II	T3	N0	M0
Stage III A	T1, T2, T3	N1	M0
Stage III A	T4	N1	M0
Stage III B	T4	N1	M0
Stage III B	Any T	N2, N3	M0
Stage IV	Any T	Any N	M1

Table 2. TNM Staging for Anal Cancer.

The gynecological examination, including cervical cancer screening is recommended for women with anal cancer. The HIV test is recommended. In case of positivity, CD4 levels should be evaluated.

The endoanal ultrasound, especially with three-dimensional view, helps in assessing the depth of tumor invasion and involvement of adjacent nodes.

7. Natural history of high grade squamous intraepithelial lesions and anal cancer

Much of the information about anal cancer, because of its low incidence, is extrapolated from cervical cancer. This extrapolation is due to the great similarity between the histology and histopathology of the tissues involved.

HPV can lead to formation of anal warts, low-grade squamous intraepithelial lesion (LSIL), high-grade squamous intraepithelial lesion (HSIL) and cancer. The mechanisms of progression of lesions in the anal canal are not fully elucidated. (Ortoski & Kell, 2011)

The development of squamous cell carcinoma of the anus appears to be similar to squamous cell carcinoma of the cervix, which means, transition from anal low-grade squamous intraepithelial lesions (LSIL) for anal high-grade squamous intraepithelial lesions (HSIL) and then to squamous cell carcinoma.

Genital warts are typically caused by serotypes of HPV that are at low risk for induction of carcinoma. LSIL can be identified in association with warts, especially those flat lesions. The presence of concomitant condylomatous lesions and HSIL is uncommon in immunocompetent patients. However, in immunocompromised patients, HSIL is usually found in association with genital warts. These patients have infections with multiple HPV types, compared with immunocompetent patients, which may explain this finding.

Both the cervix and the anal canal have regions of metaplasia replacing glandular epithelium with squamous epithelium. HPV infects the basal cells causing an interruption in the cycle of cell differentiation and maturation of precursors leading to the development of cancer.

The virus interferes with the mechanisms of the cell cycle, resulting in cell proliferation during latency. There is a loss of cell cycle inhibition through the action of two viral genes E6 and E7. The E7 interferes with the cell cycle, allowing the cell to progress from G1 to S phase. The events caused by E7 are not sufficient for malignant transformation. Accumulated genetic errors in cell replication are necessary for malignant transformation, which is consistent with the fact that chronic infection with HPV is necessary for the onset of cancer. The accumulation of genetic errors is facilitated by E6. This protein binds to p53, leading to degradation it. The p53 protein is a protein important for regulating the cell cycle that leads to apoptosis of cells with accumulated genetic errors, preventing replication errors.

Taking into account the high incidence of HSIL in HIV-positive MSM, it appears that only a minority will progress to cancer, but it is not possible to predict which lesions will progress, regress or persist.

The prevalence of high-grade squamous intraepithelial lesions (HSIL) confirmed by biopsy is very high: approximately 50% of homosexual HIV positive and 25% of HIV negative MSM.

High-grade anal dysplasia in HIV-positive men can progress to invasive cancer within a short period of time (Kreuter et al, 2010)

The role of HIV infection in anal cancer has not been elucidated. Population studies failed to show a correlation, including a study by the authors of epidemiological data in Brazil. The use of antiretroviral therapy and increased survival of HIV-positive can change this data in the future.

8. Histopathology of intraepithelial lesions and anal cancer

The classification follows the same cytological classification of cervical cytology:

ASCUS: Atypical Squamous Cells Undetermined Significance

ASCH: Atypical Squamous Cells suspicious for HSIL

ASIL: Atypical Squamous intraepithelial Lesion

LSIL: Low-grade Squamous intraepithelial Lesion

HSIL: High-grade Squamous intraepithelial Lesion

SCC: Squamous Cell Carcinoma

Histological classification terminology follows below:

AIN: Anal intraepithelial neoplasia

AIN 1: Mild dysplasia

AIN 2: Moderate dysplasia

AIN 3: Severe dysplasia / carcinoma in situ

Invasive Anal Carcinoma

The LSIL corresponds to an AIN. The HSIL corresponds to AIN2, carcinoma in situ or AIN3. The ASCUS and ASCH don`t have all the features of HSIL, but are not classified as benign.

Anal cancer is classified by degree of differentiation and histogenesis.

There are several microscopic appearances, including large-cell keratinizing, large-cell and basaloid nonkeratinizing. The term cloacogênic carcinoma is used to basaloid tumors and forms of non-keratinized squamous cell carcinoma.

Although squamous intraepithelial lesions and squamous cell carcinoma lesions are most often found, the distinction between squamous cell carcinoma poorly differentiated and other lesions such as lymphoma and melanoma can be difficult, sometimes requiring use of immunohistochemistry.

9. Screening

The screening performed in cervical cancer led to a decrease in the incidence of cancer with early detection of pre malignant lesions. Taking into account the similarity between anal cancer and cervical cancer, there are proposals for population screening for anal cancer. (Darragh & Winkler, 2011)

The goal of screening is to identify and treat cancer and early high grade squamous intraepithelial lesion (HSIL). As in cervical cancer, anal cytology is classified as atypical squamous cells of undetermined significance (ASCUS), atypical squamous cells suspicious for HSIL (ASCH), low grade squamous intraepithelial lesion (LSIL), high-grade squamous intraepithelial lesion (HSIL) or cancer.

The introduction of population screening programs for high-grade squamous intraepithelial lesion (HSIL) is limited by little evidence that interventions alter the natural history of HPV infection and progression to anal cancer. No randomized clinical trial was conducted to validate any form of screening for anal cancer. In specific groups of patients who have an increased incidence, as men who have sex with men (MSM), the screening should be performed. In this group of patients the incidence of cancer is comparable with cervical cancer where screening is routinely performed.

The simplest screening test is the digital anal-rectal exam. The lesions would be palpable, even in the absence of clinical symptoms. This technique, although inexpensive, is not commonly used.

Anal cytology has been used since 2005, but there is still a difficulty in their interpretation. The purpose of anal cytology is to take samples of all the anal canal, including the transformation zone. Samples of cells are collected by a swab inserted into the anal canal through the dentate line, thus allowing the collection of samples of the distal rectal wall. The cytology identifies intraepithelial lesions as LSIL, HSIL, and cancer in situ. The differential diagnosis of HSIL and cancer (early invasive ASCC) is difficult. Therefore biopsy for diagnostic confirmation is necessary (Bean & Chhieng, 2009).

A cost-effectiveness proposal is anal cytology testing every 1 to 2 years in HIV positive and men who have sex with men (MSM) HIV negative (Lam et al, 2011).

The hybrid capture test can complement cytology, with the identification of serotypes of HPV anal cancer precursors.

Taking into account the similarities with cervical cancer, was introduced a form of anal colposcopy, called high-resolution anoscopy (HRA). The HRA is indicated in those patients in whom cytology showed ASCUS, ASCH, LSIL or HSIL. Similar to colposcopy, adequate equipment and training are needed. An anoscope is introduced to approximately 2 cm from the anus, allowing visualization of the dentate line and the transitional zone. It is applied a solution of 3% acetic acid. Using a gynecological standard colposcope with a light source and lens with a magnification of 20 to 30 times, the examiner tries to identify areas of dysplasia. The Lugol iodine solution is then applied revealing dysplastic areas. Vascular changes such as neovascularization, venous interruption, changes in venous caliber are also suggestive of malignant tissues. Guided biopsies are performed in these abnormal areas. A biopsy is the gold standard for identification of squamous intraepithelial lesions.

10. Treatment of high grade squamous intraepithelial lesions (HSIL)

There is ample evidence that HSIL is the precursor to anal cancer, although the rate of progression to cancer is unknown.

Several treatments are recommended for the HSIL, which is a benign lesion and it takes a long time for malignant transformation.

The use of electrocautery has the advantage of being easily accessible in various surgical environments. It is less morbid than surgical excision, especially in extensive lesions. A disadvantage is that it doesn`t allows the histopathology of the lesion, and may not identify an invasive carcinoma. The recurrence with use of electrocautery is 79% in 12 months, with 100% risk at 50 months in HIV positive men. The use of high-resolution anoscopy contributes to the identification of lesions to be cleared.

A complete excision of the anal transition zone is possible, however may impair continence, being reserved for early carcinomas. Depending on the size of the lesion, the use of flaps may be necessary for the reconstruction of the skin. Surveillance anoscopy with high resolution is recommended.

In well-defined lesion with the use of Infra-Red Coagulation (IRC) can be attempted.

Topical agents may be tried. Imiquimod is an immune response modifier with potent antiviral and antitumor activity. It has been used to treat warts, basal cell carcinoma, vulvar intraepithelial neoplasia, squamous cell carcinomas of the skin, herpes and others. The application of imiquimod is safe, effective and promising in the treatment of HSIL. Topic 5% 5-fluorouracil (5FU) may be used in combination with imiquimod.

Another topical agent cidofovir is promising. This is a 1% gel used 5 days a week for 6 weeks for effective control of HPV. When used in intraepithelial lesions, this was proven effective in several cases (Snoek et al, 2000).

Liquid nitrogen, as well as cryotherapy, may be used.

11. Treatment of anal cancer

Prevention and early detection of anal cancer is of paramount importance due to the impact on survival. Patients with localized cancer of the anus have a five-year survival rate of approximately 80%. Patients with metastases have a survival rate of 30%.

The radio chemotherapy is the gold standard for treatment of anal cancer. Surgical treatment may be performed.

Surgical excision may be used in early carcinomas, well differentiated that did not exceed the submucosa. This type of treatment has a recurrence rate of 20 to 78% with a 5-year survival from 45 to 85%. This treatment should be used in selected cases. Mobile lesions smaller than 2 cm are candidates for this treatment modality.

The abdomino-perineal amputation was the most widely used form of treatment in the past. Although this treatment is aggressive, the results are not encouraging. The recurrence is 27% to 50% and 5-year survival ranges from 24% to 62% with a mortality rate of 2-6%. Currently, the abdomino-perineal amputation is reserved for those patients who do not tolerate radio chemotherapy. This operation is also indicated in cases of treatment failure by radio chemotherapy.

Treatment with radio chemotherapy was initiated in 1974 by Nigro et al. The treatment involves the use of radiotherapy combined with 5-fluorouracil (5 FU) and mitomycin C. This form of treatment proposed by Nigro was used initially as a neoadjuvant regimen for abdomino-perineal amputation. After 6 weeks the patients underwent operation. Nigro noted that a number of surgical specimens showed complete pathological response, which led him to propose exclusive radio chemotherapy treatment. Other studies have been performed comparing radiotherapy alone with radio chemotherapy, showing the superiority of radio chemotherapy. Studies have also shown a better therapeutic response with the use of mitomycin C associated with radiotherapy and 5 FU, despite its greater toxicity.

The radio chemotherapy has complications such as dermatitis, mucositis, diarrhea, fecal incontinence, bone marrow depression, cystitis, enteritis and vascular involvement.

In cases of failure to treat with radio chemotherapy, new sessions of radiation or surgical treatment of redemption can be realized.

Brachytherapy is used as an alternative to radiotherapy with the aim of preserving adjacent organs from radiation. It is still in studies to date.

HIV patients are treated with a lower dose of radio chemotherapy than for HIV-negative patients, due to increased risks of toxicity in these patients.

Metastatic disease appears in 10 to 17% of patients treated with radio chemotherapy. The most common site of metastasis is the liver. Treatment includes chemotherapy 5 FU combined with cisplatin, carboplatin, doxorubicin and semustine.

12. Prognosis

The 5-year survival for anal cancer is 80.1% for localized anal cancer, 60.7% for regional disease, and 29.4% for metastatic disease. The nodal involvement, T stage, and male are predictors of distant metastases, high rate of colostomy, and a worse survival with the use of radio chemotherapy. HIV-positive patients with low CD4 counts and high viral load has worse prognosis. (Abbas, 2010)

13. HPV vaccination

In 2006, the first U.S. FDA prophylactic vaccine against HPV was approved. The quadrivalent vaccine has proved effective in preventing infection against HPV 16, 18, 6 and 11 in healthy women. The bivalent vaccine is effective against serotypes 16 and 18. The vaccine is recommended for women from 11 to 26 years of age before the onset of sexual activity.

As for male vaccination, is still controversial. Among the benefits related to the vaccine in males, is prevention of penile cancer, beyond the indirect benefits that women have with male vaccination. In countries like the United States, only 37% of eligible women received the vaccine in 2008. Vaccinating men might increase protection against HPV in both men and women. There is a recommendation to vaccinate men from 9 to 26 years of age.

Although the vaccine is effective in preventing cervical HPV infection, is still uncertain protection of their anal infection. Studies show the prevention of intraepithelial neoplasia type 2 and 3.

There are doubts about vaccination of HIV-positive, since the vaccine response in immunocompromised patients is uncertain. (Anderson, 2009)

14. Conclusion

Anal cancer, particularly squamous cell carcinoma is a disease whose incidence is increasing. Prevention and early diagnosis is the key to reducing mortality caused by the disease. The prevalence of HPV is currently too high and its prevention and detection constitutes a major medical challenge. HPV has an important role in the pathogenesis of anal carcinoma, especially in immunocompromised patients. Risk group subjects should take precautions. The HPV vaccine can reduce the incidence of disease in the near future and contribute significantly in reducing mortality from anal cancer.

15. References

Abbas A, Yang G, Fakih M. (2010). Management of anal cancer in 2010. *Oncology* Vol. 24, No. 4, (April 2010), pp. 364-369.

Anderson JS, Hoy J, Hillman R, et al. (2009). A randomized, placebo-controlled, dose-escalation study to determine the safety, tolerability, and immunogenicity of an HPV-16 therapeutic vaccine in HIV-positive participants with oncogenic HPV infection of the anus. *J Acquir Immune Defic Syndr* Vol.52, No.3, (November 2009), pp.371-381.

Bean S, Chhieng DC. (2009). Anal-rectal cytology: a review. *Diagnostic Cytopathology* Vol.38, No.7, (2009), pp.538-546.

Chang G J, Berry J M, Jay N et al. (2002). Surgical treatment of high-grade anal squamous intraepithelial lesions. *Diseases of the colon & Rectum* Vol.45, No.4, (april 2002), pp.453-458.

Chin-Hong PV, Vittinghoff E, Cranston RD et al. (2004). Age-specific prevalence of anal human papillomavirus infection in HIV-negative sexually active men who have sex with men: the EXPLORE study. *The Journal of Infectious Diseases* Vol.190, (December 2004), pp.2070-2076

Czoski-Murray C, Karnon J, Jones R et al. (2010). Cost effectiveness of screening high-risk HIV-positive men who have sex with men(MSM) and HIV-positive women for anal cancer. *Health Technology Assessment* Vol.14, No.53, (November 2010)

Darragh TM, Winkler B. (2011). Anal cancer and cervical cancer screening: key differences. *Cancer Cytopathology* Vol.119, (February 2011), pp.5-19.

Dietz CA, Nyberg CR. (2011). Genital, oral, and anal human papillomavirus infection in men who have sex with men. *J Am Osteopath Assoc* Vol 111, Supplement 2, No3, (March 2011), pp.S19-S25.

Durães LC, Sousa JB. (2010). Anal cancer and sexually transmitted diseases: What.is the correlation? *Revista do Colégio Brasileiro de Cirurgia* Vol.37, No.4, (2010), pp.265-268.

Fox PA. (2006). Human papillomavirus and anal intraepithelial neoplasia. *Current Opinion in infectious Diseases* vol. 19, (2006), pp.62-66.

Galani E, Christodoulou C. (2009). Human papilloma viruses and cancer in the post-vaccine era. *European Society of Clinical Microbiology and Infectious Deseases* Vol.15, (2009), pp.977-981.

Garnock-Jones K, Giuliano A R. (2011). Quadrivalent human pipillomavirus (HPV) types 6,11,16,18 vaccine for the prevention of genital warts in males. *Adis Drugs Profile* Vol.71, No.5, (2011), pp.591-602.

Giuliano A R, Lee J H, Fulp W et al. (2011). Incidence and clearance of genital human papillomavirus infection in men (HIM): a cohort study. *Lancet* Vol. 377, (March 12, 2011), pp.932-940 .

Giuliano A R, Anic G, Nyitray A G. (2010). Epidemiology and pathology of HPV disease in males. *Gynecology Oncology* Vol.117, (2010), pp.s15-s19.

Gervaz P, Habnloser D, Wolff B G, et al. (2004). Molecular biology of squamous cell carcinoma of the anus: a comparison of HIV-positive and HIV-negative patients. *The Society for Surgery of the Alimentary Tract* Vol. 8, No. 8, (2004), pp.1024-1031.

Goldstone SE, Moshier E. (2010). Detection of oncogenic human papillomavirus impacts anal screening guidelines in men who have sex with men. *Diseases of the Colon & Rectum* Vol.53, (2010), pp.1135-1142.

Goodman M T, McDuffie K, Hernandez B Y et al. (2011). The influence of multiple human papillomavirus types on the risk of genotype-concordant incident infections of the anus and cervix: the Hawaii HPV cohort study. *The Journal of Infectious Diseases* Vol.203, (February 2011), pp.335-340 .

Herfs M, Hubert P, Moutschen M et al. (2011). Mucosal junctions: open doors to HPV and HIV infections? *Trends in Microbiology* Vol.19, No.3, (March 2011), pp.114-120.

http://www.seer.cancer.gov/statfacts/html/anus.html

Jemal A, Siegel R, Ward E, et al. (2009). Cancer statistics, 2009. *CA A Cancer Journal for Clinicians* Vol.59, (2009), pp.225-249.

Kreuter A, Potthoff NH, Bockmeyer T et al. (2010). Anal carcinoma in human immunodeficiency virus-positive men: results of a prospective study from Germany. *British Journal of Dermatology* Vol.162, (2010), pp.1269-1277.

Lam JMC, Hoch JS, Tinmouth J et al. (2011). Cost-effectiveness of screening for anal precancers in HIV-positive men. *AIDS* Vol.25, No.5, (2011), pp.635-642, ISSN 0269-9370.

Lu B, Viscidi RP, Lee JH et al. (2011). Human papillomavirus (HPV) 6,11,16, and 18 seroprevalence is associated with sexual practice and age: results from the multinational HPV infection in men study (HIM study). *Cancer Epidemiology, Biomarkers & Prevention* Vol.20, (May 2011), No5, pp.990-1002.

Mavrogianni P, Alexandrakis G, Stefanaki C et al. (2011). The role of cytology and HPV typing as a screening tool in patients with intraanal warts. *J Clin Gastroenterol* Vol.45, No.4, (April 2011), pp.e39-e43.

McCormack P L, Joura E A. (2010). Quadrivalent human papillomavirus (types 6,11,16,18) recombinant vaccine (Gardasil). *Adis Drugs Evaluation* Vol.70, No.18, (2010), pp.2449-2474.

Nahas C, Lin O, Weiser M R et al. (2006). Prevalence of perianal intraepithelial neoplasia in HIV-infected patients referred for high-resolution anoscopy. *Diseases of the colon & rectum* Vol.49, (October 2006), pp.1581-1586.

Nielsen A, Munk C, Kjaer S. (2011). Trends in incidence of anal cancer and high-grade anal intraepithelial neoplasia in Denmark, 1978-2008. *International Journal of Cancer* (2011), pp.1-6.

Nigro ND, Seydel HG, Considine B et al. (1983). Combined preoperative radiation and chemotherapy for squamous cell carcinoma of the anal canal. *Cancer* Vol. 51, (1983), pp.1826-1829.

Nigro ND, Vaitkevicius VK, Considine B Jr. (1974). Combined therapy for cancer of the anal canal: A preliminary report. *Diseases of the Colon and Rectum* Vol.17, (1974), pp. 354-356.

Nivatvongs S. (2006). Perianal and Anal Canal Neoplasms, In: *Neoplasms of the Colon, Rectum, and Anus 2nd edition*, Gordon PH, Nivatvongs S, pp.305-326, Informa healthcare, ISBN-13: 978-0-8247-2959-2, New York

Ortoski RA, Kell CS. (2011). Anal cancer and screening guidelines for human papillomavirus in men. *J Am Osteopath Assoc* Vol 111, Supplement 2, No3, (March 2011), pp.S35-S43.

Palefsky J. (2009). Human papillomavirus-related disease in people with HIV. *Current Opinion in HIV and AIDS* vol. 4 (2009) pp. 52-56.

Palefsky J. (2008). Human papillomavirus and anal neoplasia. *Current HIV/AIDS Reports* vol. 5, (2008), pp. 78-85.

Piketty C, Darragh TM, Costa MD et al. (2003). High prevalence of anal human papillomavirus infection and anal cancer precursors among HIV-infected persons in the absence of anal intercourse. *Annals of Internal Medicine* Vol.138, No6, (March 2003), pp.453-459.

Ramamoorthy S, Liu Y T, Loo L at al. (2010). Detection of multiple human papillomavirus genotypes in anal carcinoma. *Infectious Agents and Cancer http://www.infectagentscancer.com/content/5/1/17* Vol.5, No.17, (2010), pp.1-5.

Siegel R, Ward E, Brawley O et al. (2011). Cancer statistics, 2011. *CA A Cancer Journal for Clinicians* Vol.61, No.4, (July/August 2011), pp212-236.

Silva I T C, Gimenez F S, Galvao R S. (2011) Performance of p16 immunocytochemistry as a marker of anal squamous intraepithelial lesions. *Cancer Cytopathology* (jun 2011), pp.167-176.

Sobhani I, Vuagnat A, Walker F, et al. (2001). Prevalence of high-grade dysplasia and cancer in the anal canal in human papillomavirus-infected individuals. *Gastroenterology* Vol. 120, no. 4, (2001), pp.857-866.

Snoeck R, Noel JC, Muller C, et al. (2000). Cidofovir, a new approach for the treatment of cervix intraepithelial neoplasia grade III. *Journal Medical Virology* Vol.60, (2000), pp. 205-209.

Uronis HE, Bendell JC. (2007). Anal Cancer: An Overview. *The Oncologist* Vol.12, (2007), pp.524-534.

Veo C A R, Saad S S, Nicolau S M et al. (2008). Study on the prevalence of human papillomavirus in the anal canal of women with cervical intraepithelial neoplasia grade III. *European Journal of Obstetrics & Gynecology andReprodutive Biology* Vol. 140, (2008), pp.103-107.

Welton M L, Sharkey F E, Kahlenberg M S. (2004). The etiology and epidemiology of anal cancer. *Surgical Oncology Clinics of North America* Vol.13, (2004), pp.263-275.

Wilkin T, Lee J Y, Leasing S Y et al. (2010). Safety and immunogenicity of the quadrivalent human papillomavirus vaccine in HIV-!-infected men. *The journal of infectious diseases* Vol.202, (October 2010), pp.1246-1253.

Wong A K, Chan R C, Aggarwal N et al. (2010). Human papillomavirus genotypes in anal antraepithelial neoplasia and anal carcinoma as detected in tissue biopsies. *Modern Pathology* Vol.23, (2010), pp.144-150.

9

Recurrent Oral Squamous Papilloma in a HIV Infected Patient: Case Report

Helena Lucia Barroso dos Reis[1,*], Mauro Romero Leal Passos[1], Aluízio Antônio de Santa Helena[2], Fernanda Sampaio Cavalcante[3], Arley Silva Júnior[1] and Dennis de Carvalho Ferreira[3]

[1]Fluminense Federal University (UFF)
[2]UNIABEU University
[3]Federal University of Rio de Janeiro (UFRJ)
Brazil

1. Introduction

The Human Papillomavirus (HPV) is a DNA virus of the Papilomaviridae family that cannot be cultivated. It is a small, non-enveloped virus of about 55nm in diameter. It is comprised of 72 capsomers in one capsid of icosahedral symmetry.(1) It presents considerable tropism for epithelial and mucous tissues having a variable incubation period that can last from three weeks to an indeterminate period (2, 3). This virus may be associated to sexual transmission ranging from oral lesions to the formation of cervical cancer, constituting high-impact pathology (4).

More than 100 HPV genotypes have already been described so far and, among these, 24 genotypes have been associated with oral lesions (HPV-1, 2, 3, 4, 6, 7, 10, 11, 13, 16, 18, 30, 32, 33, 35, 45, 52, 55, 57, 59, 69, 72 e 73)(5). Terai et al (1999) in a PCR-based study on HPV prevalence highlighted the presence of HPV 18 in a normal mucous membrane, suggesting that the oral cavity may be a virus reservoir and that the association with other factors, such as alcohol and smoking, could induce the appearance of lesions(6).

Various types of HPV has been described, with oncogenic potential and associated to oral lesions: Squamous papilloma (SP), condyloma acuminatum (CA) and focal epithelial hyperplasy (FEH) are the most frequent pathological entities associated to HPV, and this virus has been identified and correlated to the lichen planus (LP), Pemphigus vulgaris (PV), squamous cell carcinoma (SCC) and verrucose carcinoma (VC) (7). Currently oral manifestations of the HPV infection have increased in patients infected with HIV/AIDS, including children patients (8).

This report discusses the vulnerability of HIV infected individuals to HPV infection as well as the knowledge required by clinicians. As such, the objective of this study is to relate a

*Corresponding Author

case of a HIV-infected patient with a recurrent oral lesion associated to HPV, monitored at the Oral Pathology department of Federal University from Rio de Janeiro (UFRJ), under informed consent of the patient.

2. Case report

A white male patient, 44 years was referred to the Department of Oral Pathology at Rio de Janeiro Federal University, complaining of swelling on tip of tongue, started seven months earlier. During anamnesis the patient related a history of multiple sexual partners, and practice of unprotected oral, vaginal and anal sex, with previous episodes of sexually-transmitted diseases (STD) (gonorrhea and syphilis) adequately treated.

The patient reported being HIV-infected for 10 years and no antiretroviral therapy. Blood evaluation showed a CD4 T lymphocyte count of 640 cells/mm^3 and viral load of 585 copies/ml. Oral examination revealed a red verrucous 3 mm diameter lesion, on the left side of the tongue, suggestive of oral SP (figure 1). An excisional biopsy was carried out, and postoperative advise given.

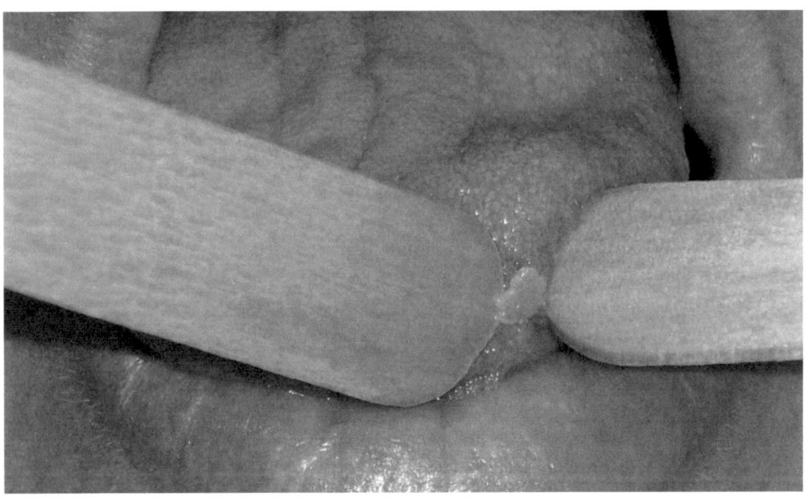

Fig. 1. Verrucose lesion on the left side of the tongue.

The histopathology showed morphology compatible with SP (figure 2), and the patient was informed about HPV infection, the risk of relapse, the risk of oral-genital transmission, and the importance of periodic monitoring. Two months after, a further vegetative 2 mm diameter verrucous lesion on the same site was revealed, indicating relapse. A repeat excisional biopsy was taken, and the histopathology indicated SP. At present the patient is under periodic clinical check-up.

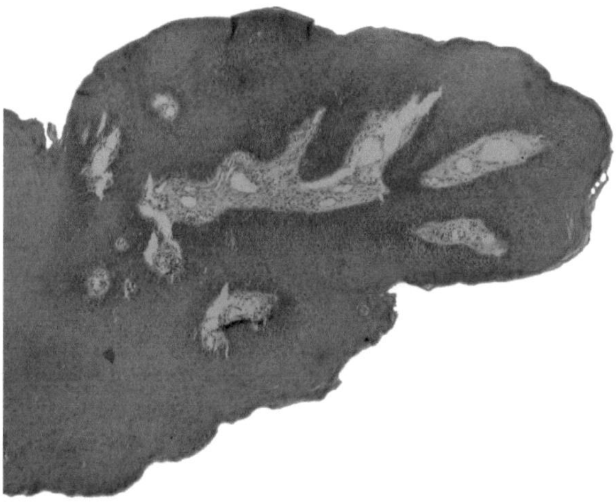

Fig. 2. Proliferative papillomatose and parakeratose lesion.

3. Discussion

The high number of different sexual partners, immunologic deficiency and STDs make the incidence of HPV infection increasingly high (2). This infection often occurs on oral mucosa and the sites most involved are labial mucosa, with 55% of cases, the palate, jugal mucosa, gums, tonsils, uvula and roof of the mouth (9). Although the tongue is not commonly affected, the case presented both lesions on the tip of this organ.

One study evaluated clinical and histopathological features in 12 oral lesions of SP - being the tongue - and found that the time development of these lesions ranged from 2 months to 20 years, being the tong the most prevalent site, with lesions about 3 mm in diameter, with rounded appearance (10). SP can be further divided into several types: isolated, solitary and multiple-recurring (11). The findings observed in this study showed that lesion development (about 7 months), in the lingual site as the most frequent and round lesion.

HPV infection can occur in three ways: transitory infection in 50% of cases; spontaneous regress lesions in 30% of cases; and persistent infections, with constant relapses. Clinically the lesions normally have a verrucous aspect that may be not detected by visual inspection, but through magnification techniques such as colposcopy. Diferent laboratory techniques for diagnosis should read as cytology, biopsy, immunohistochemistry and molecular techniques (2, 3).

The oral SP is a benign entity presented as an exophytic lesion, with a rugose red or white surface, sessile or pediculed (12). It can be granular, fingerlike and may be asymptomatic. (11). In this case both lesions were clinically considered verrucous, vegetative and sessile.

The classical manifestations of HPV infection is the CA followed by verruca vulgaris (VV) and FEH. However, the virus has been identified in other oral afflictive entities such as VP, LP and leukoplasies, probably representing a coincidence of tissue infection and not a causal factor.

As for its differential diagnosis, the literature shows that other diseases may be an oral challenge to diagnose as condyloma acuminatum, verruca vulgaris, focal epithelial hyperplasia (Heck disease), papillary hyperplasia and verruciformis, because they are among a clinically and/or histopathological the injuries that present similarities although the feature distinct, it needs an sufficient training for the health professional to perform an adequate approach to these lesions (13)

Although many oral SP appear to be of viral etiology, the infectivity of the HPV must be of a very low order. The route of transmission of the virus is unknown for oral lesions, although direct contact would be favoured as in the present case. Surgical removal is the treatment of choice by either routine excision or laser ablation. Other treatment modalities include electrocautery, cryosurgery, and intralesional injections of interferon. Recurrence is uncommon, except for lesions in patients infected with human immunodeficiency virus (HIV) (10,11).

HPV related lesions are usual in HIV infected patients, in both genital and oral sites (14). Morphologically, hyperkeratosis, koilocytosis, diskeratosis, papillomatosis and acanthosis, whenever present in papilloma lesions suggest HPV infection (15, 16). However, other benign oral lesions such as VV, CA and FEH more readily present cytopathic effects induced by HPV than papilloma (17). Papillomavirus was also found for the first time in endodontic abscesses (18).

A report showed that the prevalence of HPV in HIV-infected adults is greater (36.4%) than in HIV-negative patients (6.1%) (19). However, a study in children, showed a prevalence of 3.6% in HIV+ patients against 12.3% of those not infected (20). Therefore, more studies into HPV infection and prevalence among the HIV+ individuals are needed in order to clarify the significance of these lesions. It seems that an emphasis on HIV treatment rather than on the HIV immunosuppression has had a noticeable role in oral HPV infections in HIV + individuals. (CAMERON 2005). (21)

Owing to the oncogenic role of certain types of HPV, the relation between this virus and carcinogenesis in oral mucosa is still controversial. Various studies have identified HPV in biopsies of oral SCC and VC (4, 9, 12). Among HPV types found in the oral mucosa, types 6 and 11 are more prevalent in benign lesions on the oral epithelium and types 16 and 18 more prevalent in malignant lesions. In this case HPV identification was not done as the material sent for analysis was scarce (4, 9).

The methods of HPV identification in human tissue vary in sensitivity include electronic microplasy, immunohistochemistry, immunofluorescence, hybridization in situ, Southern blot, dot blot, reverse blot hybridization and polymerase chain reaction (PCR) (22). Morphological analysis cannot typify the virus, but can suggest its presence, being useful in public health policies (12, 23).

The table below shows HPV identification studies as well as the types most frequently found.

Methods	Number of positive cases/population evatuated	HPV types	Reference	Year
In situ DNA-hibridization	7/20	2, 6, 11	Eversole & Laipis(24)	1986
In situ DNA-hybridization applied on paraffin sections	4/7	4, 6, 11	Syrjanen, Syrjanen & Lamseng(25)	1986
PCR Dot blot	4/19 13/19	6, 11 6, 11	Ward *et al.*(26)	1995
PCR	11/27	6, 13, 16	Jimenez *et al.*(27)	2001

Table 1.

The treatment of oral SP may be clinical, by the use of keratolytic agents such as trichloroacetic acid (40 - 90%), a podophyllum 25%, 5-fluoracil and imiquimod; or surgical, by cold, electrical or laser excision. Surgical removal is recommended in few lesions presentations and when histopathological analysis is desired (2, 3, 9).

The patient should be monitored for 6 (six) months after treatment of lesions, which is a critical period for recurrence (2, 3). This data is in agreement to the present report, as relapse occurred in the second month of outpatient monitoring.

One study showed that majority of men do not seek medical care or advice when they have advanced symptoms of HPV infection, and especially when it causes some discomfort. The major concern of infected individuals is in the consequences of this infection in terms of their social and sexual lives. Fear and pain are also raising questions present feelings and anxieties, and consequently suffering. The men in general are very dependent on their sexuality and regard penis as the main organ of the body (28,29).

The patient infected by HPV has affected sex life leading to insecurity in all aspects of life, going to be afraid of losing their jobs if discovered, fear of rejection from their partner, fear of betrayal and fear of comment friends (28,29).

A nested case-control study conducted with 2194 HIV-positive patients showed no association between changes in CD4 cell count and risk of oral warts (30).

The main causes of transmission of HPV infection are the lack of prevention information, prejudices, early onset of sexual activity, multiple partners, not using condoms. Health professionals should play a role through educational activities, working with sexual health promotion and prevention information, encouraging protected sex practices, while respecting the socio-cultural needs of each individual and promoting the biopsychosocial help (28,29). At the present moment, there are two types of HPV prophylactics vaccines, a bivalent that protect against HPV-16/18 and the quadrivalent (HPV-6,11,16). These vaccines are available globally. There is no reason to believe that the vaccine don't work against HPV at the oral mucosa or another anatomical site (31,32,33).

4. Conclusion

Oral lesions may represent an important significance for professionals who treat HPV infection or other STDs. Research into oral cavity lesions should be given value by the dental surgeon or other health professionals who treat HPV infection cases or other STDs. Furthermore, prevention is the most efficient strategy for HPV infection control, including HPV vaccination for oral and genital infection, through suitable sexual guidance in order to reduce situations of vulnerability.

5. References

[1] Scheurer ME, Tortolero-Luna G, Adler-Storthz K. Human papillomavirus infection: biology, epidemiology, and prevention. Int J Gynecol Cancer 2005; 15: 727–746.

[2] Brasil. Ministério da Saúde. Secretaria de Projetos Especiais de Saúde. Coordenação de Doenças Sexualmente Transmissíveis e AIDS. Manual de Controle das Doenças Sexualmente Transmissíveis. 4 ed. Brasília:2006.

[3] Passos MRL. Deessetologia no bolso: o que deve saber um profissional que atende DST. Niterói: RQV; 2004. p. 70-5.

[4] Café MEM, Gontijo B, Silva CMR, Pereira LB. Formas de transmissão do vírus papiloma humano em lesões anogenitais na infância. Comitê de Dermatologia Pediátrica da Sociedade Mineira de Pediatria. Belo Horizonte, 2006.

[5] Oliveira MC, Soares RC, Pinto LP, Costa A de LL. HPV e carcinogênese oral: revisão bibliográfica. Rev Bras Otorrinolaringol 2003 jul/ago; 69(4): 553-9.

[6] Terai M, Hashimoto K, Yoda K, Sata T. High prevalence of human papilomavíruses in the normal oral cavity of adults. Oral Microbiol and Immunology 1999; 14:201-5.

[7] Nonnenmacher B, Breitenbach V, Villa LL, Prolla JC, Bozzetti MC. Genital human papillomavirus infection identification by molecular biology among asymptomatic women. Rev. Saúde Pública. 2002 Feb;36(1):95-100.

[8] Summersgill KF. et al. *Human papillomavirus in the oral cavities of children and adolescents. Oral Surg Oral Med Oral Pathol Oral Radiol Endod.* v.91, p.62-69, 2001.

[9] Padayachee A. Human papillomavirus (HPV) types 2 and 57 in oral verrucae demonstrated by in situ hybridization. J Oral Pathol Med 1994; 23:413-7

[10] Carneiro TE, Marinho SA, Verli FD, Mesquita AT, Lima NL, Miranda JL. Oral squamous papilloma: clinical, histologic and immunohistochemical analyses. J Oral Sci. 2009; 51(3):367-72.

[11] Jaju PP, Suvarna PV, Desai RS. Squamous Papilloma: Case Report and Review of Literature. Int J Oral Sci. 2010; 2(4): 222–225.

[12] Heard I, Palefsky JM, Kazatchkine MD. The impact of HIV antiviral therapy on human papillomavirus (HPV) infections and HPV-related diseases. Antiviral Therapy. Paris, 2004. 9:13-22.

[13] Dos Reis HB, Rabelo PC, De Santana MF, Ferreira DC, Filho AC. Oral squamous papilloma and condyloma acuminatum as manifestations of buccal-genital infection by human papillomavirus. Indian J Sex Transm Dis. 2009; 30: 40–42.

[14] Fakhry C, Sugar E, D'Souza G, Gillison M . *Two-Week versus Six-Month Sampling Interval in a Short-Term Natural History Study of Oral HPV Infection in an HIV-Positive Cohort. 2010 ; PLoS ONE* 5(7): e11918.

[15] Frega A. Human papillomavirus in virgins and behaviour at risk. Cancer Letters, v.194, p.21, 2003.

[16] Castro TPPG, Bussoloti Filho I. Prevalence of human papillomavirus (HPV) in oral cavity and oropharynx. Rev. Bras. Otorrinolaringol. 2006 Apr; 72(2): 272-282.

[17] Greenspan, J.S.; Greenspan, D.; Lenette, E.T. Replication of Epstein -Barr virus within the epithelial cells of Oral" hairy" leukoplakia an AIDS-Associated lesions N Engl J Med, v. 313, n. 25, p. 1564-71, 1985

[18] Ferreira DC, Paiva S S, Carmo FL, Rôças IN, Rosado AS, Santos KRN, Siqueira Jr. JF. Identification of herpesviruses types 1 to 8 and human papillomavirus in acute apical abscesses..Journal of Endodontics, v. 37, p. 10-16, 2011.

[19] Cameron JE, Hagensee ME. Oral HPV complications in HIV-infected patients. Curr HIV/AIDS Rep. 2008 Aug; 5(3):126-31.

[20] Jeftha AD, Dhaya D, Marais D, et al. Comparing Oral HPV types in HIV Positive and Negative Children. Annual Meeting and Exhibition of the AADR San Antonio. 2003.

[21] Cameron JE,MercanteD, Gaffiga AM,Leigh JE,Fidel PL jr,Hagensee ME. The impact of highy active antiretroterapy and immunodeficiency on human papillomavirus infection of the oral cavity of human immunodeficiency virus seropositive adults.Sex Trans Dis 2005 nov,32(11):703-9

[22] Venturi Beatriz da Rocha Miranda, Cabral Márcia Grillo, Lourenço Simone de Queiroz Chaves. Oral squamous cell carcinoma - contribution of oncogenic virus and some molecular markers in the development and prognosis of the lesion: a review. Rev. Bras. Otorrinolaringol. 2004; 70(3):385-392.

[23] Syrjänen, K. et al. Morphological and immunohistochemical evidence suggesting human papillomavirus (HPV) involvement in oral squamous cell carcinogenesis. Int. J. Oral Surg. v.12, p,418-424, 1983.

[24] Eversole LR, Laipis PJ. Oral squamous papillomas: Detection of HPV DNA by in situ hybridization.Oral Surgery, Oral Medicine, Oral Pathology. 1988; 65(5):545-550.

[25] Syrjänen SM, Syrjänen KJ, Lamberg MA. Detection of human papillomavirus DNA in oral mucosal lesions using in situ DNA-hybridization applied on paraffin sections. Oral Surgery, Oral Medicine, Oral Pathology. 1986; 62(6): 660-667.

[26] Ward KAR, Napier SS, Winter PC, Maw RD, Dinsmore WW. Detection of human papilloma virus DNA sequences in oral squamous cell papillomas by the polymerase chain reaction. Oral Surgery, Oral Medicine, Oral Pathology. 1995; 80(1): 63-66.

[27] Jimenez C, Correnti M, Salma N, Cavazza ME and Perrone M: *Detection of human papillomavirus DNA in benign oral squamous epithelial lesions in Venezuela. J Oral PatholMed*30: 385-388, 2001.

[28] Arcoverde MAM, Wall ML. Assistência "prestada ao ser" masculino portador do HPV: contribuições de enfermagem. DST - J brasileiro Doenças Sex Transm. 2005; 17(2): 133-7.

[29] Santos C, de Souza LRF, de Jesus MLA, Souza RR, Cortez EA, Veneu ACS. Nursing Performance in Health assistance and HPV prevention in man. Rev. de Pesq.: cuidado é fundamental Online 2009; 1(2): 372-383.

[30] King MD, Reznik DA, O´Daniels CM, Larsen NM, Osterbolt D, Blumberg HM. Human Papillomavirus-Associated Oral Warts among Human Immunodeficiency Virus-Seropositive Patients in the Era of Highly Active Antiretroviral Therapy: An Emerging Infection. Clin Infect Dis. (2002) 34(5): 641-648

[31] Brotherton, JML; Gertig DM. Primary prophylactic human papillomavirus vaccination programs: future perspective on global impact. *Expert Rev. Anti Infect. Ther.* 9(8), 627–639 (2011).

[32] Weiss, TW; Rosenthal, SL; Zimet ZD. Attitudes toward HPV Vaccination amongWomen Aged 27 to 45. International Scholarly Research Network ISRN Obstetrics and Gynecology Volume 2011, Article ID 670318, 6 pages.

Part 5

Epidemiology

10

Sexually Transmitted Infections Among Army Personnel in the Military Environment

Krzysztof Korzeniewski
Military Institute of Medicine, Department of Epidemiology and Tropical Medicine
Poland

1. Introduction

Sexually Transmitted Diseases (STD's) have always been a considerable problem in the military environment. The incidence of STD's among soldiers participating in combat operations dates back to the very first military conflicts (Rasnake et al., 2005; Emerson, 1997; Holmes et al., 1970). Sex industry has always thrived in the vicinity of military quarters and bases, and services of female sex workers have routinely been used by military personnel - physically active men. A French commander living in the 17th century once claimed that commercial sex workers 'killed ten times as many men as enemy fire' (Greenberg, 1972).

The incidence of STD's among military personnel in the past was divided into four periods. The first lasted until the beginning of the 20th century when the effects of venereal infections were noticed but widely ignored. The second phase, which lasted until the 1940s, covered the period of intensive scientific development (including laboratory diagnostics which made it possible to identify sexually transmitted pathogens). It was also the time of implementing certain preventive measures such as criminal procedure in the cases of prostitution. The third period started in the 1940s from the moment penicillin was introduced as a means of treating syphilis and gonorrhea on a mass scale (Greenberg, 1972). The next, fourth period in the history of STD's started in the 1980s and lasts until today. This stage is dominated by viral infections caused by *immunodeficiency virus* (HIV), *herpes simplex virus* (HSV), *human papilloma virus* (HPV) as well as bacterial infections caused by *Chlamydia trachomatis*, which all commonly occur in the whole world, both among civilians and military personnel (Gaydos et al., 1998, 2000; Fleming et al., 1997; Kotloff et al., 1998). Diseases induced by the above mentioned pathogens together with an increased incidence of gonorrhea pose a serious epidemiological risk due to a large number of asymptomatic infections, particularly among women, and ease of transmission in closed environments such as the military. Nowadays the military career is becoming increasingly popular among females. As early as in 1996-97 app. 17% of all new recruits to all military services of the United States were women (Walter Reed Army Institute Research, 1998). Screening tests for *Chlamydia* infections conducted among female U.S. Army recruits in the same period demonstrated a prevalence of 9.2% in a cohort of >13,000 women (Gaydos et al., 1998). This led to a conclusion that preventive medicine tasked with controlling STD's in the military environment can no longer focus only on transmission of STD's among female sex workers and men soldiers, but it should also concentrate on transmission among soldiers of both sexes assigned to military duty in the same time and place.

The institution which has gathered the most comprehensive data on the incidence of STD's among military personnel is undoubtedly health service of the U.S. Armed Forces. American soldiers remain the best diagnosed and medically consulted professional group in the U.S., although they represent merely 1% of working population aged 18-45 (Hodge et al., 2002). The incidence of venereal diseases diagnosed among soldiers serving in their home countries are comparable to those observed in the local civilian population. However, the situation may change drastically if troops are deployed to an area of operations overseas. The prevalence of venereal diseases in combat troops is likely to be much higher than during peacetime and it is then strictly connected with ongoing military activities in the theater operations (Malone et al., 1993; Melton, 1976).

2. Past and present scenario of STD's in army personnel

2.1 World war I

Throughout World War I venereal diseases accounted for over 6.8 million lost duty days and the discharge from active duty of more than 10,000 soldiers serving in the U.S. Army (Deller et al., 1982). STD's with dominating role of lues and gonorrhea were the second major reason for lost duty days (the first one were sanitary losses due to the influenza pandemic in the period 1918-1919) (Rasnake et al., 2005).

2.2 World war II

During World War II the incidence of STD's in all units of the U.S. Armed Forces was estimated at 43/1000 soldiers (Padget, 1963). In the period of preparations preceding the Invasion of Normandy taking place in the U.K., the prevalence of STD's was estimated at 35-40/1000 soldiers, whereas during the invasion itself the incidence dropped to 5/1000 soldiers. However, soon afterwards the prevalence of STD's increased again reaching the level of 50/1000 in combat troops. In the second part of 1945, after the ceasefire was declared and hostilities in Europe ceased, during the occupation of Germany by the U.S. Forces, the incidence rate of STD's surged (most of venereal diseases posed gonorrhea) and it was estimated at 190/1000 soldiers (Sternberg & Howard, 1960).

2.3 Korean war

Throughout the Korean War in the period 1951-55, the incidence of venereal diseases was estimated at 184/1000 soldiers (Deller et al., 1982), gonorrhea accounted for three-fourths of all STD diagnoses. In some of the U.S. Forces units the incidence rate reached up to 500 cases per 1000 person-years (p-yrs) (McNinch, 1954).

2.4 Vietnam war

An increased sexual activity and therefore higher incidence of STD's was observed in the population of American soldiers fighting in Vietnam in the 1960s and 1970s (Hart, 1973, 1974). During the Vietnam War venereal diseases were listed as the number one diagnosis in the Army's monthly morbidity reports (Deller et al., 1982). A substantial number of STD's led to the foundation of the Venereal Disease Control Branch of the U.S. Public Health Service (U.S. Department of Health, Education, and Welfare, 1962). In the period 1963-72 the prevalence of STD's among U.S. soldiers serving in Vietnam was estimated at 260 cases per 1000 p-yrs. Despite increased morbidity rates, merely 1% of patients diagnosed with STD's required hospitalization. Modern therapy of STD's, unlike medical treatment provided at the beginning of the 20th century, does not generally require a patient to be hospitalized and the majority of cases are diagnosed and treated on the outpatient basis (Deller et al., 1982; Shapiro & Breschi, 1974). Research conducted in the U.S. Air Force Hospital in Vietnam from November 1970 to June 1971 demonstrated that only 25 American soldiers were hospitalized due to venereal diseases. Whereas in all clinics (General Medicine, Dermatology, and Urology) of the same U.S. Hospital an average of 292 reported new cases of gonorrhea were treated ambulatorily per month (3202 cases from November 1970 to September 1971) (Shapiro & Breschi, 1974). The incidence of gonorrhea accounted for 90% of all STD's diagnosed in the U.S. Forces during the Vietnam War. In 1963 American troops serving in Vietnam were experiencing more than 300 cases of gonorrhea per 1000 p-yrs (Rasnake et al., 2005). In a study on a crew of a Navy aircraft carrier, the annual rate of gonorrhea was 582/1000 service members and nongonococcal urethritis was 459/1000 men (Harrison, 1974). Soldiers typically contracted an infection on a leave during port calls as a result of sexual contact with a female sex workers. During a 6-day port call in the Philippines, the average U.S. sailor had 1-2 partners and had intercourse three times. Examination post-exposure demonstrated gonorrhea in 8.2% white and 19.1% black soldiers (Holmes et al., 1970). By contrast, a recent study of U.S. soldiers in Fort Bragg, North Carolina, reported rates of 5 cases of gonorrhea per 1000 p-yrs (Sena et al., 2000).

Throughout the military conflicts conducted in Korea and Vietnam a vast number of STD's characteristic of hot climate areas were also reported. For instance, chancroid was 14- to 21-fold more common than gonorrhea in the population of American soldiers deployed to Korea (Asin, 1952). Research conducted among soldiers serving in the U.S. Forces assigned to Vietnam revealed that chancroid was the second most frequently reported venereal disease, the first one being gonorrhea (Kerber et al., 1969). Another venereal infection prevalent in hot climate areas is lymphogranuloma venereum. The disease is rare in both the U.S. and Europe but it is diagnosed in the population of sailors or soldiers returning from endemic regions in Asia, Africa, South America and the Caribbean (Perine & Osoba, 1990). Research conducted in the U.S. Forces in 1968 demonstrated 20 cases of lymphogranuloma venereum among military personnel home-bound from Vietnam or having a sexual partner returning from Asia (Abrams, 1968).

2.5 United Nations peacekeeping operations

Countries in Southeast Asia or Sub-Saharan Africa are characterized by high incidence of STD's in the local population. Soldiers deployed to military operations (usually UN peacekeeping missions) executed in the aforementioned endemic areas are at a high risk from STD's (Shafer et al., 2002). Military personnel is reported to have high rates of sexual contact with overseas nationals during deployments, ranging from 45% to 56% (Miller & Yeager, 1995; Hopperus et al., 1995). A study of Dutch soldiers deployed on five-month peacekeeping duties with the United Nations Transition Authority in Cambodia (UNTAC) found that 45% had sexual contact with prostitutes or other members of the local population during their deployment (Soeprapto et al., 1995). STD's were the most commonly reported infectious diseases for the duration of the UN peacekeeping mission in Cambodia at the beginning of the 1990s. Cases of a HIV infection were the focus of attention of military health services operating on the UNTAC peacekeeping mission largely due to the fact that the incidence of HIV/AIDS among local female sex workers was high. The research conducted in 5 different areas of Cambodia among 437 prostitutes providing services in local brothels demonstrated that up to 40.5% were HIV positive, 38.7% had a *Chlamydia* infection and/or gonorrhea, and 13.8% syphilis (Ryan et al., 1998). The risk of infection was much increased by the fact that Cambodian citizens were not using condoms (Hor et al., 2005). The research conducted among female sex workers from Siem Reap (n=140) demonstrated that 78% were using condoms during intercourse with clients, whereas only 20% of them were using condoms during intercourse with their regular partners (Wong et al., 2003). The research conducted in the population of Indonesian contingent (n=3627) demonstrated HIV infections in 12 cases (ratio 3.3/1000 soldiers). The analysis of medical records belonging to 707 Polish soldiers assigned to the UNTAC peacekeeping mission who had been treated on the 1st and 2nd level of UN medical centers from May 1992 to September 1993 revealed that 92 soldiers (13% of the studied group) developed an STD (85 cases of gonorrhea, 5 HIV infections, 1 case of syphilis). All of the infected soldiers reported sexual contact with local women. The majority of the infectees were young privates (Korzeniewski, 2008). The entire population of the Polish Military Contingent acting under the UN mandate in Cambodia in 1992-93 (n=1254) were subjected to medical examination and diagnostic tests upon their home-coming. 97 of the examined soldiers were diagnosed with imported STD's: 9 HIV infections, including 1 case of AIDS; 55 of gonorrhea, 8 of syphilis, 17 of genital warts, 5 of genital herpes, 2 of granuloma inguinale, and 1 of lymphogranuloma venereum) (Korzeniewski et al., 2003).

UNAIDS has estimated that military personnel are two to five times more likely than civilians to contract STD's including HIV (Bazergan & Easterbrook, 2003). In times of conflict, the rate of HIV/AIDS among the military can be even more than 50 times higher than in peacetime (Tripodi & Patel, 2004). In 2000, a U.S. Intelligence Council Report estimated a HIV prevalence rate of between 10 and 20% among the armed forces of the Ivory Coast and Nigeria, and even higher prevalence of 40-60% among the militaries of the war-affected countries of Angola and the Democratic Republic of the Congo (U.S. National Intelligence Council, 2000). The UN recommends that HIV-positive personnel serving in national contingents should not be deployed to peacekeeping missions (United Nations, 1999). However, internal control over military personnel assigned to the UN operations based on routinely conducted tests is still missing. As a result, actual incidence rates of HIV infections among the UN peacekeepers cannot be specified. Although reliable data is absent, it has been estimated that rates are high among peacekeepers, especially in areas where the rate of HIV infection in the entire population exceeds 5%. HIV prevalence among peacekeepers assigned to the UN mission in Sierra Leone (UNAMSIL) was estimated at 32%, 17% in the UN Mission in Ethiopia and Eritrea (UNMEE), and 8% in the UN Mission in the Democratic Republic of the Congo (MONUC) (U.S. General Accounting Office, 2001).

2.6 U.S. Armed Forces

Within the last two decades the incidence of STD's among American troops was highly irregular. For the duration of such operations as *Desert Shield/Desert Storm* (the Persian Gulf War), *Restore Hope* (Somalia) it did not exceed 1% of the total number of all diagnoses. Several factors are considered to have influenced such a huge reduction in the number of STD's infections. In the case of nearly all contemporary military operations, especially those conducted in Muslim countries, contacts with local people have always been kept to a minimum (Hyams et al., 1995; Wassermann et al., 1997). Also, alcohol is prohibited, and if soldiers are entitled to a leave it always takes place outside the zone of operations. Health prevention measures undertaken by medical services in a mission area are directed towards preventing STD's by offering soldiers unlimited access to condoms (Berg, 2005). Yet, despite all the prevention measures taken by medical services, the incidence of STD's in U.S. military personnel, especially in those under 25, has been increasing. At the beginning of the 1990s 7.4% of U.S. military personnel was diagnosed with gonorrhea and 15.6% with *Chlamydia* infections (Zenilman et al., 2002; Cecil et al., 2001). In the period 2004-2009 research on prevalence of gonorrhea and chlamydiasis was carried out in the population of American soldiers serving in Iraq and Afghanistan. Gonorrhea rates ranged from a low 5/100,000 deployed personnel in 2005 to a high 17.6/100,000 in 2008 and 2009. Much higher rates were reported among young female soldiers and among personnel who had just been deployed to Iraq and Afghanistan. *Chlamydia* infection rates increased every year, peaking in 2009 with a total rate of 246.3/100,000 deployed personnel with higher rates in females (770.9/100,000) than in men (192.6/100,000) (Aldous et al., 2011). The research carried out in the population of the U.S. Forces soldiers (n=7,000) deployed to Bagram, Afghanistan from March to August 2005 demonstrated that 17 out of 2870 admissions to the U.S. Combat Support Hospital (on an outpatient basis) were due to STD's (8 cases of chlamydiasis, 4 of gonorrhea, 2 of genital warts, 2 of genital herpes, 1 of trichomoniasis) (Korzeniewski, 2011).

The U.S. Preventive Services Task Force guidelines (Meyers et al., 2008; U.S. Preventive Services Task Force, 2007) recommend yearly gonorrhea screening for sexually active women under 25 and chlamydiasis screening for sexually active women under 25 or for those over 25 with risk factors. All the U.S. services follow these guidelines and provide routine testing for those 25 years old and younger (USACHPPM, 2007). *Chlamydia* infection and gonorrhea remain the two most commonly reported STD's in the U.S. Forces (Seung-eun, 2010). American soldiers are a high-risk group as far as the incidence of STD's is concerned. App. 40% of the U.S. Forces personnel are people aged 17-24. In contrast, the U.S. civilian population at the same age accounts for only 14% of the entire population (Armed Forces Health Surveillance Center, 2009). Untreated *Chlamydia trachomatis* and *Neisseria gonorrhoeae* infections can result in pelvic inflammatory disease which may lead to ectopic pregnancy, infertility, and low birth weight (Cates et al., 1990). A considerable number of STD's diagnosed among military personnel, such as chlamydiasis or gonorrhea are mildly symptomatic or asymptomatic and therefore they do not greatly affect combat readiness of troops (Gaydos et al., 2000). It does, however, facilitate the spread of STD's both inside and outside the military environment, which may in the future lead to some serious health complications, especially in women (Gaydos & Gaydos, 2008).

Chlamydiasis remains the most commonly reported infectious disease not only in the U.S. Armed Forces but also in the U.S. civilian population (Niebuhr et al., 2006). The incidence rates of *Chlamydia* infection registered in a military base Fort Bragg, North Carolina (one of the largest U.S. Army's units) in 1996 among male and female active duty soldiers were 3-fold to 6-fold higher than comparable rates reported in the civilian population of North Carolina and in the United States as a whole, especially among soldiers who were in the lower enlisted ranks, nonwhite and single (Sena et al., 2000). Reports prepared in the United States within the framework of the Defense Medical Surveillance System in the period 2000-2008 among non-deployed, active duty members demonstrated overall incidence of 922 cases per 100,000 person-years (392/100,000 person-years in the Navy; 1431/100,000 person-years in the Army). A total of 103,257 *Chlamydia* cases (95% lab-confirmed) were reported during the study period (Jordan et al., 2011). In the period 2000-2009 over 12,000 U.S. soldiers had recurrent diagnoses of a *Chlamydia* infection within a single year (Armed Forces Health Surveillance Center, 2010a). As opposed to gonorrhea, more than 90% of *Chlamydia trachomatis* infections in males are asymptomatic. Research in male population diagnosed with chlamydiasis demonstrated a slight increase in prostatitis and a fourfold risk of epididymitis (Trei et al., 2008).

Gonorrhea remains second, following *Chlamydia* infection, on the list of the most frequently reported venereal diseases in all services the U.S. Armed Forces. In the past gonorrhea provided a benchmark for determining morbidity rates in the military environment (Emmerson, 1997). In 2003 the incidence rate of gonorrhea in the U.S. Forces was estimated at 143 cases/100,000 in relation to 116/100,000 reported nationwide. Such high morbidity rates can be explained by a large number of asymptomatic infections, particularly among women. In male population asymptomatic infections account for 10% of all cases, whereas in female population - 50% (Niebuhr et al., 2006).

In the 1980s another STD joined the list of venereal diseases occurring in the military environment - AIDS. The HIV testing program covering donors at Army blood banks, applicants to the military, active-duty soldiers, the Army Reserves, and the National Guard was introduced in the U.S. Forces in 1985 (Brown et al., 1996). Until the end of the 1990s the number of HIV infections among the U.S. Forces personnel remained at a relatively low and constant level (Vu et al., 2002). In 1994 in the population of 378,000 active-duty soldiers who were screened, 650 were found to be HIV-positive (Renton & Whitaker, 1994). The rate of HIV seroconversion amounted to 1275 cases in all of the U.S. Forces (Renzullo et al., 2001). In recent years the number of infections has increased. 1373 new cases of HIV infections had been registered until January 2004 only among the U.S. Air Force personnel, 561 soldiers died of AIDS (Rasnake et al., 2005). Since October 1985 a HIV infection has been a medically disqualifying condition for entry to military service in the U.S. Forces. However, other STD's continue to occur at relatively high rates in the active American soldiers. Research into the incidence rates of STD's among the U.S. Forces military personnel was conducted in the period 2004-2009. Overall incidence rates of *Chlamydia* infections, *herpes simplex virus* (HSV), gonorrhea, and *human papilloma virus* (HPV) were 1056.2, 879.6, 230.8, and 2307.4 per 100,000 p-yrs, respectively (more service members were diagnosed with HPV than other STD's). The rate of syphilis was much lower than the rates of other venereal diseases (34.6 per 100,000 p-yrs). STD's rates were higher among military members who were female, in their 20s, black, in the Army, and from the southern regions of the United States (Armed Forces Health Surveillance Center, 2010b). Examination of 1737 female American soldiers preparing for deployment to *Operation Iraqi Freedom* (Iraq) and *Operation Enduring Freedom* (Afghanistan) which was conducted in Camp Doha, Kuwait at the turn of 2003 and 2004 revealed venereal infections in 44 patients (2.5% of the examined group). *Herpes simplex 2* (genital herpes), *Condyloma acuminata* (genital warts), and *Chlamydia trachomatis* were the most commonly identified infections accounting for 29.5%, 25%, and 20.5% of the diagnoses, respectively (Wright et al., 2006). The majority of women with genital herpes and genital warts are asymptomatic. Asymptomatic are also 70% women with chlamydiasis. It has been estimated that there is an 8% prevalence rate of *Chlamydia* in a non-deployed, asymptomatic active duty female army population (Catterson & Zadoo, 1993). Nevertheless, it seems that STD's incidence rates reported in the population of soldiers deployed to contemporary military operations executed in different climatic and sanitary conditions have no significant influence on military readiness (Wright et al., 2006). As far as the military environment is concerned, the largest number of STD's is observed among young soldiers (recruits and basic trainees) who enter the military service with habits and behaviors they had acquired in their home environment (Brodine & Shafer, 2003; Gaydos et al., 2003). In the United States nearly 50% of all STD's reported every year are diagnosed in the population aged 15-24 (Weinstock et al., 2004). They experience certain health problems, including asymptomatic STD's which are not subjected to introductory screening upon admission to the military service (Shafer et al., 2008). Both, male and female military personnel are at risk (Abel et al., 1996).

2.7 STD's in the world

According to the World Health Organization approximately 340 million new STD's, mainly gonorrhea, chlamydiasis, trichomoniasis and syphilis are treated in the whole world every year. In addition to this, a substantial number of viral STD's, such as HPV, HSV or HIV infections are reported annually. Although the majority of all reported STD's are found in the Third World countries, they also pose a considerable epidemiological and economic problem in highly industrialized countries. Prevalence and incidence of STD's throughout the world depend on a number of factors, such as accessibility of diagnostics and health prevention programs aimed at controlling venereal diseases, sexual behavior in local population, the standard of living, the number of female sex workers, drug addicts and other risk groups inhabiting a given territory. Morbidity rates of particular STD's vary in different regions of the world. For instance, gonorrhea is far more common in developing countries, whereas in highly industrialized countries (where the introduction of effective prevention programs led to a reduction in the number of gonorrhea cases), *Chlamydia* infections prevail (Berg, 2005).

2.8 STD's in the U.S.A.

In the United States alone up to 18.9 million new venereal diseases are diagnosed per year and an astronomical amount of 17 billion USD is allocated for medical treatment of STD's (Weinstock et al., 2000). The highest incidence of STD's is reported in the population under 25, i.e. young people who appear to be more inclined to risky behaviors (such as unprotected sex) than the older section of a society. 1.2 million cases of chlamydiasis (401.3 cases/100,000 population) and over 340,000 cases of gonorrhea (111.6/100,000 population), two most commonly occurring contagious diseases in the U.S., were reported to Centers for

Disease Control and Prevention (CDC) in 2008. The largest number of infections was diagnosed in girls and young women aged 15-24. The majority of *Chlamydia* infections prevailing in the United States remain undiagnosed. The number of chlamydiasis among American citizens is estimated at 2.8 million new cases per year (Centers for Disease Control and Prevention, 2009). In the period 2002-2008 detection of *Chlamydia* infections in male population had increased by 45%, which was largely due to the accessibility of less invasive diagnostic procedures. Although the reported number of chlamydiasis in males is lower than in females, the CDC has estimated that the current numbers of new infections in both populations are comparable (Datta et al., 2007). According to the CDC undiagnosed and untreated STD's cause infertility in at least 24,000 American women every year (Centers for Disease Control and Prevention, 2009). Untreated chlamydiasis and gonorrhea lead to pelvic inflammatory disease (PID) in 10-20% of the infected females and in consequence can cause long-term complications such as chronic pelvic pain, ectopic pregnancy, and previously mentioned infertility (Hook & Handsfield, 2008; Hillis & Wasserheit, 1996). The highest incidence rates of *Chlamydia* infections and gonorrhea in the United States are reported in the population of young African-American women, whereas the highest incidence rates of syphilis are registered among young African-American men. Afro-Americans represent merely 12% of the American population, yet 70% of gonorrhea infections are reported in this particular ethnic group. In 2008 the chlamydiasis and syphilis rates among Afro-Americans were 8 times higher than in the white population (Centers for Disease Control and Prevention, 2008).

70% of chlamydiasis and 50% of gonorrhea infections in females are asymptomatic. The CDC recommends annual screening for *Chlamydia* infections in the population of sexually active women under 25, as well as among older women with risk factors such as multiple sex partners (Centers for Disease Control and Prevention, 2006). According to different sources of the U.S. health services the number of *N. gonorrhoeae* infections in the American population is estimated at 700 000 per year (Centers for Disease Control and Prevention, 2010). Asymptomatic gonorrhea is rare in males; it is far more common in females (Brill, 2010). It has been estimated that for every case of gonorrhea diagnosed in the U.S. there are 3 cases of a *Chlamydia* infection (Centers for Disease Control and Prevention, 2009). Additionally, app. 100,000 cases of primary and secondary syphilis are diagnosed in the population of American citizens per year. The number of syphilis diagnoses account for less than 1% of the total 12 million new cases reported annually in the whole world (Centers for Disease Control and Prevention, 2006). HPV infection (genital warts) is yet another STD commonly reported in the United States. It was diagnosed in 5.6% of sexually active U.S. adults aged 18-59 (Dinh et al., 2008).

2.9 Military environment

Incidence rates of STD's reported in the military environment cannot be directly compared to the same rates registered in the civilian environment due to large demographic differences in both populations. Military personnel are predominantly young single and sexually active men. Increased incidence of venereal diseases has been reported in the population of lower ranking enlisted personnel, whereas, there is not much data on incidence rates among officers, warrant officers, and senior noncommissioned officers. It has been assessed that higher-ranking, older and better educated soldiers who follow health prevention programs (the use of condoms) rarely acquire an STD (Berg, 2005). Research conducted in the period 1989-91 among the U.S. Navy and Marine Corps male personnel (n=1744) during their on board deployment to South America and Africa revealed STD's in 10% of the crew, out of which only 10% were officers. The majority of sailors who reported sexual contact with prostitutes during port calls were young, non-white and single. 42% of the studied group reported sexual intercourse with female sex workers, of which 29% had one sexual partner, 35% 2-3, and 35% 4 or more partners. Enlisted personnel had sexual contact with prostitutes more often than officers (43% vs. 26%) (Malone et al., 1993).

The military environment represents a professional group which is at a high risk from venereal diseases, particularly on deployment to military operations conducted in different climatic and sanitary conditions. Even in the 1990s, when there was a lower number of armed conflicts with the participation of multinational coalition forces in the world, the incidence rates of STD's reported among military recruits (Gaydos et al., 1998) and other military populations were high (Brodine et al., 1998; McKee et al., 1998). A noticeable growth in the number of diagnosed STD's in the military environment is commonly reported during deployment to foreign countries. Regular sexual contact with sex workers and inconsistency in the use of condoms are considered to be the main risk behaviors for STD acquisition during deployment (Malone et al., 1993). Young, non-white, unmarried soldiers are at greatest risk from venereal diseases (Sena et al., 2000). Prevalence of STD's in the military environment is determined by a number of factors such as age, race, socioeconomic status (Coutinho, 1994). The epidemiology of STD's does differ markedly from the routes of transmission of other contagious diseases. In the case of venereal diseases a risk group usually represents only a part of the total population: young, sexually active people. Asymptomatic carriers have a dominant role in the spread of infections. The fact of having recovered from an STD does not boost immunity to venereal disease in the future; the clinical picture as well as the course of STD's may differ in each case. STD transmission rates may be characterized by such great diversity within the same population that monitoring venereal diseases in a specific study group is no mean achievement (Berg, 2005).

3. Risk factors and prevention

The most common risk factors resulting in STD's infections, both inside and outside the military environment, include risky sexual behaviors, such as sexual contact with prostitutes, casual sex with strangers, sex with multiple partners (even if a person practices serial monogamy), homosexuality, sex with partners taking drug injections, sex with a partner who has had multiple sex partners, including partners taking drug injections, sex with partners likely to be STD's carriers, unprotected sex (condoms). Another group of risk factors include early sexual initiation, delayed medical diagnostics and avoiding medical treatment. Risk markers, which indicate presence of risk factors, include marital status, race, urban residence, low socioeconomic status (Aral & Holmes, 1990).

Other variables may also function as risk factors or risk markers, e.g. age, sex, smoking, use of alcohol or drugs, previous STD's infections, lack of circumcision (Berg, 2005). However, the dominant role in the spread of STD's, especially in developing countries, belongs to female sex workers (Day, 1988; Padian, 1988). In areas of military deployment where contact among soldiers and the local people is unrestricted and where unwritten social norms do not exist, there is a specific kind of symbiosis between the population of soldiers who have money and wish to entertain themselves and the population of local female sex workers who need means of support. Prostitution is cheap and commonplace in all Third World countries. Due to low prices of sex services prostitutes need a large number of customers to earn their living, while soldiers can afford multiple sex services. In areas where multinational troops are deployed there are a large number of makeshift shops, bars, and restaurants all around military bases which provide military personnel not only with stimulants such as alcohol and drugs but also with sex services (Berg, 2005).

Another risk factor determining the occurrence of STD's in the military environment is sexual assault of women, which is experienced by 4 to 9% of female service members. 8% of Persian Gulf War veterans reported sexual abuse during *Operation Desert Shield/Operation Desert Storm* in 1990-91. Another 34% of female respondents reported a rape or attempted rape during active duty. Many had been raped more than once; 14% reported being gang raped during active duty. However, three-fourths of the women who were raped did not report the incident to a ranking officer (Valente & Wight, 2007).

The risk of acquiring an STD infection is higher in military personnel with a history of a venereal disease in the past, among soldiers who had sexual contact with men, sex workers or drug addicts, soldiers who had casual sex or multiple sex partners (Renzullo et al., 1990). Alcohol consumption by soldiers executing mandatory tasks on military operations is yet another risk factor as far as the incidence of STD's is concerned. Alcohol consumption reduces morale, and it also co-exists with sexual activity and often leads to contact with sex workers, part of whom (especially in war-affected countries with low sanitary conditions) are infected with venereal diseases. During World War II (Ratcliff, 1947; Wittkower & Cowan, 1944), similarly to the Vietnam War (Hart, 1974, 1973) alcohol was claimed to be one of the risk factors for an STD acquisition. A vast majority of STD's reported in the military environment is diagnosed among young soldiers. There is a tendency among adolescents to have unplanned casual sex with sexually active partners (Hamburg, 1986). They are well aware they are playing with fire, yet they justify their actions by saying it is a way to relieve emotional tension resulting from the dangers of military service. One of the most significant risk factors determining the occurrence of STD's in the military environment is the necessity to deploy troops to operations conducted abroad in adverse climatic and sanitary conditions - in areas where the incidence rates of STD's among the local people are particularly high and where military personnel have the possibility to spend their time off outside military bases making use of available sexual services.

Soldiers assigned to military service in different climatic regions are typically sexually active people who wish to relieve stress and emotional tension associated with the execution of mandatory tasks in the area of operations. There is a specific form of initiation which consists in familiarizing young soldiers by their older colleagues with certain amusements based on sexual services provided by prostitutes, alcohol consumption or drug use. Taking advantage of the so called 'illegal entertainment' is a common way of spending time off during holidays and on leaves among military personnel. Such forms of spending time off-duty is preferred by soldiers who are single, low-ranking, low educated or who have problems with obeying the law (Berg, 2005). Departure from the rule was the Vietnam War, where all of the military personnel in the population of American soldiers, regardless of their age, marital status or education, made use of sexual services provided by female sex workers (in a large part infected with venereal diseases). 44% of married recruits, 56% of recruits over 30 years old and 30% with high school education treated sexual contact with prostitutes as a natural way of spending their time off-duty (Hart, 1973).

Increased incidence of STD's among military personnel engaged in military operations is also determined by the absence of alternative ways of spending time off-duty, such as a gym, a cinema or a library. As a result military personnel tend to seek other forms of entertainment to fight against monotony (Ratcliff, 1947). In military bases offering off-duty entertainment to service members the number of STD's being the result of sexual contact with female sex workers has been considerably reduced (Berg, 2005). The primary task of preventive medicine, which is part of medical support provided for troops engaged in operations conducted in adverse climatic and sanitary conditions, apart from defining risk factors for STD's in the military environment and preventing the occurrence of STD's, should be regular cooperation with representatives of the local public health authorities in the aspect of controlling the number of venereal diseases in a given territory, especially among risk groups (female sex workers) who may have contact with service members. A good example in this respect is the cooperation between the U.S. Navy and the Social Hygiene Department in the Philippines in the field of diagnostics and treatment of venereal diseases in the population of registered female sex workers who had been screened for STD's (the incidence rate of gonorrhea was merely 4% in the examined group). By contrast, the incidence rate of gonorrhea among unregistered female sex workers in the same territory was estimated at 40% (Hooper et al., 1978).

4. Conclusions

Sexually transmitted diseases do not pose a serious epidemiological risk among army personnel in the military environment under the condition of regular clinical and laboratory supervision of the soldiers' health status. The risk of acquiring an infection increases drastically in cases of unprotected casual, sexual intercourse. In recent years the hazard of developing of venereal diseases in the military environment has increased due to the fact that military service has ceased to be an all-male profession. In national contingents participating in peace and stabilization operations women account for a substantial part of military population. In some units of the U.S Forces female represent up to 15% of the population, which certainly influences the fact that sexual activity among military personnel is becoming increasingly commonplace. Screening conducted among personnel of the U.S. Forces revealed clinical symptoms and/or lab-confirmed cases of STD's. The results clearly indicate that detailed tests need to be carried out among male and female soldiers, before relocating to military service overseas as well as in the theater operation. Out of sexually transmitted diseases, chlamydiasis, gonorrhea and viral infections (HSV, HPV, HIV) prevail in military personnel. Chlamydiasis remains the most frequently diagnosed venereal disease in the population of soldiers. The epidemiological services of the U.S. Army recommend screening for *Chlamydia trachomatis* in all candidates entering the U.S Forces. Other STD's, especially HIV/AIDS, also constitute a considerable epidemiological risk in the military population. Screening for HIV infections is routinely carried out in the majority of the Armed Forces. The incidence rate of STD's among soldiers surges drastically during warfare and is several times higher in comparison with peacetime. Military contingents generally consist of young, sexually active men who tend to treat contact with female sex workers as a means of stress relief. The incidence rates of venereal diseases are hugely influenced by the region of deployment. In Muslim countries lying in the Middle East and Central Asia which are burdened with a number of moral restrictions, the access to sexual services is extremely limited. Therefore, in comparison with other diseases prevalent in these areas, STD's do not pose a serious health hazard for service members. In contrast, the epidemiological situation in other parts of the world, i.e. in Southeast Asia or Sub-Saharan Africa is completely different. Unlimited access to sexual services provided by sex workers of whom a vast majority is infected with STD's results in the increased incidence rates of sexually transmitted diseases in these regions and a much higher risk of acquiring an infection by soldiers deployed to military operations. Military health services and the representatives of preventive medicine in particular, need to bear this information in mind as future military operations with the participation of the multinational coalition forces are likely to be conducted in Africa where the incidence rates of STD's are one of the highest in the world.

5. References

Abel E., Adams E., Stevenson R. (1996). Sexual risk behaviour among female army recruits. *Military Medicine*, Vol. 161, No. 8, (August 1996), pp. 491-494

Abrams, A.J. (1968). Lymphogranuloma venereum. *The Journal of the American Medical Association*, Vol. 205, No. 4, pp. 199-202

Aral, S.O. & Holmes, K.K. (1990). Epidemiology of sexual behaviour and sexually transmitted diseases. In: *Sexually Transmitted Diseases*, Holmes, K.K.; Mardh, P.A., Sparling, P.F. & Wiesner, P.J., (Ed.), pp. 19-36, McGraw-Hill, New York, USA

Armed Forces Health Surveillance Center. (2010a). Brief Report: Recurrent Chlamydia Diagnoses, Active Component, 2000-2009. *Medical Surveillance Monthly Report*, Vol. 17, No. 8, (August 2010), pp. 15-17

Armed Forces Health Surveillance Center. (2010b). Sexually Transmitted Infections, U.S. Armed Forces, 2004-2009. *Medical Surveillance Monthly Report*, Vol. 17, No. 8, (August 2010), pp. 2-10

Armed Forces Health Surveillance Center. (2009). Defense Medical Epidemiology Database, June 2009, Available from www.afhsc.mil

Aldous, W.K.; Robertson, J.L., Robinson, B.J., Hatcher, C.L., Hospenthal, D.R., Conger, N.G. & Murray, C.K. (2011). Rates of Gonorrhea and Chlamydia in U.S. Military Personnel Deployed to Iraq and Afghanistan (2004-2009). *Military Medicine*, Vol. 176, No. 6, (June 2011), pp. 705-710

Asin, J. (1952). Chancroid: A report of 1,402 cases. *American Journal of Syphilis, Gonorrhea, and Venereal Diseases*, Vol. 36, pp. 483-487

Bazergan, R. & Easterbrook, P. (2003). HIV and UN peacekeeping operations. *AIDS*, Vol. 17, No. 2, (January 2003), pp. 278-279

Berg, S.W. (2005). Sexually Transmitted Diseases and Human Immunodeficiency Virus Infection, In: *Diseases Spread by Close Personal Contact*, Grey, G.C.; Feighner, B., Trump, D.H., Berg, S.W., Zajdowicz, M.J. & Zajdowicz, T.R., (Ed.), In: *Military Preventive Medicine: Mobilization and Deployment*, Kelley, P.W., (Ed.), Vol. 2, pp.

1146-1175, Borden Institute Walter Reed Army Medical Center, Office of the Surgeon General at TMM Publications, Washington DC, USA

Brill, J.R. (2010). Diagnosis and Treatment of Urethritis in Men. *American Family Physician*, Vol. 81, No. 7, pp. 873-878

Brodine, S.K. & Shafer, M.A. (2003). Combating Chlamydia in the military: Why aren't we wining the war? *Sexually Transmitted Diseases*, Vol. 30, pp. 545-548

Brodine, S.K.; Shafer, M.A., Shaffer, R.A., Boyer, C.B., Putnam, S.D., Wignall, F.S., Thomas, R.J., Bales, B. & Schachter, J. (1998). Asymptomatic sexually transmitted disese prevalence in four military populations: application of DNA amplification assays for Chlamydia and gonorrhea screening. *The Journal of Infectious Diseases*, Vol. 178, pp. 1202-1204

Brown, A.F.; Brundage, J.F., Tomlinson, J.P. & Burke, D.S. (1996). The US Army HIV testing program: the first decade. *Military Medicine*, Vol. 161, pp. 117-122

Catterson, M.L. & Zadoo, V. (1993). Prevalence of asymptomatic chlamydial cervical infection in active duty army females. *Military Medicine*, Vol. 158, pp. 618-619

Cates, W.; Rolfs, R. & Aral S. (1990). Sexually transmitted diseases, pelvic inflammatory disease, and infertility: An epidemiologic update. *Epidemiologic Reviews*, Vol. 12, pp. 199-220

Cecil, J.A.; Howell, M.R., Tawes, J.J., Gaydos, J.C., McKee, K.T., Quinn, T.C. & Gaydos, C.A. (2001). Features of *Chlamydia trachomatis* and *Neisseria gonorrhoeae* infection in male Army recruits. *The Journal of Infectious Diseases*, Vol. 184, pp. 1216-1219

Centers for Disease Control and Prevention. (2010). Gonorrhea fact sheet, October 2010, Available from www.cdc.gov/std/gonorrhea/stdfact-gonorrhea.htm

Centers for Disease Control and Prevention. (2009). Sexually Transmitted Diseases in the United States, 2008. *National Surveillance Data for Chlamydia, Gonorrhea, and Syphilis*, November 2009, Available from www.cdc.gov/std/stats

Centers for Disease Control and Prevention. (2006). Sexually transmitted diseases treatment guidelines, 2006. *Morbidity and Mortality Weekly Report*, Vol. 55, p. 11

Coutinho, R.A. (1994). Epidemiology of sexually transmitted diseases. *Sexually Transmitted Diseases*, Vol. 21(Suppl), pp. 51-52

Datta, S.D.; Sternberg, M., Johnson, R.E., Berman, S. Papp, J.R., McQuillan, G., Weinstock, H. (2007). Gonorrhea and Chlamydia in the United States among persons 14 to 39 years of age, 1999 to 2002. *Annals of Internal Medicine*, Vol. 147, No. 2, pp. 89-96

Day, S. (1988). Prostitute women and AIDS: Anthropology. *AIDS*, Vol. 2, pp. 421-428

Deller, J.J.; Smith, D.E., English, D.T. & Southwick, E.G. (1982). Venereal diseases, In: *General Medicine and Infectious Diseases*, Ognibene, A.J. & Barett O., (Ed.), In: *Internal Medicine in Vietnam*, Ognibene, A.J., (Ed.), Vol. 2, pp. 233-255, Medical Department, U.S. Army, Office of the Surgeon General, and Center of Military History, Washington DC, USA

Dinh, T.H.; Sternberg, M., Dunne, E.F. & Markowitz, L.E. (2008). Genital warts among 18- to 59-year-olds in the United States, National Health and Nutrition Examination Survey, 199-2004. *Sexually Transmitted Diseases*, Vol. 35, No. 4, pp. 357-360

Emmerson, L.A. (1997). Sexually transmitted disease controlled in the Armed Forces, past and present. *Military Medicine*, Vol. 162, No. 2, (February 1997), pp. 87-91

Fleming, D.T. ; McQuillan, G.E., Johnson, R.E., Nahmias, A.J., Aral, S.O., Lee, F.K. & St Louis, M.E. (1997). Herpes simplex virus type 2 in the United States, 1976-1994. *The New England Journal of Medicine*, Vol. 337, (October 1997), pp. 1105-1111

Gaydos, C.A. & Gaydos, J.C. (2008). Chlamydia in the United States Military: Can We Win This War? *Sexually Transmitted Diseases*, Vol. 35, No. 3, pp. 260-262

Gaydos, C.A.; Howell, M.R., Quinn, J.C., McKee, K.T. & Gaydos, J.C. (2003). Sustained high prevalence of *Chlamydia trachomatis* infections in female army recruits. *Sexually Transmitted Diseases*, Vol. 30, pp. 539-544

Gaydos, C.A.; Quinn, T.C. & Gaydos, J.C. (2000). The challenge of Sexually Transmitted Diseases for the Military: What Has Changed? *Clinical Infectious Diseases*, Vol. 30, pp. 719-722

Gaydos, C.A.; Howell, M.R., Pare, B., Clark, K.L., Ellis, D.A., Hendrix, R.M., Gaydos, J.C., McKee, K.T. & Quinn, T.C. (1998). *Chlamydia trachomatis* infections in female military recruits. *The New England Journal of Medicine*, Vol. 339, (September 1998), pp. 739-744

Greenberg, J.H. (1972). Venereal disease in the Armed Forces. *Medical Aspects of Human Sexuality*, Vol. 6, 165-201

Hamburg, B.A. (1986). Subsets of adolescent mothers: Development, biomedical, and psychosocial issues. In: *School-Age Pregnancy and Parenthood: Biosocial Dimensions*, Lancaster, J.B. & Hamburg, R.A., pp. 115-145, Aldine De Gruyter, New York, USA

Harrison, W.O. (1974). Cohort study of venereal diseases, *Proceedings of One-hundred-second Annual Meeting of the American Public Health Association and Related Organizations*, New Orleans, USA, 20-24 October 1974

Hart, G. (1974). Factors influencing venereal infection in a war environment. *The British Journal of Venereal Diseases*, Vol. 50, pp. 68-72

Hart G. (1973). Psychological aspects of venereal disease in war environment. *Social Science & Medicine*, Vol. 7, pp. 455-467

Hillis, S.D. & Wasserheit, J.N. (1996). Screening for Chlamydia - a key to the prevention of pelvic inflammatory disease. *The New England Journal of Medicine*, Vol. 334, No. 21, pp. 1399-1401

Hoge, C.W.; Lesikar, S.E., Guevara, R., Lange J., Brundage, J.F., Engel, C.C., Messer, S.C. & Orman, D.T. (2002). Mental Disorders Among U.S. Military Personnel in the 1990s: Association With High Levels of Health Care Utilization and Early Military Attrition. *American Journal of Psychiatry*, Vol. 159, pp. 1576-1583

Holmes; K.K., Johnson, D.W. & Trostle, H.J. (1970). An estimate of the risk of men acquiring gonorrhea by sexual contact with infected females. *American Journal of Epidemiology*, Vol. 91, 170-174

Hook, E.W. & Handsfield, H.H. Gonococcal Infections in the adult. (2008). In: *Sexually Transmitted Diseases*, Holmes, K.K.; Sparling, P.F., Stamm, W.E., et al. (Ed.), 4th Edition, pp. 627-645, McGraw Hill, Inc., New York, USA

Hooper, R.R.; Reynolds, G.H., Jones O.G., Zaidi, A., Wiesner, P.J., Latimer, K.P., Lester, A., Campbell, A.F., Harrison, W.O., Karney, W.W., & Holmes, K.K. (1978). Cohort study of venereal disease: The risk of gonorrhea transmission from infected women to men. *American Journal of Epidemiology*, Vol. 108, No. 2, (August 1978), pp. 136-144

Hopperus Buma, A.P.; Veltink, R.L., van Ameijden, E.J., Tendeloo, C.H. & Coutinho, R.A. (1995). Sexual behaviour and sexually transmitted diseases in Dutch marines and naval personnel on a United Nations mission in Cambodia. *Genitourinary Medicine*, Vol. 71, pp. 172-175

Hor, L.B.; Detels, R., Heng, S. & Mun, P. (2005). The role of sex worker clients in transmission of HIV in Cambodia. *International Journal of STD & AIDS*, Vol. 16, No. 2, pp. 170-174

Hyams, K.C.; Hanson, K. & Wignall, F.S. (1995). The Impact of Infectious Diseases on the Health of U.S. Troops Deployed to the Persian Gulf During Operations Desert Shield and Desert Storm. *Clinical Infectious Diseases*, Vol. 20, pp. 1497-1504

Jordan, N.N.; Seung-eun, L., Nowak, G., Johns, N.M. & Gaydos J.C. (2011). *Chlamydia trachomatis* Reported Among U.S. Active Duty Service Members, 2000-2008. *Military Medicine*, Vol. 176, No. 3, (March 2011), pp. 312-319

Kerber, R.E.; Rowe, C.E. & Gilbert, K.R. (1969). Treatment of chancroid: A comparison of tetracycline and sulfisoxazole. *Archives of Dermatology*, Vol. 100, pp. 604-607

Korzeniewski, K. (2011). Health hazards in areas of military operations conducted in different climatic and sanitary conditions. *International Maritime Health*, Vol. 62, No. 1, pp. 41-62

Korzeniewski, K. (2008). Peacekeeping in South-East Asia. *International Journal of Health Science*, Vol. 1, No. 3, pp. 88-92

Korzeniewski, K., Kierznikowicz, B. & Olszański, R. (2003). Sexually transmitted diseases among Polish soldiers serving in the U.N. peace missions in Lebanon and Cambodia. *International Maritime Health*, Vol. 54, pp. 101-107

Kotloff, K.L.; Wassermann, S.S., Russ, K., Shapiro, S., Daniel, R., Brown, W., Frost, A., Tabara, S.O. & Shah, K. (1998). Detection of genital human papillomavirus and associated cytological abnormalities among college women. *Sexually Transmitted Diseases*, Vol. 25 (May 1998), pp. 243-250

Malone, J.D.; Hyams, K.C., Hawkins, R.E., Sharp, T.W. & Daniell, F.D. (1993). Risk factors for sexually transmitted diseases among deployed US military personnel. *Sexually Transmitted Diseases*, Vol. 20, pp. 294-298

McKee, K.T.; Burns, W.E., Russell, L.K., Jenkins, P.R., Johnson, A.E., Wong, T.L. & McLawhorn, K.B. (1998). Early syphilis in an active duty military population and the surrounding civilian community, 1985-1993. *Military Medicine*, Vol. 163, pp. 368-375

McNinch, J.H. (1954). Venereal disease problems: U.S. Army Forces, Far East 1950-1953. *Proceedings of Recent Advances in Medicine and Surgery*, 19-30 April 1954, Army Medical Service Graduate School, Walter Reed Army Medical Center, Washington DC, USA

Melton, L.J. (1976). Comparative incidence of gonorrhea and nongonococcal urethritis in the United States Navy. *American Journal of Epidemiology*, Vol. 104, pp. 535-542

Meyers, D.; Wolff, T., Gregory, K., Marion, L., Moyer, V., Nelson, H., Petiti, D. & Sawaya, G.F. (2008). USPSTF recommendations for STI screening. *American Family Physician*, Vol. 77, No. 6, pp. 819-824

Miller, N. & Yeager, R. (1995). By virtue of their occupation, soldiers and sailors are at greater risk. Special report: The military. *AIDS Analysis Africa*, Vol. 5, pp. 8-9

Niebuhr, D.W.; Tobler, S.K., Jordan, N.N. & Singer, D.E. (2006). Sexually transmitted infections among military recruits, In: *Recruit Medicine*, DeKoning, B.L., (Ed.), pp. 255-275, Borden Institute Walter Reed Army Medical Center, Office of the Surgeon General at TMM Publications, Washington DC, USA

Padget, P. (1963). Diagnosis and treatment of the venereal diseases, In: *Infectious Diseases*, Havens, W.P., (Ed.), In: *Internal Medicine in World War II*, Coates, J.B., (Ed.), Vol. 2, pp. 409-435, Medical Department, U.S. Army, Office of the Surgeon General, Washington DC, USA

Padian, N.S. (1988). Prostitute women and AIDS: Epidemiology. *AIDS*, Vol. 2, pp. 413-419

Perine, P.L. & Osoba, A.O. (1990). Lymphogranuloma venereum. In: *Sexually Transmitted Diseases*, Holmes, I.I.; Mardh, P.A., Sparling, P.F., et al. (Ed.), pp. 195-204, McGraw-Hill, New York, USA

Rasnake, M.S.; Konger, N.G., McAllister, C.K., Holmes, K.K. & Tramont, E.C. (2005). History of U.S. Military Contributions to the Study of Sexually Transmitted Diseases. *Military Medicine*, Vol. 170, No. 4, (April 2005), pp. 61-65

Ratcliff, T.A. (1947). Psychiatric and allied aspects of the problem of venereal diseases in the army. *Journal of the Royal Army Medical Corps*, Vol. 89, pp. 122-131

Renton, A.M. & Whitaker, L. (1994). Using STD occurrence to monitor AIDS prevention. *Social Science & Medicine*, Vol. 38, pp. 1153-1165

Renzullo, P.I.; Sateren, W.B., Garner, R.P., Milazzo, M.J., Birx, D.L. & McNeil, J.G. (2001). HIV-1 seroconversion in the United States Army active duty personnel, 1985-1999. *AIDS*, Vol. 15, pp. 1569-1574

Renzullo, P.I.; McNeil, J.G., Levin, L.I., Bunin, J.R., Brundage, J.F. (1990). Risk factors for prevalent human immunodeficiency virus (HIV) infection in active duty Army men who initially report no identified risk: a case-control study. *Journal of Acquired Immune Deficiency Syndromes*, Vol. 3, pp. 266-271

Ryan, C.A.; Vathiny, O.V., Gorbach, P.M., Leng, H.B., Berlioz-Arthaud, A., Whittington, W.L. & Holmes, K.K. (1998). Explosive spread of HIV-1 and sexually transmitted diseases in Cambodia. *Lancet*, Vol. 351, No. 9110, p. 1175

Sena, A.C.; Miller, W.C., Hoffman, I.F., Chakraborty, H., Cohen, M.S., Jenkins, P. & McKee, K.T. (2000). Trends of Gonorrhea and Chlamydial Infection during 1985-1996 among Active-Duty Soldiers at a United States Army Installation. *Clinical Infectious Diseases*, Vol. 30, pp. 742-748

Seung-eun, L.; Nauschuetz, W., Jordan, N., Lindler, L., Steece, R., Pfau, E. & Gaydos, J.C. (2010). Survey of Sexually Transmitted Disease Laboratory Methods in US Army Laboratories. *Sexually Transmitted Diseases*, Vol. 37, No. 1, pp. 44-48

Shafer, M.A.; Boyer, C.B., Pollack, L.M., Moncada, J., Chang, J. & Schachter, J. (2008). Acquisition of *C. trachomatis* by young women during their first year of military service. *Sexually Transmitted Diseases*, Vol. 35, pp. 255-259

Shapiro, S.R. & Breschi, L.C. (1974). Venereal disease in Vietnam: clinical experience at a major military hospital. *Military Medicine*, Vol. 139, pp. 374-379

Sternberg, H.T. & Howard E. (1960). Venereal diseases, In: *Communicable Diseases Transmitted Through Contact or By Unknown Means*, Vol. 5, In: *Preventive Medicine in World War II*, p. 139, U.S. Department of the Army, Office of the Surgeon General, Washington DC, USA

Trei, J.S.; Canas, L.C. & Gould, P.L. (2008). Reproductive tract complications associated with *Chlamydia trachomatis* infection in US Air Force males within 4 years of testing. *Sexually Transmitted Diseases*, Vol. 35, No. 9, pp. 827-833

Tripodi, P. & Patel, P. (2004). HIV/AIDS, Peacekeeping and Conflict Crises in Africa. *Medicine, Conflict and Survival*, Vol. 20, No. 3, pp. 195-208

United Nations. (1999). Medical support manual for United Nations peacekeeping operations, Ed. 2, pp. 47-48, New York, USA

USACHPPM. (2007). A Guide to Female Soldier Readiness. USACHPPM Technical Guide 281. *U.S. Army Center for Health Promotion & Preventive Medicine*, January 2007, Available from http://chppm-www.apgea.army.mil/documents/TG/TECHGUID/TG281January2007-1.pdf

U.S. Department of Health, Education, and Welfare. (1962). The eradication of syphilis: a task force report to the Surgeon General, Public Health Service, on syphilis control in the United States, *Public Health Service publication no. 918*, Washington DC, USA

U.S. General Accounting Office. (2001). UN peacekeeping: United Nations faces challenges in responding to the impact of HIV/AIDS on peacekeeping operations. *Report to the Chairman*, pp. 8-9, Committee on International Relations, House of Representatives, Washington DC, USA

U.S. National Intelligence Council. (2000). Global Infectious disease threat and its implications for the United States. *National Intelligence Council*, p. 29, Washington DC, USA

U.S. Preventive Services Task Force (2007). Screening for chlamydial infection: U.S. Preventive Services Task Force recommendation statement. *Annals of Internal Medicine*, Vol. 147, No. 2, pp. 128-134

Valente, S. & Wight C. (2007). Military Sexual Trauma: Violence and Sexual Abuse. *Military Medicine*, Vol. 172, No. 3, (March 2007), pp. 259-265

Vu, M.Q., Steketee, R.W., Valleroy, L., Weinstock, H., et al. (2002). HIV incidence in the United States, 1978-1999. *Journal of Acquired Immune Deficiency Syndromes*, Vol. 31, pp. 188-201

Walter Reed Army Institute of Research. (1998). Accession medical standards analysis and research activity. *Annual report*. Washington DC, USA

Wasserman, G.M.; Martin, B.L. & Hyams, K.C. (1997). A Survey of Outpatient Visits in a United States Army Forward Unit during Operation Desert Shield. *Military Medicine*, Vol. 162, No. 6, (June 1997), pp. 374-379

Weinstock, H.; Berman, S. & Cates, W. (2000). Sexually transmitted diseases among American youth: Incidence and prevalence estimates, 2000. *Perspectives on Sexual and Reproductive Health*, Vol. 36, pp. 6-10, 22, 59

Wittkower, E.D. & Cowan, J. (1944). Some psychological aspects of sexual promiscuity: Summary of an investigation. *Psychosomatic Medicine*, Vol. 6, pp. 287-294

Wong, M.L.; Lubek, I., Dy, B.C., Pen, S., Kros, S. & Chhit, M. (2003). Social and behavioural factors associated with condom use among direct sex workers in Siem Reap, Cambodia. *Sexually Transmitted Infections*, Vol. 79, No. 2, pp. 163-165

Wright, J.; Albright, T.S., Gehrich, A.P., Dunlow, S.G., Lettieri, C.F. & Buller, J.L. (2006). Sexually Transmitted Diseases in Operation Iraqi Freedom/Operation Enduring Freedom. *Military Medicine*, Vol. 171, No. 10, (October 2006), pp. 1024-1026

Zenilman, J.M.; Glass, G., Shields, T., Jenkins, P.R., Gaydos, J.C. & McKee, K.T. (2002). Geographic epidemiology of gonorrhoea and *Chlamydia* on a large military installation: application of a GIS system. *Sexually Transmitted Infections*, Vol. 78, pp. 40-44

11

Syphilis and Herpes Simplex Virus Type 2 Sero-Prevalence Among Female Sex Workers and Men Who Have Sex with Men in Ecuador and Andhra Pradesh (India)

Juan Pablo Gutiérrez and Erika E. Atienzo
Instituto Nacional de Salud Pública
México

1. Introduction

Sexually Transmitted Infections (STI) are a major public health issue worldwide because of their severe consequences for millions of men, women and children (World health organization [WHO], 2001, 2007). Despite of that, there is lack of data on their magnitude; the most recent estimations from the World Health Organization (WHO) are from 1999, when it was estimated that 340 million of new cases of curable STIs such as Syphilis, Neisseria gonorrhoeae, Chlamydia trachomatis and Trichomonas vaginalis occurred every year (WHO, 2001). Recent studies continue to reveal an increment in STI diagnosis across the world (Centers for Disease Control and Prevention (CDC), 2011; Cliffe et al., 2008; Herida et al., 2005; Johnston et al., 2005; Nicoll & Hamers, 2002; Uuskula et al., 2010).

Female sex workers (FSW) and men who have sex with men (MSM) has been reported as population groups with an average number of sexual partner higher than the general population. Because of this, and because their partners are from different groups in the population, FSW and MSM are key for STIs transmission dynamics. Epidemiological studies among MSM are still scarce particularly in developing regions (Caceres, C. et al., 2006). However the existent studies on the effects of HIV/STI prevention interventions highlight the fact that, for the most largely affected community in the HIV era, rigorous prevention strategies are urgently needed (Coates et al., 2008; Herbst et al., 2005; Johnson et al., 2008; Johnson et al., 2002).

FSW are still at the center of the epidemic in many countries, especially where heterosexual transmission of HIV is the main mode of transmission (Ghys et al., 2001). FSW vulnerability to STI/HIV results from diverse factors including a high rate of sexual partners, unprotected sex or inconsistent condom use and lack of access to health services (Ghys et al., 2001). Also, gender inequities, violence, exploitation, and criminalization, are all factors affecting unprotected and forced sex, which will in turn increase the risk for a FSW to contract an STI (Okal et al., 2011; Panchanadeswaran et al., 2008).

This chapter provides an overview on STI among MSM and FSW from two developing countries: Ecuador and India. We aim to present a panorama of syphilis and herpes simplex virus type 2 (HSV 2) sero-prevalence and trends during a 4 year period, in two high-level vulnerable groups from two countries with very different economies, cultural and social norms. We will explore the similarities and differences in the trends on STI in MSM and FSW, allowing the readers the reflection on individual and contextual factors that may contribute to these trends in STI sero-prevalence in each population.

The content is divided in three sections. The first section briefly reviews background information regarding STI epidemics in Ecuador and India, giving emphasis to the scarce available data for MSM and FSW in relation to syphilis and HSV-2 infection. Second section presents the results of our study, particularly those related to trends on STI and HIV sero-prevalence from 2002/3 to 2007. Finally, as discussion points, we present some reflections derived from the results, highlighting the challenges to develop effective prevention strategies for MSM and FSW, and the need for large scale survey research using biomarkers for STIs.

2. Background

Because of the HIV infections worldwide, STIs that result in genital ulcers such as syphilis and HSV-2 started to get a lot more attention since these infections predispose the risk of HIV infection (Sgaier et al., 2011). One important feature of these infections is that the effectiveness of condoms decreases in the presence of ulcers, as the right protection must not only cover body fluid exchange but also the affected areas.

In spite of the fact that syphilis is a treatable infection since antibiotics were introduced, it is still a major public health issue. Even when the use of antibiotics is evident because of the global decline in syphilis prevalence (Sgaier et al., 2011), there is some evidence showing that in the last decade there has been a reappearing in several countries, specially among high-risk population groups such as MSM (Buchacz et al., 2005; Doherty et al., 2002; Gao et al., 2009; Hopkins et al., 2004; Peterman et al., 2005). In addition, the low effectiveness of contraceptives (including condoms) to prevent infections such as syphilis, on one hand, and the indiscriminate use of antibiotics that increases the risk of resistant chains, on the other, could lead to a more complex situation regarding the eradication of this infection even when there is an effective treatment available nowadays.

At the same time, there has been an important increase in the prevalence of viral infections around the world, including HSV-2. It is known now that HSV-2 is the main cause of genital ulcers in developing countries (WHO, 2007). It has been documented that gender, race, the number of sexual partners and the place of residence are among the factors related to the prevalence of this virus (Whitley & Roizman, 2001). According to a systematic review of HSV-2 sero-prevalence studies on an international scale (Smith & Robinson, 2002), the highest prevalence found has been documented in Africa and America, and the lowest has been documented in Asia. According to the authors, the virus prevalence increases with the potential time of exposure, meaning that it consistently increases with age, especially among 15 to 24 year old women and it appears particularly in groups with a higher prevalence of risky practices. This virus is even considered as a reliable marker of high-risk sexual behavior.

Population groups such as MSM or FSW are specially vulnerable to STIs because of a higher number of sexual partners than the general population, resulting in more exposure. In addition, high-risk practices such as unprotected sex or inconsistent condom use that can be associated with a higher probability of infection among these groups have been documented.

India, in Asia, has the second highest population in the world. This country is extremely socially, economically, and culturally diverse. High marginalization conditions prevail over an important percentage of its population even when there is a growing economy. Andhra Pradesh is a southern Indian state, the fifth largest territory in the country, with a surface area that can be compared with that of Ecuador. It has a population of 80 million people and its main economic activity is agriculture, although it has had an important development in technological fields in recent years.

Ecuador, a south American country, has a population of 14 million people and an oil based economy with agriculture being the second economic activity.

Both Ecuador and Andhra Pradesh, located in opposite hemispheres, share similar economic conditions, which make them archetypes of countries with limited incomes, and with an important inequality in the income distribution. These countries are, however, countries with such a cultural diversity that they show distinctive traits. Stated below, we present a brief review of existing evidence regarding syphilis and HSV-2 sero-prevalence among FSW and MSM in Ecuador and India.

2.1 Evidence of STI in Ecuador

As in many Latin-American countries (LA), in Ecuador, STIs frequency and distribution registries provides little useful information, due partly to a sub report that has been estimated of a considerable magnitude, because of the stigma associated to these infections (Galban & Benzaken, 2007). In combination with these restrictions related to health information systems, the evidence resulting from scientific investigation and publications is limited as well. Regional research has been carried out in the Andean area (Colombia, Ecuador, Bolivia, Peru), which has provided more information to rely on. Data reported to UNAIDS indicates that regarding HIV, most countries in this region face a concentrated epidemic with HIV prevalence lower than 1%, around 0.4%, among general adult population, but with higher numbers among high-risk population groups such as MSM and among injectable drug users also in some countries (IDU) (UNAIDS/WHO, 2009).

Available data from multicentric studies carried out for several countries in the Andean area, particularly in Ecuador (Bautista et al., 2006; Bautista et al., 2004; Centers for Disease Control and Prevention (CDC), 2011; Montano et al., 2005), reveal that Ecuador has the highest HIV prevalence among FSW in the Andean area, with a 1.8-2% prevalence (Bautista et al., 2006; Montano et al., 2005). HIV prevalence among MSM in Ecuador has been found around 11 and 29% (Bastos et al., 2008; Bautista et al., 2004; Montano et al., 2005).

There is almost no available data regarding syphilis and HSV-2 epidemiological state in this country, except for a few studies reported before the year 2000 (Jaramillo & Medina, 1998; Oswaldo et al., 1993). Nevertheless, according to one study using data reported by health ministries of 19 LA countries, in 2006, Ecuador reveled 1,885 syphilis cases (Galban & Benzaken, 2007). There is no further published data regarding these two STIs among FSW and MSM.

2.2 Evidence of STI in India

Contrary to what happens in Ecuador, there is a large number of published studies regarding sero-prevalence of STIs among the Indian population, revealing a wide range of prevalence

(Das et al., 2011). Generally speaking, an important decrease in HIV prevalence in southern Indian states has been documented, where a series of strategies focusing on the prevention of new HIV infections have been put into practice (Kumar et al., 2006). According to the last UNAIDS report, in 2009 there were 2,300,000 people of 15 and up, living with HIV in India, in contrast with 2,500,000 in 2001; the HIV general prevalence among the adult population in 2009 is 0.3% (UNAIDS, 2010). An HIV prevalence of 5 to 13% specially among FSW has been reported (Pal et al., 2004; Shethwala et al., 2009; Uma et al., 2005), whereas MSM report a prevalence of 9 to 18% (Brahmam et al., 2008; Kumta et al., 2010; Solomon et al., 2010).

However syphilis and HSV-2 available data are not as specific, and results differ according to the population group and the geographic location (Sgaier et al., 2011).

Concerning the syphilis infection, studies carried out among FSW show a prevalence between a range of 6-10% (Das et al., 2011; Shethwala et al., 2009). Yet, other studies reveal higher rates, between 22-31% (Desai et al., 2003; Family Health International/Development Fund for International Development/Andhra Pradesh State AIDS Control Society, 2001; Pal et al., 2004; Wayal et al., 2011). Because of this variation, it has been suggested that a decrease in prevalence among this group has happened in the last few years. For example, in three southern Indian states, data show that from 2005 to 2009 syphilis prevalence significantly dropped among FSW population, even when this was not so clear among its clients (Adhikary et al., 2011).

In relation to MSM, there is a lot less reported regarding STIs; however some of the studies report a syphilis prevalence between 6 and 17% (Brahmam et al., 2008; Gupta et al., 2006; Kumta et al., 2010; Setia et al., 2006; Solomon et al., 2010). Just as for FSW population, one study show that in a ten years time, syphilis prevalence significantly dropped in a MSM sample group (Gupta et al., 2006).

There is even less information regarding the spread of HSV-2 than for other STIs. However, in the last few years, this infection has been placed among the most common in high-risk population groups in India (Kumarasamy et al., 2008). Data taken from FSW sample groups show that a high percentage of them are infected with HSV-2, reporting a prevalence of 56 to 73% (Shahmanesh et al., 2009; Uma et al., 2005; Wayal et al., 2011). MSM studies show elevated prevalence as well. For example, a study carried out with a MSM sample group in 8 Indian cities showed a HSV-2 prevalence of 26% (Solomon et al., 2010), whereas another study carried out with MSM in Mumbai clinics show a 40% prevalence (Setia et al., 2006).

2.3 The Frontiers Prevention Project (FPP)

Data for this analysis are from the evaluation of a large HIV prevention intervention, the Frontiers Prevention Project (FPP). The FPP was implemented globally by the International HIV/AIDS Alliance. As part of the FPP evaluation, sero-surveys of MSM and FSW were conducted between 2002/2003 and 2007 in sites from 8 cities in Ecuador and 24 geographical sites in India. Potential sites of concentration of MSM and FSW were identified through interviews with key informants and mapping exercises that were conducted in each city. At selected sites, MSM and FSW were contacted and recruited by members of the same key population.

For the 2007 survey, a second mapping/identification exercise was carried out in each city to identify new meeting sites. MSM and FSW were recruited using the same strategy from

2002/2003. At both years, capillary blood samples were taken for assays on serological antibodies to herpes simplex virus type 2 using Focus Diagnostics HerpeSelect 2™, and Trepanostika™ from bioMerieux for the diagnosis of syphilis. For this work we use information collected at all the sites both in Ecuador and India, but controlling for the potential effect of the FPP prevention package. HerpeSelect 2 for sexually active adults has a sensibility of 96.1% and a specificity of 97% (Focus Diagnostics, n.d.). Trepanostika manufacturer reported 100% sensitivity and specificity (BioMérieux, n.d.).

This study was approved by the Ethics and Research Committee at the National Institute of Public Health of Mexico, the Ecuador National Health Board, the Administrative Staff College of India, the Indian Health Ministry's Screening Committee and the International HIV/AIDS Alliance.

3. Results

During these two periods (2003 and 2007), biological samples of 11,272 participants were collected: 7,178 provided biological samples between 2002/2003 (baseline data) and 4,584 in 2007. In 2003 information from 3,995 key populations (FSW and MSM) members in Ecuador and 2,524 in India was collected, whereas in 2007 the sample consisted of 2,060 members in Ecuador and 2,524 in India. Table 1 shows the population distribution according to group, country and time period.

Group		Country				Total
		Ecuador		India		
		2003	2007	2003	2007	
	MSM	1,933	1,004	1,755	1,143	5,835
	FSW	2,062	1,056	1,428	1,381	5,927
Total by year		3,995	2,060	3,183	2,524	
Total by country		6,055		5,707		11,762

Table 1. Study sample size by country, year and group.

For the analysis presented here, we fitted a probit model including three dummy variables and their pairwise and triple interaction. Interacted variables are time (2003 vs 2007), country (Ecuador vs India) and group (MSM vs FSW). We obtained the marginal effects of such interaction using inteff3 command in Stata (V. 10), controlling for the potential effect of the FPP prevention package. Dependant variables are syphilis and HSV-2 sero-prevalence, and the co-infection between both.

Hereafter, the most important aspects of prevalence found for each population group in both countries is described, followed by the results of the multivariate analysis, presenting syphilis results first and HSV-2 data next. The proneness of co-infection between both STIs is also concisely pointed out. In order to thoroughly analyze the characteristics of these FSW and MSM sample groups, previous publications can be consulted (Dandona, L. et al., 2005; Dandona, R. et al., 2005; Dandona et al., 2006; Gutierrez et al., 2010; Gutierrez et al., 2006a; Gutierrez et al., 2006b; Kumar, G.A. et al., 2006).

3.1 Syphilis sero-prevalence

Regarding the presence of syphilis, Ecuador´s data show an overall prevalence increase between 2003 and 2007, so that in 2007 general prevalence was twice as much (8%) as in 2003 (4%). While increase in prevalence is observed in Ecuador, the opposite findings were noted in India, meaning that in this country, syphilis prevalence decreased between 2003 and 2007, with an overall prevalence of 18% and 8% respectively for each year.

Even though this is the overall trend at a country level, this trend appears in different extents for each group in each country (Fig.1). It also shows that in both, Ecuador and India, syphilis prevalence is higher among MSM when compared with FSW, a condition that persists from the baseline to the follow-up. While in 2003 Ecuador has a syphilis prevalence of 5% and 3% among MSM and FSW respectively, in India this prevalence is 21% and 15%. It is interesting to notice that in 2007, both groups in the two countries tend to bare a syphilis prevalence of around 8%.

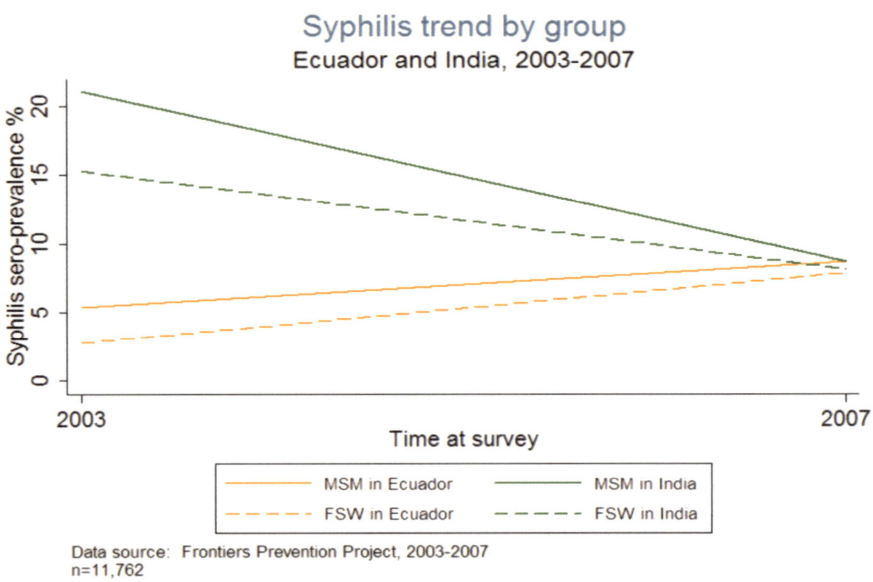

Fig. 1. Syphilis trend among men who have sex with men (MSM) and female sex workers (FSW) in Ecuador and India, 2003-2007.

The results from the multivariate analysis show that in 2003, the probability of a FSW of being syphilis sero-positive in Ecuador is 2.3 percentage points below when compared to MSM in that same country ($p \leq 0.01$). In India, FSW have a probability of 5.7 percentage points below MSM of a syphilis sero-positive diagnosis in 2003 ($p \leq 0.01$). In 2007 there are no significant differences when comparing FSW to MSM in either country.

The difference among these two groups in terms of their vulnerability is clearly shown when analyzing the effect of time in the probability of a syphilis positive diagnosis. For MSM in Ecuador, the time trend is shown in a 3 percentage points increase in syphilis probability ($p \leq 0.01$). This effect is of a greater magnitude among FSW in this country, since it shows an increase of near 5 percentage points in syphilis probability between 2003 and 2007 ($p \leq 0.01$).

For Indian population, in contrast, the trend in time shows that the probability of syphilis sero-positive diagnosis among MSM decreased 12 percentage points in time ($p \leq 0.01$), whereas for FSW there was a 6.8 percentage points decrease ($p \leq 0.01$).

3.2 Herpes simplex virus type 2

Regarding HSV-2, the overall prevalence in both countries is high, nevertheless, there is a similar trend to the one that takes place with syphilis prevalence. As an increase in HSV-2 prevalence is perceived in Ecuador between 2003 (61%) and 2007 (87%), a decrease is observed in India, going from an overall prevalence of 43% in 2003 to a 20% in 2007.

As shown in figure 2, HSV-2 prevalence during 2003 among MSM was similar in both countries, with a prevalence around 37-38%. Also in both countries, but in contrast to the syphilis situation, the FSW group shows the highest HSV-2 prevalence, particularly in Ecuador. In this country the STIs prevalence among FSW is 83%, whereas in India it is documented to be 50%. By 2007 MSM show an important increase in the prevalence of this virus in Ecuador (80%), reaching a more similar prevalence to that documented for FSW in this same country in 2007 (92%). In India, there is a similar decrease for FSW and MSM from 2003 to 2007, showing a prevalence of 14% and 24% respectively in 2007.

The most significant variation in HSV-2 prevalence was observed among MSM in Ecuador. According to the multivariate analysis, the HSV-2 sero-positive probability is 43 percentage points higher for FSW in Ecuador in contrast with MSM ($p \leq 0.01$), but in 2007 this difference narrows down so that the probability of infection is only 10 percentage points higher for FSW ($p \leq 0.01$). In other words, in the follow-up, prevalence in both groups tend to resemble. In India, the risk for FSW in contrast with MSM is comparatively similar from 2003 to 2007; at baseline, the probability of an HSV-2 diagnosis is 13 percentage points higher for FSW in contrast with MSM ($p \leq 0.01$), whereas at follow-up, the difference is only 10 percentage points ($p \leq 0.01$), close to that of Ecuador (Fig. 2).

In terms of the time trend over the probability of a HSV-2 positive diagnosis, we found that time increases this probability 41 percentage points among the MSM population in Ecuador ($p \leq 0.01$), whereas among the FSW population in the same country, the probability increases only 8 percentage points ($p \leq 0.01$). On the other hand, the effect of time for the Indian population is closer between MSM and FSW, as HSV-2 sero-positive probability decreased 23 percentage points for MSM ($p \leq 0.01$) and 26 points for FWS ($p \leq 0.01$) from 2003 to 2007.

3.3 Syphilis and HSV-2 co-infection

Finally, it is important to look into the co-infection trend shown among these two STIs. In terms of overall prevalence, in 2003 in Ecuador, 3% of the sample was positive for both syphilis and HSV-2 infection, while in India it was 13%. In 2007 the prevalence of co-infection in Ecuador reached 7%, while in India it decreased to come at 3%.

At a group level it is clear that the co-infection pattern tends to be similar among MSM and FSW in each country, and this is evident both in 2003 and 2007 (Fig. 3). In 2003, the co-infection prevalence in Ecuador among MSM was 4.5%, while for FSW it was 2.6%. The same year, in India, the co-infection prevalence was 13% for MSM and 12% for FSW. During the follow-up, in Ecuador around 7% of these groups show a co-infection of these two STIs, meanwhile, in India, a co-infection among both groups is documented in around 3-4% (Fig. 3). There is no evidence of a significant difference regarding co-infection when comparing MSM and FSW in each country and year.

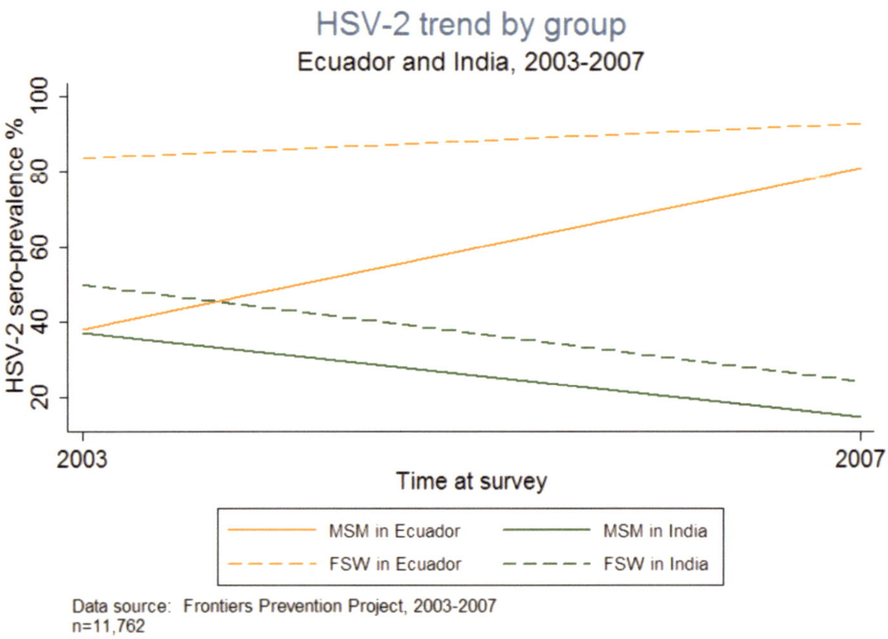

Fig. 2. Herpes simplex virus type 2 (HSV-2) trend among men who have sex with men (MSM) and female sex workers (FSW) in Ecuador and India, 2003-2007.

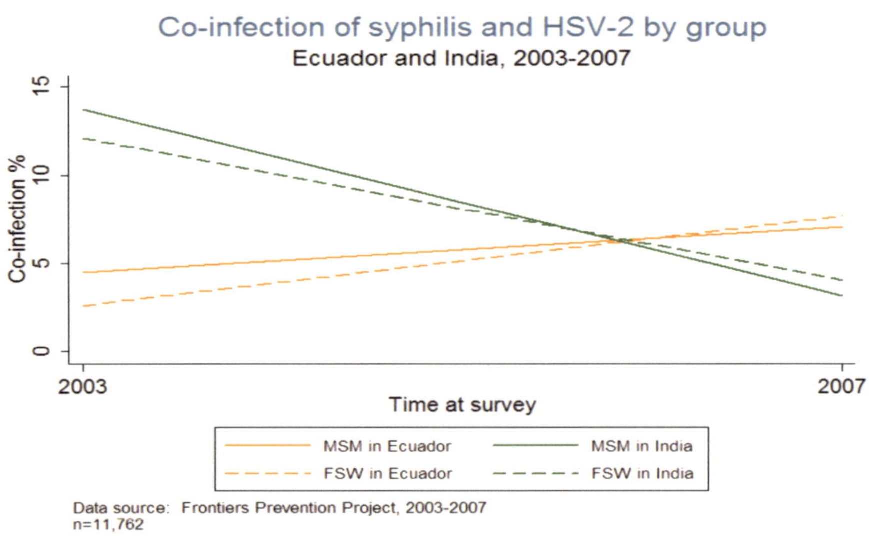

Fig. 3. Syphilis and Herpes simplex virus type 2 (HSV-2) co-infection among men who have sex with men (MSM) and female sex workers (FSW) in Ecuador and India, 2003-2007.

Regarding co-infection among both STIs at the country level, we found the same trend that is identified for each particular STI. In other words, while in Ecuador there is an increasing trend for both STIs co-infection, in India the trend is decreasing. For example, the results from the multivariate analysis show that the trend in time is that the probability of co-infection among MSM increases 2.5 percentage points ($p \leq 0.01$) in Ecuador, in the mean time, it increases 5 points among FSW in that same country ($p \leq 0.01$). In contrast, in India, the probability of co-infection among MSM from 2003 to 2007 decreases 10 percentage points ($p \leq 0.01$), whereas for FSW it decreases as far as 7 percentage points ($p \leq 0.01$).

4. Conclusion

This chapter presents the results of a research conducted to explore syphilis and HSV-2 prevalence among MSM and FSW population groups in Ecuadorean and Indian sites, with data collected from 2003 to 2007. According to our results, there is an important presence of both STIs among these population groups, each one affecting to a different extent each one of the groups. Consistent with other published studies, the results show a reduction of syphilis and herpes sero-prevalence among high-risk population groups in India. On the other hand, an important STI increase was reported in Ecuador during the same time period among FSW and MSM. This breakdown shows, first of all, that there is no uniform behavior of STIs around the world, and secondly, that the extent of these infections is clearly related to the specific context.

Another contribution of this research is the fact that the data come from a much larger sample than the one usually reported in STIs studies in these countries. In addition, the research allows the examination of the co-infection pattern among these two STIs, bringing in extremely original data about a rarely published topic, specially in developing countries (Lama et al., 2006). According to this, the co-infection of these STIs show the same trend as when addressed individually, in other words, there is an increase in Ecuador´s case, but a decrease in India.

In India, there has been great mobilization towards the creation and execution of HIV prevention strategies intended for different population groups in the last few years (Gangopadhyay et al., 2005; Guinness, 2011; Kumar et al., 2011; Reza-Paul et al., 2008; Verma et al., 2010). In our study, when comparing both countries, Ecuador´s scenario is less favorable since for both MSM and FSW, prevalence of these STIs tends to increase in time. On the other hand, in India the prevalence of these infections shows a significant decrease. In this sense, it can be suggested from our results that the important effort carried out in AP (India) regarding control of HIV could have favored a decrease in high-risk behavior. This means that the documented reduction of HIV in India (Rao et al., 2009) may be due to a decrease in high-risk behavior that, at the same time, reduces other STIs infection such as syphilis and HSV-2, although this cannot be completely sustained for infections that cause ulcers, considering their high prevalence reported in this study. What seems evident is that even with such efforts, the number of infected people in AP is extremely elevated.

In Ecuador, there is no evidence regarding the implementation of prevention strategies, nevertheless, it is clear that on an overall scale, in the LA area, the few documented prevention efforts have been intended primarily for the general population, excluding more vulnerable population groups such as MSM and FSW (Caceres, C.F., 2004; Huedo-Medina et al., 2010). The results shown here, could symbolize the great need for the creation and execution of massive efforts focusing on these vulnerable population groups in the LA area.

The relationship between genital herpes and HIV infection has been thoroughly described in publications, pointing out that the risk of getting HIV is twice as much for a person infected with HSV-2 (Wald & Link, 2002). It is also known that syphilis infection assists HIV transmission as well (Buchacz et al., 2005). In this sense, prevention and treatment of other STIs can play a part in the reduction of risk of HIV transmission in a population group with a high rate of sexual partners, such as FSW and MSM (WHO, 2007).

International publications point out that in developing countries HSV-2 sero-positivity is mostly among women when compared to men. On the other hand, at an international scale, a syphilis outbreak has been reported particularly among MSM population groups (Buchacz et al., 2005; Doherty et al., 2002; Gao et al., 2009; Hopkins et al., 2004; Peterman et al., 2005). In accordance with this, the results of this research show that for both countries, syphilis prevalence in 2003 is higher among MSM, whereas HSV-2 mostly affects FSW population groups. Nevertheless, the time trend shows that in Ecuador´s case, the most significant increase of HSV-2 prevalence happens among MSM, while syphilis increases affecting mostly FSW. In contrast, as stated before, in India the general trend is a decrease in syphilis infection, although such decrease was lesser among FSW.

MSM and FSW are a stigmatized and hard to reach population. Frequently, FSW are threatened by legal frameworks that criminalize sex work (Operario et al., 2008; Vandepitte et al., 2006). At the same time, in many developing countries MSM face social and cultural stigma and discrimination (Beyrer, 2008). These are factors that affect surveillance and research directed toward these populations, thus limiting the comprehension on how the STI epidemic is being driven in a specific group or country (Beyrer, 2008).

As stated earlier, available information related to syphilis and HSV-2 prevalence in these two countries is very scarce, particularly in Ecuador. So, the present study is a valuable contribution regarding the presence of STIs among two very vulnerable groups, allowing to detail the syphilis and HSV-2 prevalence trend for each one of these groups. Because of the profile described here for these STIs, the need to create and execute specific strategies for each one of these populations is evident.

It is important to mention that according to the manufacturer, the assay used for syphilis, Trepanostika, has a 100% sensitivity and specificity (BioMérieux, n.d.). HerpeSelect 2 has 96% sensibility and 97% specificity (Focus Diagnostics, n.d.). Both assays are therefore highly precise given the level of the prevalences.

The lack of data regarding STI distribution and magnitude remains as a problem in the HIV epidemic. Without such information, the size of the population being affected by STI may stay largely unknown as well as their health needs (Shahmanesh et al., 2008). An understanding of STI levels and its distribution across a geographical region would allow the planning of effective prevention efforts that correctly address the needs of most vulnerable groups (Dhawan & Khandpur, 2009; Jain et al., 2008). At the same time, the information provided by serological surveys can be used for evaluation purpose, allowing to assess the impact of preventive programs at a large scale in a given country (Smith & Robinson, 2002).

To conclude, the information provided in this research has a meaningful impact in terms of STI and HIV prevention. Syphilis and HSV-2 opportune detection is important in order to prevent HIV infection among vulnerable and affected groups, which translates in the need to execute effective interventions that include STI detection, treatment and control (Setia et al., 2006).

5. Acknowledgment

We thank all participants from India and Ecuador for their valuable information. We also like to thank to the International HIV/AIDS Alliance, and their local implementing partners, Kimirina in Ecuador and the India HIV/AIDS Alliance in AP. The FPP was supported by a grant from the Bill and Melinda Gates Foundation.

6. References

Adhikary, R., Ramanathan, S., Gautam, A., Goswami, P., Ramakrishnan, L., Kallam, S., Mainkar, M.M., Brahmam, G.N.V., Subramanaian, T. & Paranjape, R.S. (2011). Epidemiology oral session 8: STIs and HIV in female sex workers: Recent trends in STIs and HIV among female sex workers and their clients in India: results from repeated cross-sectional surveys. Abstract no. O1-S08.05, *19th biennial conference of the International Society for sexually transmitted diseases Research*, Québec, July 10-13, 2011.

Bastos, F.I., Caceres, C., Galvao, J., Veras, M.A. & Castilho, E.A. (2008). AIDS in Latin America: assessing the current status of the epidemic and the ongoing response. *Int J Epidemiol*, Vol. 37, No. 4, pp. (729-737), ISBN 1464-3685.

Bautista, C.T., Sanchez, J.L., Montano, S.M., Laguna-Torres, V.A., Lama, J.R., Kusunoki, L., Manrique, H., Acosta, J., Montoya, O., Tambare, A.M., Avila, M.M., Vinoles, J., Aguayo, N., Olson, J.G. & Carr, J.K. (2004). Seroprevalence of and risk factors for HIV-1 infection among South American men who have sex with men. *Sex Transm Infect*, Vol. 80, No. 6, pp. (498-504), ISBN 1368-4973.

Bautista, C.T., Sanchez, J.L., Montano, S.M., Laguna-Torres, A., Suarez, L., Sanchez, J., Campos, P., Gallardo, C., Mosquera, C., Villafane, M., Aguayo, N., Avila, M.M., Weissenbacher, M., Ramirez, E., Child, R., Serra, M., Aponte, C., Mejia, A., Velazques, N., Gianella, A., Perez, J., Olson, J.G. & Carr, J.K. (2006). Seroprevalence of and risk factors for HIV-1 infection among female commercial sex workers in South America. *Sex Transm Infect*, Vol. 82, No. 4, pp. (311-316), ISBN 1368-4973.

BioMérieux. (No date). Trepanostika™ TP recombinant, 10.09.2011, Avaible from: http://www.biomerieux-diagnostics.com/servlet/srt/bio/clinical-diagnostics/dynPage?open=CNL_CLN_PRD&doc=CNL_PRD_CPL_G_PRD_CLN_41&pubparams.sform=2&lang=en

Beyrer, C. (2008). Hidden yet happening: the epidemics of sexually transmitted infections and HIV among men who have sex with men in developing countries. *Sex Transm Infect*, Vol. 84, No. 6, pp. (410-412), ISBN 1472-3263.

Brahmam, G.N., Kodavalla, V., Rajkumar, H., Rachakulla, H.K., Kallam, S., Myakala, S.P., Paranjape, R.S., Gupte, M.D., Ramakrishnan, L., Kohli, A. & Ramesh, B.M. (2008). Sexual practices, HIV and sexually transmitted infections among self-identified men who have sex with men in four high HIV prevalence states of India. *AIDS*, Vol. 22 Suppl 5, pp. (S45-57), ISBN 1473-5571.

Buchacz, K., Greenberg, A., Onorato, I. & Janssen, R. (2005). Syphilis epidemics and human immunodeficiency virus (HIV) incidence among men who have sex with men in the United States: implications for HIV prevention. *Sex Transm Dis*, Vol. 32, No. 10 Suppl, pp. (S73-79), ISBN 0148-5717.

Caceres, C., Konda, K., Pecheny, M., Chatterjee, A. & Lyerla, R. (2006). Estimating the number of men who have sex with men in low and middle income countries. *Sex Transm Infect*, Vol. 82 Suppl 3, pp. (iii3-9), ISBN 1368-4973.

Caceres, C.F. (2004). [Interventions for HIV/STD prevention in Latin America and the Caribbean: a review of the regional experience]. *Cad Saude Publica*, Vol. 20, No. 6, pp. (1468-1485), ISBN 0102-311X.

Centers for Disease Control and Prevention (CDC). (2011). CDC Grand Rounds: Chlamydia Prevention: Challenges and Strategies for Reducing Disease Burden and Sequelae. *MMWR Morb Mortal Wkly Rep*, Vol. 60, No. 12, pp. (370-373), ISBN 1545-861X.

Cliffe, S.J., Tabrizi, S. & Sullivan, E.A. (2008). Chlamydia in the Pacific region, the silent epidemic. *Sex Transm Dis*, Vol. 35, No. 9, pp. (801-806), ISBN 1537-4521.

Coates, T.J., Richter, L. & Caceres, C. (2008). Behavioural strategies to reduce HIV transmission: how to make them work better. *Lancet*, Vol. 372, No. 9639, pp. (669-684), ISBN 1474-547X.

Dandona, L., Dandona, R., Gutierrez, J.P., Kumar, G.A., McPherson, S. & Bertozzi, S.M. (2005). Sex behaviour of men who have sex with men and risk of HIV in Andhra Pradesh, India. *AIDS*, Vol. 19, No. 6, pp. (611-619), ISBN 0269-9370.

Dandona, R., Dandona, L., Gutierrez, J.P., Kumar, A.G., McPherson, S., Samuels, F. & Bertozzi, S.M. (2005). High risk of HIV in non-brothel based female sex workers in India. *BMC Public Health*, Vol. 5, pp. (87), ISBN 1471-2458.

Dandona, R., Dandona, L., Kumar, G.A., Gutierrez, J.P., McPherson, S., Samuels, F. & Bertozzi, S.M. (2006). Demography and sex work characteristics of female sex workers in India. *BMC Int Health Hum Rights*, Vol. 6, pp. (5), ISBN 1472-698X.

Das, A., Prabhakar, P., Narayanan, P., Neilsen, G., Wi, T., Kumta, S., Rao, G., Gangakhedkar, R. & Risbud, A. (2011). Prevalence and Assessment of Clinical Management of Sexually Transmitted Infections among Female Sex Workers in Two Cities of India. *Infect Dis Obstet Gynecol*, Vol. 2011, pp. (494769), ISBN 1098-0997.

Desai, V.K., Kosambiya, J.K., Thakor, H.G., Umrigar, D.D., Khandwala, B.R. & Bhuyan, K.K. (2003). Prevalence of sexually transmitted infections and performance of STI syndromes against aetiological diagnosis, in female sex workers of red light area in Surat, India. *Sex Transm Infect*, Vol. 79, No. 2, pp. (111-115), ISBN 1368-4973.

Dhawan, J. & Khandpur, S. (2009). Emerging trends in viral sexually transmitted infections in India. *Indian J Dermatol Venereol Leprol*, Vol. 75, No. 6, pp. (561-565), ISBN 0973-3922

Doherty, L., Fenton, K.A., Jones, J., Paine, T.C., Higgins, S.P., Williams, D. & Palfreeman, A. (2002). Syphilis: old problem, new strategy. *BMJ*, Vol. 325, No. 7356, pp. (153-156), ISBN 1468-5833.

Family Health International/Development Fund for International Development/Andhra Pradesh State AIDS Control Society. (2001). *Prevalence of Sexually Transmitted Infections and HIV among Female Sex Workers of Kakinada and Peddapuram, Andhra Pradesh, India*, Family Health International/Development Fund for International Development/Andhra Pradesh State AIDS Control Society, New Delhi.

Focus Diagnostics. (No date). HerpeSelect Type-Specific HSV-1 and HSV-2 IgG Diagnostic Test Kits, 10.09.2011, Available from http://www.focusdx.com/techsheets/HSV1_2TypeSpecific.pdf

Galban, E. & Benzaken, A.S. (2007). Syphilis situation in 20 latin american and caribbean countries: Year 2006. *Jornal brasileiro de doenças sexualmente transmissíveis*, Vol. 19, No. (3-4), pp. (166-172), ISBN 0103-4065

Gangopadhyay, D.N., Chanda, M., Sarkar, K., Niyogi, S.K., Chakraborty, S., Saha, M.K., Manna, B., Jana, S., Ray, P., Bhattacharya, S.K. & Detels, R. (2005). Evaluation of sexually transmitted diseases/human immunodeficiency virus intervention programs for sex workers in Calcutta, India. *Sex Transm Dis*, Vol. 32, No. 11, pp. (680-684), ISBN 0148-5717.

Gao, L., Zhang, L. & Jin, Q. (2009). Meta-analysis: prevalence of HIV infection and syphilis among MSM in China. *Sex Transm Infect*, Vol. 85, No. 5, pp. (354-358), ISBN 1472-3263.

Ghys, P.D., Jenkins, C. & Pisani, E. (2001). HIV surveillance among female sex workers. *AIDS*, Vol. 15 Suppl 3, pp. (S33-40), ISBN 0269-9370.

Guinness, L. (2011). What can transaction costs tell us about governance in the delivery of large scale HIV prevention programmes in southern India? *Soc Sci Med*, Vol. 72, No. 12, pp. (1939-1947), ISBN 1873-5347.

Gupta, A., Mehta, S., Godbole, S.V., Sahay, S., Walshe, L., Reynolds, S.J., Ghate, M., Gangakhedkar, R.R., Divekar, A.D., Risbud, A.R., Mehendale, S.M. & Bollinger, R.C. (2006). Same-sex behavior and high rates of HIV among men attending sexually transmitted infection clinics in Pune, India (1993-2002). *J Acquir Immune Defic Syndr*, Vol. 43, No. 4, pp. (483-490), ISBN 1525-4135.

Gutierrez, J.P., Molina-Yepez, D., Morrison, K., Samuels, F. & Bertozzi, S.M. (2006a). Correlates of condom use in a sample of MSM in Ecuador. *BMC Public Health*, Vol. 6, pp. (152), ISBN 1471-2458.

Gutierrez, J.P., Molina-Yepez, D., Samuels, F. & Bertozzi, S.M. (2006b). [Inconsistent condom use among sexual workers in Ecuador: results from a behavior survey]. *Salud Publica Mex*, Vol. 48, No. 2, pp. (104-112), ISBN 0036-3634.

Gutierrez, J.P., McPherson, S., Fakoya, A., Matheou, A. & Bertozzi, S.M. (2010). Community-based prevention leads to an increase in condom use and a reduction in sexually transmitted infections (STIs) among men who have sex with men (MSM) and female sex workers (FSW): the Frontiers Prevention Project (FPP) evaluation results. *BMC Public Health*, Vol. 10, pp. (497), ISBN 1471-2458.

Herbst, J.H., Sherba, R.T., Crepaz, N., Deluca, J.B., Zohrabyan, L., Stall, R.D. & Lyles, C.M. (2005). A meta-analytic review of HIV behavioral interventions for reducing sexual risk behavior of men who have sex with men. *J Acquir Immune Defic Syndr*, Vol. 39, No. 2, pp. (228-241), ISBN 1525-4135.

Herida, M., Michel, A., Goulet, V., Janier, M., Sednaoui, P., Dupin, N., de Barbeyrac, B. & Semaille, C. (2005). [Epidemiology of sexually transmitted infections in France]. *Med Mal Infect*, Vol. 35, No. 5, pp. (281-289), ISBN 0399-077X.

Hopkins, S., Lyons, F., Coleman, C., Courtney, G., Bergin, C. & Mulcahy, F. (2004). Resurgence in infectious syphilis in Ireland: an epidemiological study. *Sex Transm Dis*, Vol. 31, No. 5, pp. (317-321), ISBN 0148-5717.

Huedo-Medina, T.B., Boynton, M.H., Warren, M.R., Lacroix, J.M., Carey, M.P. & Johnson, B.T. (2010). Efficacy of HIV prevention interventions in Latin American and Caribbean nations, 1995-2008: a meta-analysis. *AIDS Behav*, Vol. 14, No. 6, pp. (1237-1251), ISBN 1573-3254.

Jain, V.K., Dayal, S., Aggarwal, K. & Jain, S. (2008). Changing trends of sexually transmitted diseases at Rohtak. *Indian Journal of sexually transmitted diseases and AIDS*, Vol. 29, No. 1, pp. (23-25), ISBN 0253-7184.

Jaramillo, G. & Medina, M. (1998). Panorama epidemiológico de las enfermedas de transmisión sexual en el Ecuador. *Revista CIEZT*, Vol. 3, No. 1, pp. (46-67), ISBN 1390-0927.

Johnson, W.D., Hedges, L.V., Ramirez, G., Semaan, S., Norman, L.R., Sogolow, E., Sweat, M.D. & Diaz, R.M. (2002). HIV prevention research for men who have sex with men: a systematic review and meta-analysis. *J Acquir Immune Defic Syndr*, Vol. 30 Suppl 1, pp. (S118-129), ISBN 1525-4135.

Johnson, W.D., Diaz, R.M., Flanders, W.D., Goodman, M., Hill, A.N., Holtgrave, D., Malow, R. & McClellan, W.M. (2008). Behavioral interventions to reduce risk for sexual transmission of HIV among men who have sex with men. *Cochrane Database Syst Rev*, Vol., No. 3, pp. (CD001230), ISBN 1469-493X.

Johnston, A., Fernando, D. & MacBride-Stewart, G. (2005). Sexually transmitted infections in New Zealand in 2003. *N Z Med J*, Vol. 118, No. 1211, pp. (U1347), ISBN 1175-8716.

Kumar, G.A., Dandona, R., Gutierrez, J.P., McPherson, S., Bertozzi, S.M. & Dandona, L. (2006). Access to condoms for female sex workers in Andhra Pradesh. *Natl Med J India*, Vol. 19, No. 6, pp. (306-312), ISBN 0970-258X.

Kumar, R., Jha, P., Arora, P., Mony, P., Bhatia, P., Millson, P., Dhingra, N., Bhattacharya, M., Remis, R.S. & Nagelkerke, N. (2006). Trends in HIV-1 in young adults in south India from 2000 to 2004: a prevalence study. *Lancet*, Vol. 367, No. 9517, pp. (1164-1172), ISBN 1474-547X.

Kumar, R., Mehendale, S.M., Panda, S., Venkatesh, S., Lakshmi, P., Kaur, M., Prinja, S., Singh, T., Virdi, N.K., Bahuguna, P., Sharma, A.K., Singh, S., Godbole, S.V., Risbud, A., Manna, B., Thirumagal, V., Roy, T., Sogarwal, R. & Pawar, N.D. (2011). Impact of Targeted Interventions on Heterosexual Transmission of HIV in India. *BMC Public Health*, Vol. 11, No. 1, pp. (549), ISBN 1471-2458.

Kumarasamy, N., Balakrishnan, P., Venkatesh, K.K., Srikrishnan, A.K., Cecelia, A.J., Thamburaj, E., Solomon, S. & Mayer, K.H. (2008). Prevalence and incidence of sexually transmitted infections among South Indians at increased risk of HIV infection. *AIDS Patient Care STDS*, Vol. 22, No. 8, pp. (677-682), ISBN 1557-7449.

Kumta, S., Lurie, M., Weitzen, S., Jerajani, H., Gogate, A., Row-kavi, A., Anand, V., Makadon, H. & Mayer, K.H. (2010). Bisexuality, sexual risk taking, and HIV prevalence among men who have sex with men accessing voluntary counseling and testing services in Mumbai, India. *J Acquir Immune Defic Syndr*, Vol. 53, No. 2, pp. (227-233), ISBN 1944-7884.

Lama, J.R., Lucchetti, A., Suarez, L., Laguna-Torres, V.A., Guanira, J.V., Pun, M., Montano, S.M., Celum, C.L., Carr, J.K., Sanchez, J., Bautista, C.T. & Sanchez, J.L. (2006). Association of herpes simplex virus type 2 infection and syphilis with human immunodeficiency virus infection among men who have sex with men in Peru. *J Infect Dis*, Vol. 194, No. 10, pp. (1459-1466), ISBN 0022-1899.

Montano, S.M., Sanchez, J.L., Laguna-Torres, A., Cuchi, P., Avila, M.M., Weissenbacher, M., Serra, M., Vinoles, J., Russi, J.C., Aguayo, N., Galeano, A.H., Gianella, A., Andrade, R., Arredondo, A., Ramirez, E., Acosta, M.E., Alava, A., Montoya, O., Guevara, A., Manrique, H., Lama, J.R., de la Hoz, F., Sanchez, G.I., Ayala, C., Pacheco, M.E., Carrion, G., Chauca, G., Perez, J.J., Negrete, M., Russell, K.L., Bautista, C.T., Olson, J.G., Watts, D.M., Birx, D.L. & Carr, J.K. (2005). Prevalences, genotypes, and risk factors for HIV transmission in South America. *J Acquir Immune Defic Syndr*, Vol. 40, No. 1, pp. (57-64), ISBN 1525-4135.

Nicoll, A. & Hamers, F.F. (2002). Are trends in HIV, gonorrhoea, and syphilis worsening in western Europe? *BMJ*, Vol. 324, No. 7349, pp. (1324-1327), ISBN 1468-5833.

Okal, J., Chersich, M.F., Tsui, S., Sutherland, E., Temmerman, M. & Luchters, S. (2011). Sexual and physical violence against female sex workers in Kenya: a qualitative enquiry. *AIDS Care*, Vol., pp. (1-7), ISBN 1360-0451.

Operario, D., Soma, T. & Underhill, K. (2008). Sex work and HIV status among transgender women: systematic review and meta-analysis. *J Acquir Immune Defic Syndr*, Vol. 48, No. 1, pp. (97-103), ISBN 1525-4135.

Oswaldo, R., Leoro, G., Aguilar, M., Jara, R., Moncayo, L. & Hearst, N. (1993). Sentinel serosurveillance for HIV in STD patients, Quito, Ecuador, 1991-1992, *International Conference on AIDS*, Berlin, Jun 6-11, 1993.

Pal, D., Raut, D.K. & Das, A. (2004). A study of HIV/STD infections amongst commercial sex workers in Kolkata. (India) Part-IV laboratory investigation of STD and HIV infections. *J Commun Dis*, Vol. 36, No. 1, pp. (12-16), ISBN 0019-5138.

Panchanadeswaran, S., Johnson, S.C., Sivaram, S., Srikrishnan, A.K., Latkin, C., Bentley, M.E., Solomon, S., Go, V.F. & Celentano, D. (2008). Intimate partner violence is as important as client violence in increasing street-based female sex workers' vulnerability to HIV in India. *Int J Drug Policy*, Vol. 19, No. 2, pp. (106-112), ISBN 1873-4758.

Peterman, T.A., Heffelfinger, J.D., Swint, E.B. & Groseclose, S.L. (2005). The changing epidemiology of syphilis. *Sex Transm Dis*, Vol. 32, No. 10 Suppl, pp. (S4-10), ISBN 0148-5717.

Rao, A.S., Thomas, K., Sudhakar, K. & Maini, P.K. (2009). HIV/AIDS epidemic in India and predicting the impact of the national response: mathematical modeling and analysis. *Math Biosci Eng*, Vol. 6, No. 4, pp. (779-813), ISBN 1547-1063.

Reza-Paul, S., Beattie, T., Syed, H.U., Venukumar, K.T., Venugopal, M.S., Fathima, M.P., Raghavendra, H.R., Akram, P., Manjula, R., Lakshmi, M., Isac, S., Ramesh, B.M., Washington, R., Mahagaonkar, S.B., Glynn, J.R., Blanchard, J.F. & Moses, S. (2008). Declines in risk behaviour and sexually transmitted infection prevalence following a community-led HIV preventive intervention among female sex workers in Mysore, India. *AIDS*, Vol. 22 Suppl 5, pp. (S91-100), ISBN 1473-5571.

Setia, M.S., Lindan, C., Jerajani, H.R., Kumta, S., Ekstrand, M., Mathur, M., Gogate, A., Kavi, A.R., Anand, V. & Klausner, J.D. (2006). Men who have sex with men and transgenders in Mumbai, India: an emerging risk group for STIs and HIV. *Indian J Dermatol Venereol Leprol*, Vol. 72, No. 6, pp. (425-431), ISBN 0973-3922.

Sgaier, S.K., Mony, P., Jayakumar, S., McLaughlin, C., Arora, P., Kumar, R., Bhatia, P. & Jha, P. (2011). Prevalence and correlates of Herpes Simplex Virus-2 and syphilis infections in the general population in India. *Sex Transm Infect*, Vol. 87, No. 2, pp. (94-100), ISBN 1472-3263.

Shahmanesh, M., Patel, V., Mabey, D. & Cowan, F. (2008). Effectiveness of interventions for the prevention of HIV and other sexually transmitted infections in female sex workers in resource poor setting: a systematic review. *Trop Med Int Health*, Vol. 13, No. 5, pp. (659-679), ISBN 1365-3156.

Shahmanesh, M., Cowan, F., Wayal, S., Copas, A., Patel, V. & Mabey, D. (2009). The burden and determinants of HIV and sexually transmitted infections in a population-based sample of female sex workers in Goa, India. *Sex Transm Infect*, Vol. 85, No. 1, pp. (50-59), ISBN 1472-3263.

Shethwala, N.D., Mulla, S.A., Kosambiya, J.K. & Desai, V.K. (2009). Sexually transmitted infections and reproductive tract infections in female sex workers. *Indian J Pathol Microbiol*, Vol. 52, No. 2, pp. (198-199), ISBN 0974-5130.

Smith, J.S. & Robinson, N.J. (2002). Age-specific prevalence of infection with herpes simplex virus types 2 and 1: a global review. *J Infect Dis*, Vol. 186 Suppl 1, pp. (S3-28), ISBN 0022-1899.

Solomon, S.S., Srikrishnan, A.K., Sifakis, F., Mehta, S.H., Vasudevan, C.K., Balakrishnan, P., Mayer, K.H., Solomon, S. & Celentano, D.D. (2010). The emerging HIV epidemic among men who have sex with men in Tamil Nadu, India: geographic diffusion and bisexual concurrency. *AIDS Behav*, Vol. 14, No. 5, pp. (1001-1010), ISBN 1573-3254.

Uma, S., Balakrishnan, P., Murugavel, K.G., Srikrishnan, A.K., Kumarasamy, N., Cecelia, J.A., Anand, S., Mayer, K.H., Celentano, D., Thyagarajan, S.P. & Solomon, S. (2005). Bacterial vaginosis in female sex workers in Chennai, India. *Sex Health*, Vol. 2, No. 4, pp. (261-262), ISBN 1448-5028.

UNAIDS. (2010). *Global report: UNAIDS report on the global AIDS epidemic 2010*, ISBN 978-92-9173-871-7, Geneva.

UNAIDS/WHO. Epidemiological fact sheet on HIV and AIDS, update 2009. Ecuador, In: UNAIDS, January 2011, Available from: http://www.unaids.org/en/

Uuskula, A., Puur, A., Toompere, K. & DeHovitz, J. (2010). Trends in the epidemiology of bacterial sexually transmitted infections in eastern Europe, 1995-2005. *Sex Transm Infect*, Vol. 86, No. 1, pp. (6-14), ISBN 1472-3263.

Vandepitte, J., Lyerla, R., Dallabetta, G., Crabbe, F., Alary, M. & Buve, A. (2006). Estimates of the number of female sex workers in different regions of the world. *Sex Transm Infect*, Vol. 82 Suppl 3, pp. (iii18-25), ISBN 1368-4973.

Verma, R., Shekhar, A., Khobragade, S., Adhikary, R., George, B., Ramesh, B.M., Ranebennur, V., Mondal, S., Patra, R.K., Srinivasan, S., Vijayaraman, A., Paul, S.R. & Bohidar, N. (2010). Scale-up and coverage of Avahan: a large-scale HIV-prevention programme among female sex workers and men who have sex with men in four Indian states. *Sex Transm Infect*, Vol. 86 Suppl 1, pp. (i76-82), ISBN 1472-3263.

Wald, A. & Link, K. (2002). Risk of human immunodeficiency virus infection in herpes simplex virus type 2-seropositive persons: a meta-analysis. *J Infect Dis*, Vol. 185, No. 1, pp. (45-52), ISBN 0022-1899.

Wayal, S., Cowan, F., Warner, P., Copas, A., Mabey, D. & Shahmanesh, M. (2011). Contraceptive practices, sexual and reproductive health needs of HIV-positive and negative female sex workers in Goa, India. *Sex Transm Infect*, Vol. 87, No. 1, pp. (58-64), ISBN 1472-3263.

Whitley, R.J. & Roizman, B. (2001). Herpes simplex virus infections. *Lancet*, Vol. 357, No. 9267, pp. (1513-1518), ISBN 0140-6736.

WHO. (2001). *Global prevalence and incidence of curable STIs*, World Health Organization, Geneva.

WHO. (2007). *Global strategy for the prevention and control of sexually transmitted infections: 2006 - 2015: breaking the chain of transmission*, World Health Organization, ISBN 978 92 4 156347 5, Geneva.

12

Knowledge, Attitude and Behaviour Related to Sexually Transmitted Infections in Portuguese School (Adolescent) and College Students

Lúcia Ramiro, Marta Reis,
Margarida Gaspar de Matos and José Alves Diniz
Projecto Aventura Social - Faculdade de Motricidade Humana / Universidade Técnica de Lisboa, Cruz Quebrada
CMDT-LA/UNL - Centro de Malária e Doenças Tropicais, Laboratório Associado
Instituto de Higiene e Medicina Tropical, Universidade Nova de Lisboa, Lisboa
Portugal

1. Introduction

Many adolescents in Portugal experience serious health and social problems related to sexually transmitted infections (STIs). Sexually transmitted infections are spread by sexual contact. Treatment is available for most STIs but prevention of these diseases is the preferable option, since they can have serious, long-term, health and social implications. Prevention is the way to control STIs.

The goals of this chapter are to analyze knowledge, attitudes and behaviours related to sexually transmitted infections in Portuguese school (adolescent) and college students.

1.1 STIs: Why is it a problem?

Globally, over 100 million STIs occur each year in people under the age of 25 years old (UNAIDS, 2008), and an estimated 11.8 million people aged 15-24 were living with HIV by mid-2002. Further, about half of all new HIV infections worldwide, or nearly 6,000 cases per day, occur in young people (UNAIDS, 2008).

The latest Portuguese report from the national monitoring center of sexually transmitted diseases (CVEDT, 2009) states that the total number of cumulative cases of HIV/AIDS was about 35 thousand with about 15 thousand of these being cases of AIDS. From the analysis of the distribution of the cases of AIDS according to the transmission categories, it appears that 40% are cases associated with heterosexual transmission. In fact, statistics suggest that the cases of AIDS confirm the epidemiological pattern recorded annually since 2000, that is, there is a proportional increase in the number of cases of heterosexual transmission.

Young people are particularly vulnerable to STIs and consequent health problems because:

- They lack information about how to prevent STIs;

- They are less likely to seek proper information or treatment due to fear, ignorance, shyness or inexperience;
- Early sexual experience can result in trauma to vaginal tissue, increasing adolescent women's vulnerability to STIs;
- Adolescents who begin sexual activity early are more likely to have a greater number of lifetime sexual partners.

Other risk factors for adolescents are:

- Unprotected sex (without condoms).
- Sex with multiple (sequential) partners.
- Having a partner who has other sex partners.
- Having a partner with STI symptoms.
- Sex with a new partner or more than one partner in the last three months.
- Sex with strangers or sex in exchange for money.
- Vulnerability to sexual violence, coercion and abuse.

According to UNAIDS (2008), some strategies to reduce STIs:

- Provide teens with the information, skills, and support they need to practice safe sexual behaviour. This programme should be tailored to youths' needs and age appropriate, culturally sensitive and teach sexual and reproductive options. Build on current knowledge of best practices by emphasizing communication, skill-building activities, and role-playing.
- Educate adolescents and young people about the risks of sexually transmitted diseases, including HIV/AIDS. Incorporate promising strategies into comprehensive STIs prevention programs including: individual and peer education, counseling, case management, after school activities, and building support systems and relationships with caring adults.
- Increase access to reproductive health care. Encourage all health care providers who provide care to youth to include comprehensive, age-appropriate information on sexual health issues, including prevention of STIs. Make confidential STI screening and treatment services easily accessible to teenagers along with culturally sensitive counseling and education regarding the use of available protective measures.

1.2 Sexual behaviour, knowledge and attitudes

Many adolescents and young adults engage in sexual intercourse, often with multiple (sequential) sex partners and without using condom. In 2006, 22.7% of high school students in Portugal reported having had sexual intercourse (Reis et al., 2011), with a majority (71.1%) reporting having had sexual intercourse for the first time at 14 years old or later. In a US research, 47.8% of high school students reported having had sexual intercourse (Eaton et al., 2008), with 7.1% reporting having had sexual intercourse for the first time before age 13. Early initiation of sexual activity has been pinpointed as an important indicator in terms of sexual health (Centers for Disease Control and Prevention, 2010; UNAIDS, 2010; WHO, 2010). Some studies even report that early sexual activity is associated with other risk behaviours, such as substance use (Madkour et al., 2010).

Although most adolescents do not have concurrent sex partners at any given point in time, the number of sex partners cumulates over time. Moreover, among sexually active young adults, only 81.3% (Portuguese survey) and 61.5% (U.S. survey) reported using a condom the last time they had sexual intercourse (Reis et al., 2011; Eaton et al., 2008). In spite of the fact that many have used condoms at some time during an episode of sexual intercourse, comparatively few report using them every time they have sex (Reis et al, 2011; Eaton et al., 2008). Thus, young adults engage in sexual behaviours that place them at risk for acquiring STIs, including HIV.

According to literature, if young people possess knowledge, information and motivation on safe sexual behaviour, they may change their attitudes and their behaviours (Synovitz et al., 2002; Thompson et al., 1999). Improving knowledge related to HIV prevention and attitudes about people living with HIV are other important aims of sexual and reproductive health. Some theories claim that being well informed about transmission/preventive behaviours regarding HIV and other STIs and developing a positive attitude towards people infected with HIV are crucial to change people's behaviours.

2. Study 1: HBSC - Health Behavior in School-aged Children

The Health Behavior in School-aged Children (HBSC) is a collaborative WHO study, developed by 44 countries in order to study school-aged behaviour regarding health and risk behaviours in adolescence. Portugal is part of this group since 1996 (Currie et al, 2000).

2.1 Method

2.1.1 Sample

The 2010 study provides national representative data of 5050 Portuguese adolescents, randomly chosen from those attending 6th, 8th and 10th grade of high school. The sample included 52.3% girls and 47.7% males, whose mean age was 13.98 years (standard deviation 1.85). The majority of adolescents are of Portuguese nationality (94.4%), 30.8% attended the 6th grade, 31.6% attended the 8th grade and 37.6% attended the 10th grade. This study uses a subset of 8th and 10th graders (n=3494). This sample included 53.6% girls and 46.4% boys, whose mean age was 14.94 years (standard deviation 1.30) (table 1).

	2010 Total sample (N=5050)		2010 Subset (N=3494)	
	N	%	*N*	%
Gender				
Male	2407	47.7	1621	46.4
Female	2643	52.3	1873	53.6
Grade				
6th grade	1556	30.8	-	-
8th grade	1594	31.6	1594	45.6
10th grade	1900	37.6	1900	54.4
Nationality[1]				
Portuguese	4562	94.4	3145	94.2
Other	269	5.6	193	5.8
	M	*SD*	*M*	*SD*
Age	13.98	1.85	14.94	1.30

[1] The total numbers differ considering that some adolescents have not replied to nationality.

Table 1. Socio demographic characteristics of total sample (N=5050) and subset (N=3494).

2.1.2 Procedure (study 1 and 2)

The procedure followed for school and college students was similar. Data were collected through a self-administered questionnaire. In study 1, data were collected from the Portuguese sample of the Health Behavior in School-aged Children (HBSC) and all procedures were followed according to the international research protocol. Study 2 - the Sexual and Reproductive Health in University Students (HBSC / SRHCS) – is an extension of the HBSC. The sampling unit used in these surveys was the class. The 139 schools/19 colleges in the samples were randomly selected from the official national list of schools/colleges, stratified by region (North, Center, Lisbon and Tagus Valley, Alentejo and the Algarve) in the mainland. In each school /college, classes were randomly selected in order to meet the required number of students for each grade. The surveys are nationwide and were conducted in 2010 for the Ministry of Portuguese Health and for the National Coordination for HIV/AIDS Infection by the Technical University of Lisbon. These studies have the approval of a scientific committee, the Ethics National Committee and the National Commission for Data Protection and followed strictly all the guidelines for human rights protection.

2.2 Measures (study 1 and 2)

For the purpose of these studies, the following parameters were assessed as detailed below:

Risky sexual behaviour was measured through the following behaviours - ever had sexual intercourse (Yes/No), age, condom use at first sexual intercourse (Yes/No). Condom use at last sexual intercourse (Yes/No) was also measured in adolescents. Another four behaviours were measured in college students: usual condom use (Yes/No), condom use last 12 months (Always/other options), occasional partners (Yes/No) and having had a sexually transmitted infection (Yes/No). As for having had sexual intercourse with alcohol (Yes/No) and drugs (Yes/No), it was measured separately in college students and jointly in adolescents. As documented in literature, having ever had sexual intercourse, occasional partners, an STI and sexual intercourse after having drunk too much alcohol or taken drugs, answer "Yes" was the one considered risky behaviour. As for condom use (first and last sexual intercourse), answer "No" was considered risky behaviour.

Knowledge regarding HIV/AIDS transmission/prevention – Adolescents and young adults were asked to respond to nine statements about HIV/AIDS transmission/prevention: 1. «it is possible to become infected with HIV/AIDS by sharing needles»; 2. «it is possible to become infected with HIV/Aids from coughing and sneezing»; 3. «an HIV infected pregnant woman may pass the virus to her baby»; 4. «it is possible to become infected with HIV/AIDS by hugging someone infected»; 5. «the oral contraceptive can protect against HIV/AIDS infection»; 6. «it is possible to become infected with HIV/AIDS by engaging in unprotected sexual intercourse with someone just once»; 7. «someone who looks healthy can be HIV infected»; 8. «it is possible to become infected with HIV/AIDS by sharing a glass, fork/spoon»; 9. «it is possible to become infected with HIV/AIDS by blood transfusion in a Portuguese hospital». Items were rated on a three response options (1= Yes, 2= No and 3= I do not know). Only responses that showed correct information scored and so final scores ranged from 0 to 9, with high scores suggesting more positive knowledge/more information.

Attitudes towards HIV/AIDS infected people. Young people were asked to respond to five statements about attitudes towards HIV-infected people: 1. «I wouldn't be a friend of someone if he had AIDS», 2. «Adolescents with AIDS should be allowed to go to school», 3. «I would sit near an infected student in classroom», 4. «I would visit a friend if he or she had AIDS» and 5. «HIV infected people should live apart of the rest of people». Items were rated on a 3-point rating scale (1= disagree to 3= agree). After recoding items 1 and 5, final scores ranged from 5 to 15, with high scores suggesting more positive attitudes.

Attitudes towards condom use. Adolescents and young adults were asked to respond to four statements: 1. « It would be embarrassing to buy condoms in a store», 2. « It would feel uncomfortable carrying condoms with me.», 3. «It would be wrong to carry a condom with me because it would mean that I' m planning to have sex» and 4. « It would feel uncomfortable to ask for condoms at health care services.». Items were rated on a 3-point rating scale (1= disagree to 3= agree). After recoding all items, final scores ranged from 4 to 12, with high scores suggesting more positive attitudes.

2.3 Results

Analyses and statistical procedures were carried out in the *Statistical Package for Social Sciences* program (SPSS, version 19.0 for Windows). The total numbers differ according to sample use (8th and 10th grade sample; 8th and 10th grade adolescents who reported having had their first sexual intercourse) and considering that some adolescents have not replied to some parameters.

Overall, questionnaires were responded by the subset of 8th and 10th graders (3494 participants), between 13 and 21 years old. Findings show the majority is not sexually active (78.2%). There is significant variation by gender since boys more often have had sexual intercourse than girls ($\chi^2(1) = 57.31$; $p = .000$). Of the ones that refer having already had their first sexual intercourse, 68.9% referred that it happened when they were 14 or more. The results showed that, despite both the majority of boys (63.1%) and girls (77.1%) having had their first sexual intercourse at the age of 14 or later, boys more often claim to have started younger (at 11 or less and between 12 and 13) ($\chi^2(2) = 19.63$; $p = .000$). 93.8% refer having used the condom in the first sexual intercourse. As for the last sexual intercourse, 95.2% refer they have used condom. Significant variation was obtained between genders in relation to condom use in first sexual intercourse ($\chi^2(1) = 4.19$; $p = .041$) with girls referring more frequent use of the condom (96.2%) than boys (91.9%). Results showed that the majority (87.3%) did not have sexual intercourse under the effect of alcohol and drugs. Yet, boys did it more frequently than girls ($\chi^2(1) = 11.76$; $p = .001$), see table 2.

The total mean score of general HIV/AIDS knowledge was 5.32 (out of 9 points), with girls (M = 5.58, SD=2.49) showing significantly more knowledge than boys [(M = 5.02, SD=2.69 (t (2902) = -5.941, p< 0.000)] (see table 3).

The mean total score in relation to attitudes towards HIV-infected people was 12.84 (SD= 2.24), with boys showing significantly less positive attitudes (M = 12.42, SD=2.35) than girls [(M = 13.19, SD=2.09 (t (2854) = -9,690, p< 0.000)] (see table 4).

	Boys (N=1588)		Girls (N=1848)		Total[1] (N=3436)		χ^2
	N	%	N	%	N	%	
Ever had sexual intercourse							57.309***
Yes	437	**27.5**	311	16.8	748	21.8	
No	1151	72.5	1537	**83.1**	2688	78.2	

Only adolescents who reported having had their first sexual intercourse (N=748)

	Boys		Girls		Total[1]		χ^2
	N	%	N	%	N	%	
Age of 1st sexual intercourse (N=731)							19.628***
Age 11 or less	43	**10.1**	11	3.6	54	7.4	
Ages 12 and 13	114	**26.8**	59	19.3	173	23.7	
Ages 14 or more	268	63.1	236	**77.1**	504	68.9	
Condom use (% of people who responded yes)							
1st sexual intercourse (N=511)	284	91.9	227	**96.2**	511	93.8	4.185*
last sexual intercourse (N=554)	302	94.1	252	96.6	554	95.2	1.919
Having had sexual intercourse under the influence of alcohol or drugs (N=693)							11.756***
Yes	66	**16.4**	22	7.6	88	12.7	
No	337	83.6	268	**92.4**	605	87.3	

[1] The total numbers differ considering that some adolescents have not replied to some paremeters.

* p< .05; ** p< .01; *** p< .001

In bold – values that correspond to an adjusted residual ≥ |1.9|

Table 2. Differences between gender and risky *sexual behaviours.*

	Boys		Girls		Total[1]		χ^2
	N	%	N	%			
It is possible to become infected with HIV/AIDS by sharing needles (N=3201)							15.970***
Yes	1135	76.9	1423	**82.5**	2558		
No	88	**6.0**	71	4.1	159		
I do not Know	253	**17.1**	231	13.4	484		
It is possible to become infected with HIV/Aids from coughing and sneezing (N=3187)							8.821*
Yes	239	**16.2**	225	13.1	464		
No	773	52.5	978	**57.1**	1751		
I do not Know	461	31.3	511	29.8	972		
An HIV-infected pregnant woman may pass the virus to her baby (N=3187)							46.559***
Yes	930	63.3	1264	**73.6**	2194		
No	126	**8.6**	75	4.4	201		
I do not Know	414	**28.2**	378	22	792		
It is possible to become infected with HIV/AIDS by hugging someone infected (N=3187)							53.203***
Yes	150	**10.2**	104	6.1	254		
No	954	64.7	1308	**76.4**	2262		
I do not Know	370	**25.1**	301	17.6	671		
The oral contraceptive can protect against HIV/AIDS infection (N=3178)							13.210**
Yes	213	14.5	216	12.6	429		
No	776	52.9	1016	**59.3**	1792		
I do not Know	477	**32.5**	480	28	957		
It is possible to become infected with HIV/AIDS by engaging in unprotected sexual intercourse with someone just once (N=3172)							41.314***
Yes	1040	71.1	1374	**80.4**	2414		
No	110	**7.5**	67	3.9	177		
I do not Know	313	**21.4**	268	15.7	581		
Someone who looks healthy can be HIV infected (N=3171)							17.175***
Yes	934	63.8	1190	**69.7**	2124		
No	142	**9.7**	109	6.4	251		
I do not Know	388	26.5	408	23.9	796		
It is possible to become infected with HIV/AIDS by sharing a glass, fork /spoon (N=3170)							10.029**
Yes	356	**24.3**	345	20.2	701		
No	578	39.5	752	**44.1**	1330		
I do not Know	531	36.2	608	35.7	1139		
It is possible to become infected with HIV/AIDS by blood transfusion in a Portuguese hospital (N=3177)							4.447
Yes	778	53	969	56.7	1747		
No	189	12,9	198	11.6	387		
I do not Know	501	34.1	542	31.7	1043		
	Boys		Girls		Total		
	M	SD	M	SD	M	SD	t
Total scale (0-9)	**5.02**	2.69	**5.58**	2.49	**5.32**	2.60	-5.941***

[1] The total numbers differ considering that some adolescents have not replied to some paremeters.
*p≤0.05; **p≤0.01; ***p≤0.001
In bold – values that correspond to an adjusted residual ≥ |1.9|

Table 3. Differences between gender and knowledge regarding HIV/AIDS transmission/prevention.

	Boys N	Boys %	Girls N	Girls %	Total[1]	χ^2
I wouldn't be a friend of someone if he had AIDS (N=3151)						53.546***
Agree	147	**10.2**	88	5.1	235	
I'm not sure	324	**22.5**	284	16.6	608	
Disagree	970	67.3	1338	**78.2**	2308	
Adolescents with AIDS should be allowed to go to school (N=3144)						27.160***
Agree	813	56.5	1115	**65.4**	1928	
I'm not sure	368	**25.6**	359	21.1	727	
Disagree	259	**18.0**	230	13.5	489	
I would sit near an infected student in classroom (N=3143)						47.805***
Agree	746	51.9	1089	**63.9**	1835	
I'm not sure	480	**33.4**	447	26.2	927	
Disagree	212	**14.7**	169	9.9	381	
I would visit a friend if he or she had AIDS (N=3145)						58.630***
Agree	920	63.9	1286	**75.4**	2206	
I'm not sure	347	**24.1**	320	18.8	667	
Disagree	172	**12.0**	100	5.9	272	
HIV infected people should live apart of the rest of people (N=3132)						48.082***
Agree	175	**12.2**	155	9.1	330	
I'm not sure	293	**20.4**	216	12.7	509	
Disagree	965	67.3	1328	**78.2**	2293	

	Boys M	Boys SD	Girls M	Girls SD	Total M	Total SD	t
Total scale	**12.42**	2.35	**13.19**	2.09	**12.84**	2.24	-9.690***

[1] The total numbers differ considering that some adolescents have not replied to some paremeters.
*p≤0.05; **p≤0.01; ***p≤0.001
In bold – values that correspond to an adjusted residual ≥ |1.9|

Table 4. Differences between gender and attitudes towards HIV-infected people.

The mean total score in relation to attitudes towards condoms was 8.73 (SD= 2.50), with boys showing significantly more positive attitude (M = 8.86, SD=2.53) than girls [(M = 8.63, SD=2.46 (t (3081) = -2,546, p< 0.011)] (see table 5).

	Boys		Girls		Total[1]		χ^2
	N	%	N	%			
It would be embarrassing to buy condoms in a store. (N=3158)							17.796***
Disagree	579	**40.0**	560	32.8	1139		
Neither agree nor disagree	350	24.2	474	**27.7**	824		
Agree	520	35.9	675	**39.5**	1195		
It would feel uncomfortable carrying condoms with me. (N=3146)							48.526***
Disagree	793	**55.0**	725	42.5	1518		
Neither agree nor disagree	324	22.5	482	**28.3**	806		
Agree	325	22.5	497	29.2	822		
It would be wrong to carry a condom with me because it would mean that I' m planning to have sex. (N=3134)							11.031**
Disagree	719	50.1	951	**56.0**	1670		
Neither agree nor disagree	379	**26.4**	397	23.4	776		
Agree	338	**23.5**	350	20.6	668		
It would feel uncomfortable to ask for condoms at the health care services (N=3112)							4.962
Disagree	698	49.1	799	47.3	1497		
Neither agree nor disagree	321	22.6	440	26.0	761		
Agree	402	28.3	452	26.7	854		
	Boys		Girls		Total		
	M	SD	M	SD	M	SD	t
Total scale	**8.86**	2.53	**8.63**	2.46	8.73	2.50	2.546*

[1] The total numbers differ considering that some adolescents have not replied to some paremeters.
*p≤0.05; **p≤0.01; ***p≤0.001
In bold - values that correspond to an adjusted residual ≥ |1.9|

Table 5. Differences between gender and attitudes towards condoms.

3. Study 2: Sexual and Reproductive Health in University Students (HBSC / SRHCS)

A nationwide survey was conducted for the Ministry of Portuguese Health and for the National Coordination for HIV/AIDS Infection to assess HIV/AIDS-related knowledge, attitudes, and practices among the population aged 18-35 years. The aim of this research was to identify those behaviours that put young people at risk of HIV infection. Disseminating the findings is also crucial since it may potentiate an advocacy tool in order to mainstream HIV/ AIDS prevention programs at university level. Therefore it is also expected that it can help catalyze a more effective role for universities to fight against diseases as well as contribute to build intervention strategies that raise public awareness.

3.1 Method

3.1.1 Sample

The sample is composed of 3278 Portuguese college students, between 18 and 35 years old, randomly chosen from those attending university during the academic year of 2009/2010. Data were collected through a self-administered questionnaire. The sample included 70%women and 30% men. The mean age was 21 years old (standard deviation 3). The majority of students are Portuguese (97.3%), single (95.5%), catholic (71.9%), heterosexual (96.4%) and were proportionally distributed among all the educational Portuguese regions, see table 6.

		N	%	M	SD
Gender	Male	993	30.3	-	-
	Female	2285	69.7	-	-
Age		3278		21.01	3.00
Nationality					
	Portuguese	3189	97.3		
	European countries	45	1.4		
	Brazilian	25	0.8		
	African countries	19	0.6		
Marital Status					
	Single	3131	95.5	-	-
	Married	84	2.6	-	-
	Unmarried cohabitation	51	1.6	-	-
	Divorced	12	0.4	-	-
Religious affiliation					
	Catholic	2357	71.9	-	-
	Protestant	40	1.3	-	-
	Buddhist	7	0.2	-	-
	Orthodox	7	0.2	-	-
	None	860	26.2	-	-
	Other	7	0.2	-	-
Sexual Orientation[1]					
	Heterosexual	2754	96.4	-	-
	Homosexual	79	2.8	-	-
	Bisexual	22	0.8	-	-

[1] The total numbers differ considering that some young adults have not replied to sexual orientation.

Table 6. Socio demographic characteristics.

3.2 Results

Analyses and statistical procedures were carried out in the *Statistical Package for Social Sciences* program (SPSS, version 19.0 for Windows). The total numbers differ according to sample use (complete sample; young adults who reported having had their first sexual intercourse) and considering that some young adults have not replied to some parameters.

Structured self-reported questionnaires were responded by 3278 participants, between 18 and 35 years old. From the total sample, 83.3% (N=2730) young people have already begun their sexual life. Men reported more often than women having had sexual intercourse ($\chi^2(1) = 29.15$; $p = .000$). Of these, 79.2% referred that they have had their first sexual intercourse at the age of 16 or later and 86.8% used the condom in their first sexual intercourse. The results showed that, despite both the majority of men (72%) and women (82.5%) having had their first sexual intercourse at the age of 16 or later, men most often claim to have started younger (at 11 or less, between 12 and 13, and between 14 and 15) ($\chi^2(3) = 60.05$; $p = .000$). Men reported more often having used condom in the first sexual intercourse than women ($\chi^2(1) = 18.56$; $p = .000$). It was also observed that among the students who already have sexual intercourse, 69% use condom usually. Significant variation was obtained between genders in relation to usual condom use ($\chi^2(1) = 4.41$; $p = .036$). Regarding genders, men refer more frequent usual use of condom (71.7%) than women (67.7%). When asked about frequency of condom use on last 12 months, only 32.6% refer using it always. Results showed that the majority of men (57.4%, 53.1%, 10.7%) have occasional sexual partners and sexual relations under the effect of alcohol and drugs. And they do it more frequently than women [($\chi^2(1)$ = 333.11; p = .000); ($\chi^2(1)$ = 166.52; p = .000); ($\chi^2(1)$ = 57.22; p = .000), respectively]. Regarding STIs, 3.3% reported having already had an STI (see table 7).

	Male (N=993)		Female (N=2285)		Total (N=3278)		χ^2
	N	%	N	%	N	%	
Ever had sexual intercourse							29.153***
Yes	880	**88.6**	1850	81.0	2730	83.3	
No	113	11.4	435	**19.0**	548	16.7	
Only young adults who reported having had their first sexual intercourse (N=2730)							
	Male		Female		Total[1]		χ^2
	N	%	N	%	N	%	
Age of 1st sexual intercourse (N=2730)							60.05***
Age 11 or less	14	**1.6**	2	0.1	16	0.6	
Ages 12 and 13	44	**5**	39	2.1	83	3.0	
Ages 14 and 15	188	**21.4**	282	15.2	470	17.2	
Age 16 and more	634	72	1527	**82.5**	2161	79.2	
Condom use (% of people who responded yes)							
1st sexual intercourse(N=2369)	728	**82.7**	1641	88.7	2369	86.8	18.56***
Usually (by the participant or partner)(N=1884)	631	**71.7**	1253	67.7	1884	69.0	4.41*
Always on last 12 months (N=842)	283	34.5	559	31.7	842	32.6	2.03
Occasional sexual partners (N=2669)							333.11***
Yes	484	**57.4**	396	21.7	880	33	
No	359	42.6	1430	**78.3**	1789	67	
Have sexual intercourse under the influence of alcohol (N=2658)							166.52***
Yes	446	**53.1**	497	27.3	943	35.5	
No	394	46.9	1321	**72.7**	1715	64.5	
Have sexual intercourse under the influence of drugs (N=2565)							57.22***
Yes	88	**10.7**	58	3.3	146	5.7	
No	731	89.3	1688	**96.7**	2419	94.3	
Have you had an STI (N=2647)							0.02
Yes	28	3.4	59	3.3	87	3.3	
No	807	96.6	1753	96.7	2560	96.7	

[1] The total numbers differ considering that some young adults have not replied to some parameters.
* p< .05; ** p< .01; *** p< .001
In bold - values that correspond to an adjusted residual ≥ |1.9|

Table 7. Differences between gender and risky *sexual behaviours.*

Knowledge regarding HIV/AIDS transmission/prevention: the distribution of each item is shown in Table 8. The level of general HIV/AIDS knowledge among young adults was high, as indicated by a total mean score of general HIV/AIDS knowledge of 7.82 out of 9 points, with females (M = 7.90, SD=0.90) showing significantly more knowledge than males [(M = 7.65, SD=1.33 (t (3215) = 421.30, p< 0.000)].

	Male		Female		Total[1]	χ^2
	N	%	N	%		
It is possible to become infected with HIV/AIDS by sharing needles (N=3264)						13.554**
Yes	963	97.9	2259	**99.1**	3222	
No	8	0.8	15	0.7	23	
I do not Know	13	**1.3**	6	0.3	19	
It is possible to become infected with HIV/Aids from coughing and sneezing (N=3253)						27.417***
Yes	64	**6.5**	75	3.3	139	
No	848	86.5	2097	**92.3**	2945	
I do not Know	68	6.9	101	4.4	169	
An HIV-infected pregnant woman may pass the virus to her baby (N=3256)						47.621***
Yes	876	89.3	2174	**95.6**	3050	
No	43	**4.4**	51	2.2	94	
I do not Know	62	**6.3**	50	2.2	112	
It is possible to become infected with HIV/AIDS by hugging someone infected(N=3254)						27.491***
Yes	29	3	50	2.2	79	
No	931	95.2	2221	**97.6**	3152	
I do not Know	18	**1.8**	5	0.2	23	
The oral contraceptive can protect against HIV/AIDS infection (N=3255)						20.861***
Yes	16	1.6	30	1.3	46	
No	929	95	2222	**97.6**	3151	
I do not Know	33	**3.4**	25	1.1	58	
It is possible to become infected with HIV/AIDS by engaging in unprotected sexual intercourse with someone just once(N=3257)						19.914***
Yes	953	97.1	2255	**99.1**	3208	
No	14	**1.4**	15	0.7	29	
I do not Know	14	**1.4**	6	0.3	20	
Someone who looks healthy can be HIV infected(N=3249)						16.347***
Yes	937	95.7	2223	**97.9**	3160	
No	12	1.2	22	1	34	
I do not Know	30	**3.1**	25	1.1	55	
It is possible to become infected with HIV/AIDS by sharing a glass, fork /spoon (N=3246)						29.658***
Yes	163	**16.7**	242	10.7	405	
No	712	72.8	1839	**81.1**	2551	
I do not Know	103	10.5	187	8.2	290	
It is possible to become infected with HIV/AIDS by blood transfusion in a Portuguese hospital (N=3249)						5.438
Yes	552	56.3	1374	60.6	1926	
No	331	33.7	681	30	1012	
I do not Know	98	10	213	9.4	311	

	Male		Female		Total		
	M	SD	M	SD	M	SD	t
Total scale	**7.65**	1.33	**7.90**	0.90	**7.82**	1.05	421.30***

[1] The total numbers differ considering that some young adults have not replied to some parameters.
*p≤0.05; **p≤0.01; ***p≤0.001
In bold - values that correspond to an adjusted residual ≥ |1.9|

Table 8. Differences between gender and knowledge regarding HIV/AIDS transmission/prevention.

Attitudes towards HIV-infected people: the distribution of each item is shown in Table 9. The mean total score in relation to attitudes towards HIV-infected people was 14.61 (SD= 1.03), with males showing significantly less positive attitudes (M = 14.42, SD=1.28) than females [(M = 14.69, SD=0.90 (t (3247) = 805.20, p< 0.000)].

	Male		Female		Total[1]	χ^2
	N	%	N	%		
I wouldn't be a friend of someone if he had AIDS (N=3266)						35.349***
Agree	20	**2**	14	0.6	34	
I'm not sure	92	**9.3**	116	5.1	208	
Disagree	872	88.6	2152	**94.3**	3024	
Adolescents with AIDS should be allowed to go to school (N=3263)						58.208***
Agree	855	87.2	2161	**94.7**	3016	
I'm not sure	86	**8.8**	72	3.2	158	
Disagree	40	**4.1**	49	2.1	89	
I would sit near an infected student in classroom (N=3259)						28.106***
Agree	853	87	2104	**92.3**	2957	
I'm not sure	98	**10**	115	5	213	
Disagree	29	3	60	2.7	89	
I would visit a friend if he or she had AIDS (N=3262)						11.184**
Agree	934	95	2215	**97.2**	3149	
I'm not sure	41	**4.2**	48	2.1	89	
Disagree	8	0.8	16	0.7	24	
HIV infected people should live apart of the rest of people (N=3265)						28.091***
Agree	12	1.2	31	1.4	43	
I'm not sure	34	**3.5**	20	0.9	54	
Disagree	939	95.3	2229	**97.8**	3168	

	Male		Female		Total		
	M	SD	M	SD	M	SD	t
Total scale	**14.42**	1.28	**14.69**	0.90	**14.61**	1.03	805.20***

[1] The total numbers differ considering that some young adults have not replied to some parameters.
*p≤0.05; **p≤0.01; ***p≤0.001
In bold – values that correspond to an adjusted residual ≥ |1.9|

Table 9. Differences between gender and attitudes towards HIV-infected people.

The mean total score in relation to attitudes towards condoms was 10.10 (SD= 2.08). There was no statistically significant difference between genders (t (1961) =.1.567, p< 0.117) (see table 10).

	Male		Female		Total[1]		χ^2
	N	%	N	%			
It would be embarrassing to buy condoms in a store. (N=3196)							36.390***
Disagree	649	**67.6**	1287	57.6	1936		
Neither agree nor disagree	207	21.6	540	24.2	747		
Agree	104	10.8	409	**18.3**	513		
It would feel uncomfortable carrying condoms with me. (N=3188)							14.904***
Disagree	706	**73.9**	1543	69.1	2249		
Neither agree nor disagree	183	19.2	439	19.7	622		
Agree	66	6.9	251	**11.2**	317		
It would be wrong to carry a condom with me because it would mean that I' m planning to have sex. (N=3188)							22.653***
Disagree	548	57.4	1468	**65.7**	2016		
Neither agree nor disagree	256	**26.8**	520	23.3	776		
Agree	150	**15.7**	246	11.0	396		
It would feel uncomfortable to ask for condoms at health care services.(N=3189)							7.791*
Disagree	620	65.0	1512	**67.7**	2132		
Neither agree nor disagree	222	**23.3**	426	19.1	648		
Agree	112	11.7	297	13.3	409		
	Male		Female		Total		
	M	SD	M	SD	M	SD	t
Total scale	**10.19**	1.94	**10.07**	2.13	**10.10**	2.08	1.567

[1] The total numbers differ considering that some young adults have not replied to some parameters.
*p≤0.05; **p≤0.01; ***p≤0.001
In bold – values that correspond to an adjusted residual ≥ |1.9|

Table 10. Differences between gender and attitudes towards condoms.

4. Conclusions

Regarding sexual behaviours, overall, findings show the majority of Portuguese adolescents (13-21 years old) is not sexually active (78.2%), while the majority of Portuguese young adults are (83.3%). Young Portuguese adults (18 – 35 years old) reported having had their first sexual intercourse at 16 years old or later. As for Portuguese adolescents, they reported it happened at 14 or more. This suggests that there is a tendency for anticipating time of sexual initiation. These results are comparable to those that have been found in a similar nationwide US research, the Youth Risk Behavior Surveillance, with 64% of young Americans (10 – 24 years old) referring not being sexually active (CDC, 2010). These may be considered similar since the age interval is broader, therefore lowering frequency of sexual activity. As for age of sexual onset, the average age for 16-20 year-olds in European countries in 2004 was 16.5 (Global Sex Survey, 2005), thus confirming our results regarding young adults. In a more recent research, 16-19 year old Brazilians reported their sexual debut to have been at 14.9 years old. (Paiva, V.; Calazans, G.; Venturi, G.; Dias, R.; & Grupo de Estudos em População, Sexualidade e AIDS, 2008.)

The rates of condom use during first sexual intercourse were very high among both Portuguese adolescents (93.8%) and young adults (86.8%). Yet, they clearly are not consistent since only 69% of young adults claim using the condom usually and only 32.6% refer using it always on last 12 months. Therefore, this suggests that protective behaviours are abandoned over time. These results seem much more promising than those of a Brazilian research (Paiva, V.; Calazans, G.; Venturi, G.; Dias, R.; & Grupo de Estudos em População, Sexualidade e AIDS, 2008), where only 65.6% of adolescents reported having used condom during first sexual intercourse.

Considering other risky behaviours, such as having had occasional sexual partners, 33% (this was asked to college students only) of young Portuguese adults reported it. These results represent higher risk than those presented by an American study (Eisenberg, Ackard, Resnick & Neumark-Sztainer, 2009) with 21.5% of young adults (median age 20.5) reporting having had occasional sexual partners.

Results showed that the majority (87.3%) of Portuguese adolescents did not have sexual intercourse under the effect of alcohol and drugs, whereas the majority of young adults (53.1%) reported the situation, considering alcohol alone. The findings related to Portuguese adolescents are confirmed in the YRSB research (CDC, 2010), with 78.4% stating not having had sexual intercourse under the effect of alcohol and drugs. As for having sexual intercourse under the effect of drugs alone, the frequency of young Portuguese adults who reported it is lower (10.7%), though serious. It was also asked to young adults if they had ever had an STI and 3.3% reported having already had an STI.

In both Portuguese studies, there is significant variation by gender since boys and men more often have had sexual intercourse, claim to have started their sexual life younger, reported having had occasional partners (young adults), having had sexual intercourse under the influence of alcohol or drugs than girls and women. Conversely, in relation to condom use in first sexual intercourse, Portuguese adolescent girls referred more frequent use of the condom (96.2%) than Portuguese boys (91.9%), which was not observed in the young adults' study. These variations by gender suggest boys and men engage in risky sexual behaviours more often than girls and women. These findings are confirmed in other studies: American boys and men initiated their sexual life younger (16.9 years old) than girls and women (17.4 years old) and stated more often (29% Vs. 14%) having had occasional partners (NSSHB, 2010; Eisenberg, Ackard, Resnick & Neumark-Sztainer, 2009).

As for knowledge regarding HIV/AIDS transmission/prevention, the total mean score of general HIV/AIDS knowledge was 5.32 among Portuguese adolescents and 7.82 among Portuguese young adults, out of 9 points. The results reveal significant variation in responses by gender: girls ($M = 5.58$, $SD = 2.49$) and young women ($M = 7.90$, $SD=0.90$) demonstrated significantly more knowledge than boys ($M = 5.02$, $SD = 2.69$) and young men ($M = 7.65$, $SD=1.33$). So, overall, results revealed the majority has a moderate/high level of knowledge but boys and young men showed bigger risk acceptance, while girls demonstrated better knowledge in relation to risk-taking. Overall, most studies reveal a moderate / high level of knowledge: in a South African study (Bana et al., 2010), 56% of 15-24 year-olds reported good knowledge level about HIV/AIDS transmission and in an Iranian study, the knowledge level was considered moderately high (Tavoosi, Zaferani, Enzevaei, Tajik & Ahmadinezhad, 2004).

In relation to attitudes towards HIV infected people, the mean total score was 12.84 (SD= 2.24) among Portuguese adolescents and 14.61 (SD= 1.03) among Portuguese young adults. Final scores ranged from 5 to 15 points. The results reveal significant variation in responses by gender, with boys (M = 12.42, SD=2.35) and young men (M = 14.42, SD=1.28) showing significantly less positive attitudes than girls (M = 13.19, SD=2.09) and young women (M = 14.69, SD=0.90). So, overall, results revealed the majority has a moderate/very positive attitude towards HIV infected people but boys and young men showed less tolerance, while girls demonstrated more tolerant attitude. Results are much higher than in an Iranian research with 15 - 17 year old students, where an intolerant attitude towards HIV infected people, especially when boys were concerned, was observed (Tavoosi, Zaferani, Enzevaei, Tajik & Ahmadinezhad, 2004).

As for attitudes towards condoms, the mean total score was 8.73 (SD= 2.50), among Portuguese adolescents and 10.10 (SD= 2.08) among Portuguese young adults. Final scores ranged from 4 to 12 points. The results revealed significant variation in responses by gender among adolescents, with boys showing significantly more positive attitude (M = 8.86, SD=2.53) than girls [(M = 8.63, SD=2.46). So, overall, results revealed the majority has a moderate/very positive attitude towards asking for, buying and carrying condoms but girls showed more difficulty in those behaviours than boys, who demonstrated a more proactive attitude. The Portuguese results are corroborated in the HBSC Scottish national sample, both in relation to overall attitude towards condom and for gender differences (Kirby, van der Sluijs & Currie, 2010).

STI and HIV infections in adolescents are at epidemic levels worldwide. As long as adolescents continue to engage in sexual behaviours that place them at risk for STI/HIV (e.g., sex without a condom and with multiple sequential sex partners), they will be vulnerable to these health threats. For reasons outlined above, a few of which are amenable to change, adolescents may be especially susceptible to STI/HIV. It is a public health imperative that we incorporate successfully demonstrated strategies from past prevention efforts into current adolescent STI/HIV prevention programs and that we also continue to search for new ways to protect our youth, as well as teach them to protect themselves from STI/HIV infections.

One of the most important facts is that condoms provide the best protection from STIs, including HIV. Condoms must be used consistently and correctly in each act of intercourse (DGS, 2004).

Researchers (Mueller, Gavin & Kulkarni, 2008) advocate that sexual activity during adolescence years may be a risk behaviour since adolescents are still going through their maturity (physical, emotional and psychological) process and therefore it should be part of intervention programs (mainly through sex education) to postpone the initiation of sexual activity.

As a result, it is also acknowledged the potential contribution of sex education to increase condom use (Kirby, Laris & Rolleri, 2007; Mueller, Gavin & Kulkarni, 2008) as well as decrease sexual intercourse associated to alcohol or drugs (Madkour et al., 2010).

Because the rates of HIV/AIDS, particularly in young people, have always been on the top concerns (UNAIDS, 2010), increasing the level of knowledge related to HIV transmission routes and prevention and developing positive attitudes towards HIV infected people have similarly been prioritized as sex education goals (Kirby, Laris & Rolleri, 2007). These studies show that both adolescents and young adults have reasonable knowledge regarding HIV/AIDS transmission/prevention and show positive attitudes towards HIV infected people.

Overall, sexual health is a topic that requires intervention. During the last decades, since AIDS has revealed itself as a major world problem, governments, including the Portuguese, have dedicated time and money to promote safer sexual and reproductive health. The implementation of sex education may be an important part of the solution for this problem. Our analyses suggest that overall the Portuguese youth have safe sexual behaviours, but there is still a need to improve since not all refer having protective behaviours, therefore putting themselves at risk of major negative consequences in terms of public health (Ramiro, Reis, Matos, Diniz, & Simões, 2011). The data from these two studies also clearly show the existence of a set of factors that determine individual differences in the performance of preventive sexual behaviours. It seems that boys and young adult males have a higher probability to get involved in risky sexual behaviours.

One of the most frequently studied factors is STI's knowledge, namely regarding HIV and AIDS. Though most studies reveal that knowledge is crucial, being informed is not enough in order to change people's behaviours. Beliefs related to condom use (such as "decreasing sexual pleasure"), attitudes (positive or negative), the perception of support from meaningful people (relatives, peers, among others), parental attitudes and behavioral skills related to communication, assertiveness, negotiation, self-efficacy) and the intention of having preventive sexual behaviours always are extremely important conditions when trying to explain differences in behaviours (Matos et al., 2010; Carvalho, & Baptista, 2006; Kirby, 2001). A crucial issue on this subject is the perception of risk that young people have, in other words, the least they consider they are at risk (somehow an extension of the sense of invulnerability which is characteristic of adolescence) and therefore the potential consequences of their behaviours, the greatest the likelihood of getting involved in risky behaviours.

Figures regarding the variety of sexual risky behaviours and the variety of factors involved in the performance of preventive sexual behaviours increase the importance of implementing programs and campaigns that aim specifically to change behaviours and promoting sexual and reproductive health (Matos, 2008; Matos et al, 2011). Most programs have youth as target population regardless genders and they are designed to be implemented in school context. In some cases, teachers and parents are also considered as important agents in youth change and peers may be used as opinion leaders (Matos, 2008).

It is fundamental to comprehend sexuality within the context of adolescence if we want to avoid unwanted or unplanned pregnancy in adolescence, abortion and STIs in general and HIV/AIDS in particular. Sexuality has an important role in adolescents' growth and development so their guidance is essential to enhance a positive, harmonious and responsible adolescence (Matos et al., 2011).

In order to fully understand adolescence, one has to consider the social, family and individual contexts where the adolescent interacts as well as the ways individuals organize sexual experiences. This means that the way adolescents relate sexually to others is deeply influenced by family and social models.

Considering that primary prevention is the one that aims to change behaviours, the evaluation of specific needs must consider the importance of social norms and peer groups, and the development of cognitive and behavioral skills that are essential to promoting and maintaining change. Sex education in health education context requires that the agents involved, whether direct or indirectly (family, schools, communities, institutions, NGOs, city councils, public and private institutes, and places of leisure and entertainment) gain awareness of their importance in young people's development.

Discussing sexuality with a youth audience is not an easy task. Overall, there's a huge difference between what they want to discuss and what adults consider is adequate or important to discuss with them. The main problem of sexuality in adolescence is lack of dialogue because some of the most important issues for them, such as the discovery of their own body, pleasure and their inner self are still taboo matters.

In order to enhance communication with adolescents and young people in general, both in school and university context, it must be developed an environment of understanding, empathy, truthfulness and genuine acceptance and respect for the adolescent/ young adult and his /her doubts, free from judgments. Therefore, the key point identified by experts is meaningful dialogue.

5. References

Aquilino, M.; & Bragadottir, H. (2000). Adolescent pregnancy: Teen perspectives on prevention. *American Journal of Maternal Child Nursing. 25,* 4, 192-197.

Bana, A.; Bhat, V.; Godlwana, X.; Libazi, S.; Maholwana, Y.; Marafungana, N.; Mona, K.; Mbonisweni, A.; Mbulawa, N.; Mofuka, J.; Mohlajoa, N.; Nondula, N.; Qubekile, Y.; & Ramnaran, B. (2010). Knowledge, attitudes and behaviours of adolescents in relation to STIs, pregnancy, contraceptive utilization and substance abuse in the Mhlakulo region, Eastern Cape. *South African Family Practice , 52,* 2, 154-158.

Carvalho, M.; & Baptista, A. (2006). Modelos explicativos dos determinantes dos comportamentos preventivos associados à transmissão do Vírus da Imunodeficiência Humana. [Explanatory models of the determinants of preventive behaviors associated with transmission of Human Immunodeficiency Virus.] *Revista Lusófona de Ciências da Mente e do Comportamento, 8,* 163-192.

Currie C.; Hurrelmann K.; Settertobulte W.; Smith R.; & Todd J. (2000). *Health and health behavior among young people.* Copenhagen: World Health Organization.

Centers for Disease Control and Prevention. (2010). Youth Risk Behavior Surveillance - United States, 2009: Surveillance Summaries. Department of Health and Human Services. *MMWR,* 59.

CVEDT - Centro de Vigilância das Doenças Sexualmente Transmissíveis. Infecção VIH / SIDA. A situação em Portugal a 31 de Dezembro de 2008. [HIV/AIDS. The situation in Portugal on December 31, 2008] (2009). Lisboa: INSA.

DGS- Direcção Geral de Saúde (2004). Orientações estratégicas. Plano Nacional de Saúde 2004-2010: mais saúde para todos. [Strategic guidelines. National Health Plan 2004-2010: better health for all.]- Lisboa: Direcção-Geral da Saúde.

Durex, Give and Receive. (2005) Global Sex Survey Results. Retrieved from internet on 19th September, 2011 from: www.durex.com/gss

Eaton, D.; Kann, L.; Kinchen, S.; Shanklin, S.; Ross, J.; Hawkins, J.; Harris, W.; Lowry, R.; McManus, T.; Cheyen D.; Lim C.; Brener, N.; & Wechsler, H. (2008). Youth risk behavior surveillance, United 3. States, 2007. *MMWR 57*(SS-4), 1-136.

Eisenberg, M. E.; Ackard, D. M.; Resnick, M. D.,& Neumark-Sztainer, D. (2009). Casual sex and psychological health among young adults: Is having "friends with benefits" emotionally damaging? *Perspectives on Sexual and Reproductive Health,* 41(4), 231-237.

Kirby, D. (2001). *Emerging Answers: Research Findings on Programs to Reduce Teen Pregnancy.* Washington, DC: National Campaign to Prevent Teen Pregnancy.

Kirby, D.; Laris, B.A.; & Rolleri, L. (2007). Sex and HIV education programs: Their impact on sexual behaviors of young people throughout the world. *Journal of Adolescent Health, 40,* 206-217.

Kirby, J.; van der Sluijs, W.; & Currie, C.; (2010). HBSC Briefing Supplement 18b: Attitudes towards condom use among young people. Child and Adolescent Health Research Unit. The University of Edinburgh. HBSC Briefing Paper Series.

Paiva, V.; Calazans, G.; Venturi, G.; Dias, R.; & Grupo de Estudos em População, Sexualidade e AIDS. Idade e uso de preservativo na iniciação sexual de adolescentes brasileiros. [Age and condom use at first sexual intercourse of Brazilian adolescents.] *Revista Saúde Pública.* 2008, vol.42, suppl.1, pp. 45-53.

Madkour, A.; Farhat, T.; Halpern, C.; Godeau, E.; & Gabhainn, S. (2010). Early Adolescent Sexual Initiation as a Problem Behavior: A Comparative Study of Five Nations. *Journal of Adolescent Health,* 47(4): 389-398.

Matos, M.G. et al. (2010). Sexualidade, cultura e saúde sexual em Portugal e na América Latina em M. Matos (coord), Sexualidade, Afectos e Cultura - Gestão de problemas de saúde em meio escolar. [Sexuality, affects and culture - Management of health problems in school.] Coisas de Ler, p. 159-175.

Matos, M.G. (ed) (2008). *Sexualidade, Segurança e SIDA,* [Sexuality, Safetiness andAids.] Lisboa: IHMT/FMH/FCT.

Matos, M.; Simões, C.; Tomé, G.; Pereira, S.; Diniz, J.; & Equipa do Aventura Social (2006). *Comportamento Sexual e Conhecimentos, Crenças e Atitudes Face ao VIH/SIDA - Relatório Preliminar,* [Sexual Behavior, Knowledge, Beliefs and Attitudes towards HIV/AIDS - Preliminar Report.] Dezembro 2006. Web site: www.fmh.utl.pt/aventurasocial; www.aventurasocial.com.

Matos, M.G.; Simões, C.; Tomé, G.; Camacho, I.; Ferreira, M.; Ramiro, L.; Reis, M.; & Equipa Aventura Social (2011). *A Saúde dos Adolescentes Portugueses - Relatório do Estudo HBSC 2010.* [The Health of Portuguese adolescents - HBSC Study Report 2010.] ACS/FMH/UTL/CMDT-UNL.

Matos, M.G.; Reis, M.; Ramiro, L.; & Equipa Aventura Social (2011). *Saúde Sexual e Reprodutiva dos Estudantes do Ensino Superior – Relatório do Estudo* [Sexual Reproductive Health of Collegue Students - Study Report] *HBSC/SSREU*. ACS/FMH/UTL/CMDT-UNL.

Mueller, T.E.; Gavin, L.E.; & Kulkarni, A. (2008) The association between sex education and youth's engagement in sexual intercourse, age at first intercourse, and birth control use at first sexual intercourse. *Journal of Adolescent Health*, 42, 89-96.

National Survey of Sexual Health and Behavior (NSSHB). (2010). Findings from the National Survey of Sexual Health and Behavior, Centre for Sexual Health Promotion, Indiana University. *Journal of Sexual Medicine, 7*, Supplement 5.

Ramiro, L.; Reis, M.; Matos, M.G.; Diniz, J.; & Simões, C. (2011). Educação Sexual, Conhecimentos, Crenças, Atitudes e Comportamentos nos adolescentes. [Sexual Education, Knowledge, Beliefs, Attitudes and Behaviors among adolescents.] *Revista Portuguesa de Saúde Pública, 29 (1)*:11-21.

Reis, M.; Ramiro, L.; Matos, M.G.; Diniz, J. A; & Simões, C. (2011). Information and attitudes about HIV/Aids in Portuguese adolescents: state of art and changes in a four year period. *Psicothema, 23(2)*, 260-266.

Reis, M.; Ramiro, L.; Carvalho; M. & Pereira, S. (2009). A sexualidade, o corpo e os amores em M. Matos & D. Sampaio (coord), Jovens com Saúde - Diálogo com uma Geração, [Youth with Health - Dialogue with a Generation.] Lisboa. Texto Editora, p. 265-282.

Synovitz, L.; Herbert, E.; Kelley, R.; & Carlson, G. (2002). Sexual knowledge of college students in a southern state: Relationship to sexuality education results of Louisianna college student study shows need for sexuality programs. *American Journal of Health Studies*. Retrieved from www.findarticles.com.

Tavoosi, A.; Zaferani, A.; Enzevaei, A.; Tajik, P.; & Ahmadinezhad, Z. (2004). Knowledge and attitude towards HIV/Aids among Iranian students. *BMC Public Health, 4*, 17.

Thompson, C.; Currie, C.; Todd, J.; & Elton, R. (1999). Changes in HIV/AIDS education, knowledge and attitudes among Scottish 15-16 years old, 1990-1994 findings from WHO: Health Behaviour in School-aged Children Study (HBSC). *Health Education Research, 14*, 357-370.

UNAIDS. (2008). Joint United Nations Programme on HIV/AIDS. Report on the global HIV/AIDS epidemic.

UNAIDS. (2010). Global Report: UNAIDS report on the Global Aids epidemic 2010. Joint United Nations Programme on HIV/Aids. WHO Library Catalogue-in-Publication Data.

WHO. (2010). Position paper on mainstreaming adolescent pregnancy in efforts to make pregnancy safer. Department of Making Pregnancy Safer. WHO Document Production Services, Geneva, Switzerland.

13

Knowledge, Attitude, Behavior, and Practice of the UNIFIL Peacekeepers on Human Immunodeficiency Virus

Abdo R. Jurjus[1,2], Inaya Abdallah Hajj Hussein[1] and Alice A. Gerges[2]
[1]*American University of Beirut*
[2]*Lebanese AIDS Society*
Lebanon

1. Introduction

1.1 Global scenario of Human Immunodeficiency Virus (HIV) and sexually transmitted diseases

Since the first report in June 1981, the Human Immunodeficiency Virus (HIV) continues to be a serious health, social, economic and even security challenge to both leaders and populations at large (CDC, 1981). About 7000 new HIV infections occur per day, and according to the UN declaration on AIDS, in June 2011, prevention remains the corner stone of all responses to the epidemic (worldstats.htm, June 2011). Despite reports of a marked progress in stabilizing the overall growth at the global level, about 27% increase in the number of people living with HIV (PLWHIV) was recorded in ten years, 26.2 million in 1999 to 33.3 million in 2009 (UNAIDS, 2010).

It is well established that the HIV epidemic patterns vary between and within countries. They are mostly linked to paid sex, drug use, and sex between men. Countries in Eastern Europe and Central Asia reported high rates of HIV transmission in networks of injecting drug users (IDUs) and their sexual partners. In such countries, PLWHIV had almost tripled since 2000, leading to the largest regional increase (UNAIDS, 2010). In addition, the total numbers of PLWHIV in North America and Western and Central Europe kept increasing from 2001, by a rate of 30%, to reach 2.3 million in 2009. Unprotected sex between men continues to dominate the patterns of HIV transmission in these regions. Men outnumber women among PLWHIV; women comprised about 26% in North America and 29% in Western and Central Europe in 2009 (Ebrahim et al., 2005; The Well Project STD, 2009; UNAIDS, 2010).

On the other hand, sexually transmitted diseases (STDs), more than 30 different types, represent a major global health threat to all sexually active individuals including army personnel (WHO-STI, 2007; De Waal, 2010). The world statistics about STDs showed an overall worldwide increase in the rates over the years among people aged 25 years or younger from an estimate of 333 million in 1997 to 340 million in 1999 new cases (Adib et al.,

2002). These infections have predominantly increased among young people and are correlated with a marked increase in sexual promiscuity in the past 30 years.

However, racial, ethnic and regional disparities persist. The complications of these diseases underscore their burden and impact on society. Consequences of undiagnosed and untreated STD's include adverse pregnancy, infertility, cancers of the reproductive tract, and increased likelihood of HIV acquisition and transmission (Gaydos et al. 2000; WHO-STI, 2007). Multiple studies have also demonstrated that HIV epidemic has become intimately associated with the increased transmission of other STD's, both biologically and behaviorally (STDstatisticsworldwide, 2011; Lazenby, 2011). The gravity of the situation necessitated the international health agencies to establish the month of April 2011 as the STD awareness month. It aimed to promote STD testing among young people and encouraged them to talk to their partners, health care providers, and parents about STD prevention (Bolan, 2011).

1.2 HIV/AIDS and sexually transmitted infections in the Middle East and North Africa region

Despite a fair amount of progress on understanding HIV and STDs epidemiology globally, knowledge of the epidemic continues to be very limited in the Middle East and North Africa (MENA) region. It has already reached all corners of the region and IDUs, men who have sex with men (MSM), and female sex workers (FSW), are documented to exist in all MENA countries (Abu-Raddad et al.,2010).

There is an increase in the numbers of PLWHIV from 2001 (180,000) to 2008 (310,000) and to 2009 (460,000) with a doubling of the average incidence from 0.1% in 2001 to 0.2% in 2009. In addition, 26,000 young people in the MENA region acquired HIV in 2009 (UNAIDS & WHO Report, 2008; UNAIDS, 2010)

Other reports showed that the prevalence of HIV in the MENA region has witnessed an increase and heterosexual transmission accounted for 80% of the cumulative total number of reported AIDS cases, while the use of non-sterile needles among injecting drug users accounted for 10%. On the other hand, transmission through blood and blood products decreased from 12% in 1993 to 0.4% in 2003 (Kim, 2002; UNAIDS & WHO Report, 2008).

Moreover, for the MENA region, an increase in STDs can be expected as provision of education and services to both young men and women are inadequate. Studies have shown moderate to high incidence rates of males engaging in sex before marriage, starting very early in adolescence, and in extramarital sex, with data indicating rates of 56.6% and 20.8%, respectively (Tawilah et al., 2002). Furthermore, other data sources showed moderate to high frequency for commercial sex work at 47.2%; moderate prevalence for men who have sex with men at 18.9%; and a close frequency for injecting drug users at 22.6% (Abu Raddad et al., 2010).

1.3 HIV/AIDS and STDs in Lebanon

In Lebanon, the number of reported HIV and AIDS cases has been steadily increasing since 1984, when the first AIDS case in the country was reported (Mokhbat et al., 1985). While the first cases of HIV/AIDS were diagnosed among emigrant Lebanese men visiting or returning home, recent data indicated that local transmission and spread of the disease were increasing and becoming a significant mode of disease acquisition, accounting for almost 29% of the HIV/AIDS cases in the country. By 2010, a cumulative number of 1,354 cases were reported to the National AIDS Program (NAP), with 83 new cases diagnosed and reported in 2009. About half of the newly reported cases were in the AIDS stage, which highlighted the late diagnosis of the disease in Lebanon and, hence, the need to encourage early detection, and to promote early testing. It is also noteworthy that women constituted around 11% of the reported cumulative cases and 37 per cent of the newly reported cases in 2009, which indicated an increasing incidence of HIV/AIDS among the Lebanese women population (NAP website, 2011).

Sexual relations remain the major mode of HIV transmission in Lebanon, accounting for 76.3 per cent, with heterosexual and homosexual relations accounting for 64.4% and 19.35%, respectively. Although testing of transfused blood for HIV has been mandatory since the 1980s, 6.4% of the HIV/AIDS cases have resulted from blood transfusion, which might be related to transfusions received prior to the implementation of universal blood screening. Other modes of HIV transmission in Lebanon included intravenous drug use, accounting for 6%, and mother-to-child transmission, accounting for 2%. It is noteworthy that an increasing trend of newly reported infections was noticed among the young population aged between 15 and 29 years, compared to a horizontal trend in other age groups (NAP website, 2011).

Concerning STDs, several published and unpublished reports on STDs in Lebanon were identified and reviewed; however, the overall approach is still fragmented and not comprehensive. Some reports showed that the rate of self-reported STDs was 11.5% in 2004, with only 35% of them seeking medical treatment (Kahhaleh et al., 2009). A cross-sectional study of 118,230 endocervical swabs from Lebanese women attending clinics and hospitals in five districts of Lebanon, over a five-year period 2002-2005, showed: (a) a rise in frequencies of abnormal Pap tests by 12.2%, (b) a 6.7-fold increase of the diagnosis of atypical squamous cells of undetermined significance (ASCUS), and (c) an increase of bacterial vaginitis by 1.4% (Karam et al., 2005).

1.3.1 Knowledge, attitudes, beliefs and practices of the Lebanese youth regarding HIV/AIDS and STDs

In Lebanon, several knowledge, attitude, beliefs and practices (KABP) studies regarding HIV/AIDS including STDs have been conducted among different groups. Such studies targeted the general population, the Lebanese Army, the Military Academy, the out of school youth, as well as, school students among others. They showed various levels of deficiencies in knowledge about modes of transmission and of prevention along with a wide range of misconceptions and risky sexual practices (Jurjus & Tohme, 2008). In this chapter, only one selected study pertaining to out-of-school youth groups, in the region of the United Nations Interim Forces in Lebanon (UNIFIL) will be highlighted.

This study conducted by Jurjus and Watfa in the South, in the aftermath of the July 2006 war, revealed that 30% of the targeted youth were unaware of HIV or AIDS, with higher proportions among girls than boys. Few knew that persons living with HIV/AIDS can look healthy and are therefore difficult to identify by just their physical appearance. Over half of the respondents could list at least two modes of transmission, including blood and sexual relations with commercial sex workers. On the other hand, high rates of misconceptions about transmission were revealed. Very few had an adequate knowledge about prevention measures, with the majority stressing cleanliness and testing of blood as important preventive measures, while only some mentioned condoms or abstinence. It is to be noted that peer pressure was a major driver for sexual activities. Young girls were at a higher risk, being in a disadvantaged situation as they perceived sex as doing whatever their partner wanted. They were unequipped with skills to negotiate condom use or refuse coerced sex. Moreover, girls in that region showed signs of depression, anxiety and lack of security. On the other hand, a majority of 60%, mainly boys, engaged in casual sex at a very early age and as many as 40% believed that anal sex was a safe practice (Jurjus & Watfa, 2008).

1.4 STDs, HIV and the army

STDs have continuously posed a significant health and security threat, and an important challenge, to military personnel throughout history (Gaydos et al., 2000). Several reports have been published regarding outbreaks of sexually transmitted diseases in armies. Such outbreaks were devastating and sometimes were determining factors for the gain or loss of a war, in particular, before the discovery of antibiotics in the nineteen fourties (Emerson, 1997).

The first well recorded outbreak of STDs among the military occurred among French troops, besieging Naples, in 1494, and killing more than 5 million people across Europe (Oriel, 1994). Another serious situation occurred at the siege of Nuremberg, between 1632 and 1648; there were about 40,000 soldiers in the Bavarian Armies compared 140,000 prostitutes and camp followers. This increase in transactional sex in the armies has led a French general to say that prostitutes "killed ten times as many men as enemy fire" (Greenberg, 1972).

In the USA, medical records from the revolutionary war indicate that STDs had a remarkable impact in term of lost person-days among members of the Continental Army. In 1776, veneral shancres, genital ulcers and gonorrhea were described by the Swedish physician Van Swieten in a book on STDs "Published, for Use of Military and Naval Surgeons in America" (Kampeier, 1982; Rasnake, 2005). During World Wars I and II the high rates of syphilis among draftees led to deferral of a large number of military personnel. However, there was a decreasing prevalence of 4.5% in 1942 due to the Penicillin therapy. On the other hand, during the Korean War in Southeast Asia, there was a surge in gonorrhea rates, they accounted for 75% of all STDs diagnosed. The rates reached as high as 500 cases per thousand person-years (py). Moreover, in 1965, troops in Vietnam were experiencing more than 300 cases of gonorrhea per 1000 py, and in Thailand 500 cases per 1000 py (Gilbert and Greenberg, 1967). In 2008, data from 21 African military forces showed that HIV prevalence was elevated compared to the general population (Ba et al., 2008).

War and deployment of army personnel, especially in foreign countries, as peacekeepers or otherwise have put soldiers at risk for contracting STDs, mostly gonorrhea, syphilis and

HIV. Today gonorrhea and syphilis are curable diseases, they rarely cause significant morbidity or lost duty time. HIV, however, represents a grave threat to infected army members and is being aggravated by the likelihood of HIV/STDs co-infection (Ebrahim et al., 2005; Lazenby, 2011).

HIV, first reported in 1981, is being considered as a significant threat to armies. In 1984, the first recognized military HIV case was recognized in a US Army recruit. He was diagnosed and died 18 months later. In 1985, in the USA, a policy was formulated whereby all recruits were tested upon entry into military service. Personnel testing positive, and were already on active duty, were retained but prohibited from overseas assignments and deployments. The army rate declined from 0.43 sera conversion per 1000 per year (py) in 1985 to 0.08 per 1000 py in 1999 and currently stands about 0.08 per 1000 py. Contact with commercial sex workers was identified as a common risk factor among certain army groups. Actually, the global movement of army personnel broadens the variety of HIV strains to which service members are exposed; from Thailand, Iraq, Afghanistan, Kenya, Uganda, and other countries. Several studies emphasized the importance of "bridge population" in the spread of such infectious diseases (Rasnake et al., 2005; kershaw, 2008; De Wall, 2010; UNAIDS, 2010).

Two remarkable events have impacted the history of STD; the use of Penicillin in the mid fourties and the reporting of HIV/AIDS in the early eighties. Experts in the field divided the history of STDs in the military into five periods. The first included the period of European Sieges and American Revolution up to 1909, the beginning of the twentieth century. It was a time when STDs were deplored and affected people stigmatized. The second period goes from 1909 to 1945. During this period, scientific knowledge and palliative treatment have flourished but not enough to cure STDs. It was not until the third period began in 1945, when the use of penicillin provided cure and other approaches to control STDs were questioned. However, the reporting of HIV in the early 1980s opened a new fourth era. During this period, new and old STDs coming from bacteria, viruses, parasites and others were relatively easily detected and screened. After the nineties, a modern era started with the advent of diagnostic molecular techniques allowing less invasive or noninvasive screening of new recruits for asymptomatic STDs and HIV and the use of new generations of drugs for cure and therapy (Gaydos et al., 2000; Rasnake et al., 2005).

Recent data show that HIV and STDs prevalences among armed forces are complex and highly variable, sometimes comparable and most of the times significantly elevated compared to the general population (Bazergan 2006; Ba et al., 2008). Actually, the prevalence differentials within armies, among armies and between armies and the civilian population depend upon multiple factors, including the demographic composition of armed forces, alcohol and drug use, local versus foreign military deployments, ethos, military policy regarding HIV and STDs in general, and availability and effectiveness of health services and prevention programs. In some cases, the behavior of young, sexually active soldiers may be governed mostly by peer pressure. In some other cases, soldiers are indicted into hyper-masculine cultures that reward risk taking, in which sex is considered a sign of virility or a compensation for the lack of emotions of professional military life (Shuper et al., 2009; Baliunas et al., 2010; UNAIDS, 2010).Moreover, soldiers deployed in foreign countries are often well paid, sometimes lonely and bored. They may attract surrounding civilian populations as well as sex workers, a situation that could lead to higher levels of transactional sex (Family Health International, 2005; Baliunas et al., 2010; UNAIDS, 2010).

Through the years, data show that STDs and HIV rates continue to rise dramatically in the military. In 2006, comparative studies of sexual behavior in Europe and the USA have shown that military personnel, both career and conscripted soldiers, have a much higher risk of HIV infection than groups of equivalent age and sex in the civilian population. Armed forces in other parts of the world like Angola, India and Uganda reflect the same phenomenon. A 1995 estimate of HIV in Zimbabwe, for instance, place the infection rate for army personnel at three to four times higher than that for the civilian population (Bazergan, 2006; European Center, 2009; UNAIDS, 2010).

The history of STDs and HIV in the military has largely focused on infection acquired by men while deployed. However, the expanding role of women in the military service added a new variable to this equation, the impact of which will be known only with time. HIV and STDs affect both men and women, but in many cases, the health problems they cause can be more severe for women. In this regard, a number of UN resolutions have addressed this topic and included gender sensitive issues in their policies (UN, 2000 resolution 1325; WHO & Global Coalition on Women and AIDS, 2004; UNFPA-Fact sheet, 2009).

1.5 HIV as a global security issue

At the turn of the millennium, the United Nations Security Council felt the global gravity of HIV/AIDS and considered it as a major public health issue and a potential threat to international peace and security (Barnett & Prins, 2006). They were partly driven by fears of high disease burdens and the attrition of military human resources. There was also a specific concern with peacekeeping, emphasizing the threats posed by HIV and AIDS to peacekeepers and peacekeeping operations, and the fear that peacekeepers might become vectors to HIV transmission (Barnett & Prins, 2006; Kershaw R, 2008). As a result, the Security Council affirmed its commitment by the resolution 1308 adopted in the year 2000, and reaffirmed a stronger commitment at multiple occasions, and most recently in 2011 by unanimously adopting the 1960 resolution encouraging more the inclusion of HIV prevention, treatment, care and support, as an integral part of peace-keeping mandates. They conceived the UN troops as part of prevention and care rather than vectors of HIV and STD transmission to civilians, especially that such troops are being involved in community based programs and interventions (Sing & Banerjee, 2006; UNAIDS Global Report, 2010; UNDP, 2010).

The consecutive commitments were adopted in response to a surge in peacekeeping, and an increase in numbers of unstable locations which have required a significantly increased deployment of peacekeepers around the world. In 2000, the number of peacekeepers worldwide was 37,000, but by 2011, there were 98,837 international peacekeepers. This increase has been matched by a growing number of countries contributing troops, up to 115 countries. Among these, some countries have HIV prevalence higher than 1% in the general population. Consequently, the percentage of international uniformed personnel reported to be living with HIV varied between missions and was in the range of 1.0% to 2.4%. Available data from selected countries indicate that the HIV prevalence varied from a low of 0.6% among recruits in Vietnam to 10.1% for recruits in Equatorial Guinea (Whiteside et al., 2006; Bing et al., 2008; Lowicki-Zucca et al., 2009; UNAIDS Global Report, 2010).

A 2007 survey of 48,116 peacekeeping personnel in three missions found that, from August 2001 to June 2007, 25 peacekeepers from the three missions had died from AIDS-related causes, and 105 had been repatriated for HIV-related reasons. Most of these repatriations were from two troop-contributing countries that did not practice pre-deployment HIV testing; only 3 were women (UNAIDS, 2011).

Nowadays, it is well known that the HIV prevalence within the uniformed services is related to a range of factors and increases with age, time in service, the maturity of the epidemic, the repertoires of violence, and the policies and activities of the command (AIDS, Security and Conflict Initiative, 2011). Surveys are planned or underway in 22 countries, they should help provide a more complete picture of the HIV epidemic among military populations by the end of 2011 (United States Department of Defense HIV/AIDS Prevention Program, 2011).

This chapter comes at a time when the global AIDS response is at a crossroads. It has been 30 years since the AIDS epidemic was first reported, and 10 years since the United Nations Security Council adopted the resolution 1308 on HIV/AIDS. Since then, significant progress has been made in providing access to HIV prevention, treatment, care and support services for all sections of society, and more so for peacekeepers and other uniformed services personnel. This chapter reviewed briefly the status of HIV and STDs in the army, in general, and UN forces, in particular. It also reported the results of a KABP survey targeting the UNIFIL in Lebanon regarding HIV, STDs, and gender sensitive issues.

2. Methods

2.1 Instrument

The study took place between 2007 and 2008 after approval of the institutional research board of the Lebanese Health Society. The instrument was a self-administered anonymous locally developed questionnaire, available in three languages, (English, French and Arabic), and distributed to six contingents. It consisted of seven sections and a total of 53 questions. It was modified and several sensitive questions, pertaining to sexual practices and STDs, although very relevant, were omitted after recommendations from the UNIFIL chief medical officer, the UNIFIL medical planning officer, and the medical officers within the selected contingents. The final questionnaire included the following seven sections:

Section one collected socio-demographic data (age, gender, nationality, marital status, educational level and military rank) as well as information on deployment history. Section two addressed, through a mixture of open-ended and closed ended questions, the general knowledge of the respondents regarding HIV/AIDS, prevention and transmission methods, the attitudes towards people living with HIV, and their perception of their own risk to catching HIV. Section three assessed the use of condoms, inquired about the availability and previous exposure to female condoms. Section four measured the frequency and amount of alcohol drinking and its association with engaging in sexual relations under influence. Section five assessed the health seeking behavior of UNIFIL forces in case of a suspected STD as well as previous history and attitude towards testing for HIV, and receiving counseling. Section six assessed the knowledge of UNIFIL members about the local population, the status women, and about problems faced by UNIFIL members when communicating with women. Section seven asked about the preferred sources of information on STDs including HIV, and inquired about the trust of UNIFIL members in Peer Leaders. This section also asked about previous training on HIV/AIDS before deployment and knowledge or hearing about the UNSCR 1308 and 1325.

2.2 Target population and sample size

The target population consisted of countries being able to speak English, French or Arabic as identified following a consultation with UNIFIL commanders. The sample size was calculated using a probability sample proportional to the total number of selected troops and based on their age, gender, and rank distribution. A total sample size of 200 individuals was targeted. It represented 8.5% of the total number of troops included in the study (N=2335). The questionnaires were randomly distributed by the medical components of each battalion and were handed back, two weeks after distribution for cleaning and data entry.

2.3 Data analysis

Frequency distributions were performed for all the variables and mean and standard deviations (± SD) were computed for age. Significant findings by nationality were also highlighted, where appropriate, and chi-square tests were used to report associations between categorical variables such as frequency of alcohol drinking and frequency of engaging in sexual relations under influence. The statistical package for social sciences (SPSS) v.16 was used for data entry and analysis. A p-value <0.05 was considered statistically significant.

3. Results

3.1 Peacekeepers profile

A total of 200 members of the UNIFIL peacekeepers proportionately distributed among six battalions from 5 different countries were selected for the study. The overall response rate was 94% with wide disparities between the battalions.

Table 1 depicts the general socio-demographic characteristics of the respondents. The mean age of the respondents was 28.4 ± 7, ranging between 19 and 51 years old. The majority (60.3%) were young adults aged between 20 and 30 years old. Men constituted almost 77.84% of the study sample. The sample size was proportionately distributed along the different nationalities and battalions with the (As) constituting half of the sampled respondents and the other nationalities having a close distribution about 13%, with a 7% for the (Es), it is connected to their low response rate. Almost half of the respondents were single while more than one third (36%) were married, and the rest being either divorced, widowed or living with a partner. Overall, 16.3% had some kind of university education including military academy, however, rates varied between 3.6% among the (Bs) and 35.6% among the (Es) with the rest having prevalence rates of university education close to the overall percentage. Almost 40% of the respondents did not complete their high school education with the highest rates being among the (Bs) (85.6%) and the lowest among the (Es) (0%).

Characteristic	Number (n=189)	Percentage
Gender		
Men	147	77.8
Women	28	14.8
Unspecified	14	7.4
Age		
mean ± SD	28.4± 7	
19-24	59	31.2
25-29	55	29.1
30-40	42	22.2
41-51	13	6.9
unspecified	20	10.6
Nationality		
A	96	50.8
B	28	14.8
C	25	13.2
D	23	12.2
E	14	7.4
Unspecified	3	1.6
Marital Status		
Single	92	48.7
Married	69	36.5
Divorced	12	6.3
Widowed	1	0.5
Unspecified	15	7.9
Educational Level		
Incomplete high school	67	36.6
Completed high school	48	26.2
Specialty education (vocational or technical school)	38	20.8
Military academy	9	4.9
Incomplete university	13	7.1
University & higher	8	4.3
Military Rank		
Soldier	111	59.4
Non-commissioned officer	28	15.0
Warrant officer	31	16.6
Officer	15	8.0
Unspecified	2	1.1

* Sometimes numbers do not add up to 189 because of missing responses

Table 1. General socio-demographic characteristics of UNIFIL respondents.

All military ranks were represented based on a proportionate distribution with soldiers constituting 60% of the respondents, non-commissioned officers (15%), warrant officers (16.6%), and the rest were just officers.

The majority of the respondents (70%) have been present in Lebanon for one to three months and more than half will be staying in Lebanon for more than four months. Almost 20% of the respondents were previously deployed on a United Nations Peacekeeping mission overseas with 60% of them having served in at least one mission (Table 2).

Characteristic	Number	Percentage
Presence in Lebanon		
Less than one month	38	20.5
One to three months	127	68.6
Four to six months	12	6.5
More than six months	8	4.3
Duration of stay		
Less than one month	4	2.1
One to three months	80	42.6
Four to six months	103	54.8
More than six months	1	.5
Previous UN deployment overseas		
Yes	37	19.7
Number of missions		
One	22	59.5
Two	8	21.6
Three	5	13.5
≥ Four	2	5.4

* Sometimes numbers do not add up to 189 because of missing responses.

Table 2. Deployment history in Lebanon and overseas.

3.2 Knowledge about HIV/ AIDS

The survey measured levels of knowledge through a series of open-ended (unprompted) questions and close-ended questions (yes, no, don't know) to asses knowledge on prevention and transmission methods as well as misconceptions regarding transmission of HIV. Based on the close-ended questions (Table 3), the majority (88.9%) of the respondents knew that AIDS is caused by a virus. However, half of them did not know that AIDS and HIV represent different stages of the disease. More than 80% agreed that condoms and staying faithful to one uninfected partner can protect from HIV infection, and almost 90% approved that using non-sterile needles might transmit HIV. Nevertheless, 47.6% did not know that HIV could be transmitted by an infected mother to her baby during breastfeeding. Regarding knowledge about HIV cases in Lebanon, the vast majority (70.1%) had no idea about the status of HIV/AIDS in the country.

	Yes	No	Don't know
AIDS is caused by a virus	88.9	4.8	6.3
HIV and AIDS are the same thing	50.8	41.2	8.0
Lebanon is known for not having reported/ registered any HIV infection	4.8	25.1	70.1
It is possible to protect yourself from HIV infection by using condoms during sexual contacts	82.4	10.7	7.0
People can get an HIV-infection by using non-sterile needles for injections	89.9	7.4	2.6
HIV-infected woman can pass on the virus to her newborn baby during breastfeeding	52.4	29.1	18.5
An HIV-infected UNIFIL soldier can be legally dismissed from the military service	33.2	31.0	35.8
Staying with one faithful partner who is not infected is one of the ways to prevent HIV infection	83.4	11.8	4.8
Do you think there is a cure for HIV/ AIDS?	8.5	79.3	12.2
Can you tell whether a person is infected with HIV by just looking at him/ her?	4.8	88.3	6.9

Correct answers are written in blue while noteworthy incorrect answers are written in red.

Table 3. Knowledge of HIV/ AIDS (%).

In addition, almost all the respondents did not have a clear idea about the legal procedures followed if a person is known to be infected with HIV among peacekeeping forces as only 31% knew that an infected UNIFIL soldier cannot be legally dismissed from the military service (Table, 3). The majority, 79.3%, knew that HIV/AIDS cannot be cured; and about 12% incorrectly answered the question regarding the ability to recognize a person living with HIV from his/her appearance. Furthermore, participants were asked whether they believe that women are at a higher risk of exposure to HIV infection compared to men. Only a minority of the respondents (16.1%) knew that women are at increased risk for becoming infected with HIV and few (6/189) could mention the correct reasons behind the increased vulnerability of women including physiological reasons, rape, and inability of women to negotiate condom use.

In unprompted questions, 72%, 39%, and 24% of the respondents, respectively, stated condoms, abstinence and staying faithful to one partner as modes of prevention from HIV (Fig. 1). Using sterile needles and avoiding drug use was mentioned by 33% of the respondents while avoiding contact with blood products and transfusions was identified as a prevention measure by only 24% of the respondents. Only 32.8% of the respondents correctly listed three prevention measures while 39.7% knew only two prevention measures, and 11.1% did not know any prevention measure from HIV (Fig. 2).

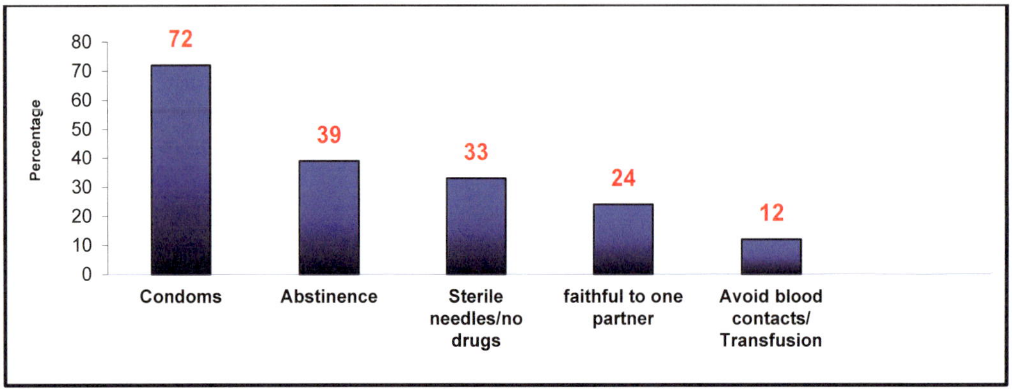

Fig. 1. Prevention methods from HIV/AIDS as listed by respondents (%).

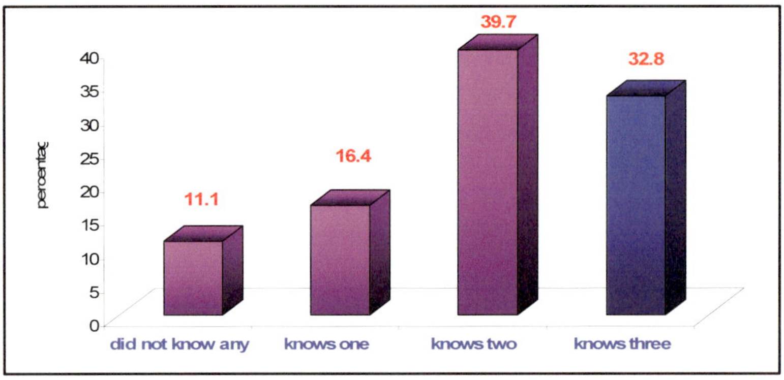

Fig. 2. Distribution of the total number of correct prevention measures listed (%).

Concerning modes of transmission, as depicted in Fig. 3, the vast majority (91%) listed unprotected sexual relations, while 62.2% mentioned infected blood and 57.5% use of non-sterile needles as modes of transmission. It is noteworthy that only 7.4% listed mother to child as a means of transmission.

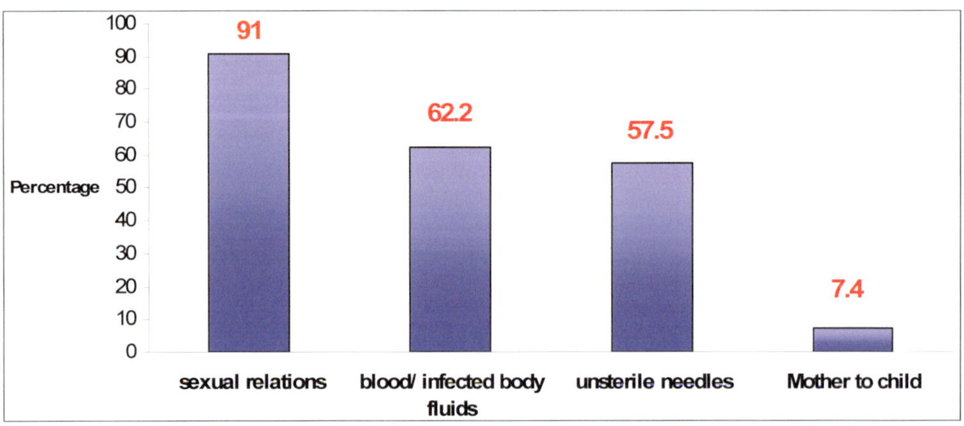

Fig. 3. Transmission methods of HIV as listed by the respondents (%).

Overall, only 48.1% of the respondents correctly listed three transmission methods while 31.7% and 7.4% knew two or one transmission method, respectively, and 12.7% of the respondents did not recognize any transmission method.

Concerning the misconceptions regarding HIV/AIDS transmission, a high prevalence was noticed among the respondents (Table 4). More than one third believed that mosquitoes and drinking contaminated water could transmit HIV; almost one fourth thought that HIV could be transmitted by sharing food or use of public toilets, and 15.3% assumed that HIV could be transmitted by sharing plates and dishes with an infected person. In addition, a common belief was that frequent testing of oneself and partner for HIV is a way of prevention which denotes the false perception that testing is a solution and highlights the fact that many do not know that the HIV test is negative for the first 6 weeks after the infection although the person is highly infective at this stage.

In brief, a comprehensive knowledge of HIV/AIDS was assumed to be present when all the following criteria were met: (a) Having at least 5 correct answers on the closed-ended questions, (b) Correctly stating three prevention measures against HIV, and (c) Rejecting four misconceptions regarding HIV transmission.

	Yes/ Don't' know	No
One can get an HIV infection when bitten by mosquito	35.9	64.2
People can get an HIV-infection by sharing plates and dishes with an HIV-infected person	15.3	84.7
You can protect yourself from HIV-infection by avoiding public toilets	24.4	75.7
People can protect themselves from HIV-infection by avoiding sharing food with a person who has HIV	23.3	76.7
People can protect themselves from HIV-infection by avoiding drinking contaminated water	36.7	63.3

Table 4. Misconceptions regarding HIV/ AIDS transmission (%).

In total, 61% of the respondents had a comprehensive knowledge about HIV/AIDS. However, rates significantly varied between nationalities as the (Cs) had the highest rates of knowledge (92%), while only 39.3% of the (Bs) had good knowledge. Concerning other nationalities, rates of good comprehensive knowledge were 69.6%, 58.3% and 57.1% for the (Ds), (As) and (Es), respectively.

3.3 Attitudes towards people living with HIV

Almost 40% of the respondents believed that persons living with HIV should be allowed to keep their work in the UNIFIL, while 32% did not believe so, and almost 20% did not know what would be the appropriate decision. Significant variations in the attitudes towards people living with HIV were noted between nationalities ($p<0.001$). The (Bs) had the least favorable attitudes as 85.7% of them believed that an HIV infected UNIFIL member should not be allowed to continue his/her work, while 74% and 70% of the (Ds) and (As), respectively reported that a UNIFIL member living with HIV should be allowed to keep his/her work. The (Es) and the (Cs) who had a positive attitude towards UNIFIL members living with HIV reached 57% and 32%, respectively. In addition, more than two thirds of the respondents (72%) reported that persons living with HIV should reveal their disease status with (Es), (Ds) and (Cs) having the highest rates ranging between 83% and 93%. On the other hand, almost half (46.6%) of the (Bs) agreed that people can keep their infection secret compared to an overall rate of 12.4% reported by the total sample.

3.4 Risk perception

About half of the respondents (44.6%) considered themselves to be at no risk of acquiring HIV (Fig. 4), while almost one third classified themselves to be at low risk, and almost 15% considered themselves to have a moderate or high risk of acquiring HIV.

Risk perception significantly ($p<0.001$) varied by nationality with two thirds (65.2%) of the (Ds) and more than half (57.1%) of the (Es) perceiving themselves at no risk, and low risk, respectively. On the other hand, 72% of the (Cs) tended to classify themselves at risk for acquiring HIV and almost one third of the (As, Bs and Es) considered themselves at high risk of catching HIV.

The majority of the (Ds) and (Es) reported that UNIFIL members are at no risk for HIV infection which agrees with the distribution of self-perception of risk reported. Similarly, the (Cs) and (Bs) had almost the same rates of perceived risk of UNIFIL members and self-perceived risk towards HIV infection with (Cs) reporting the highest risk (72%) (Fig. 5).

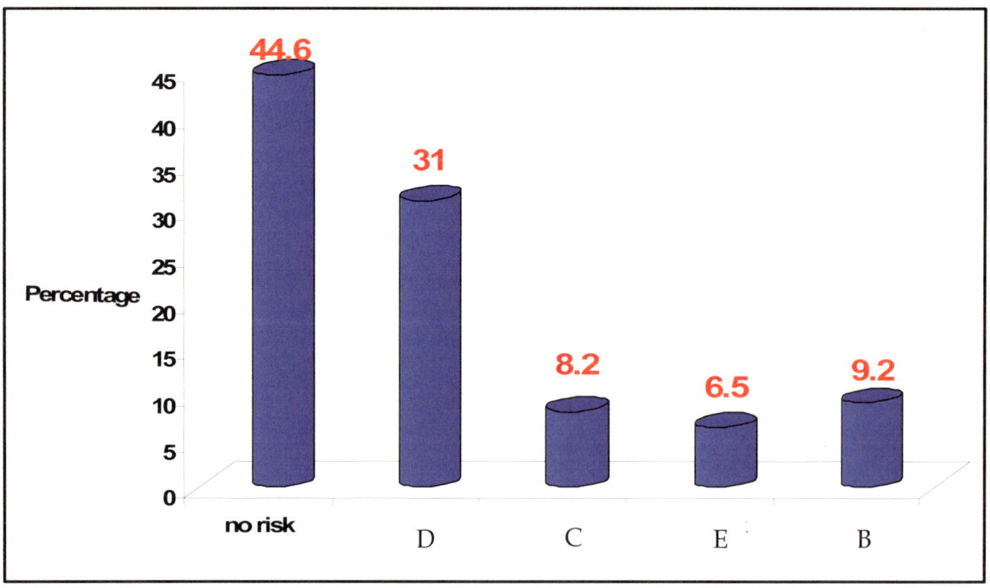

Fig. 4. Self-perception of risk of acquiring HIV among all respondents.

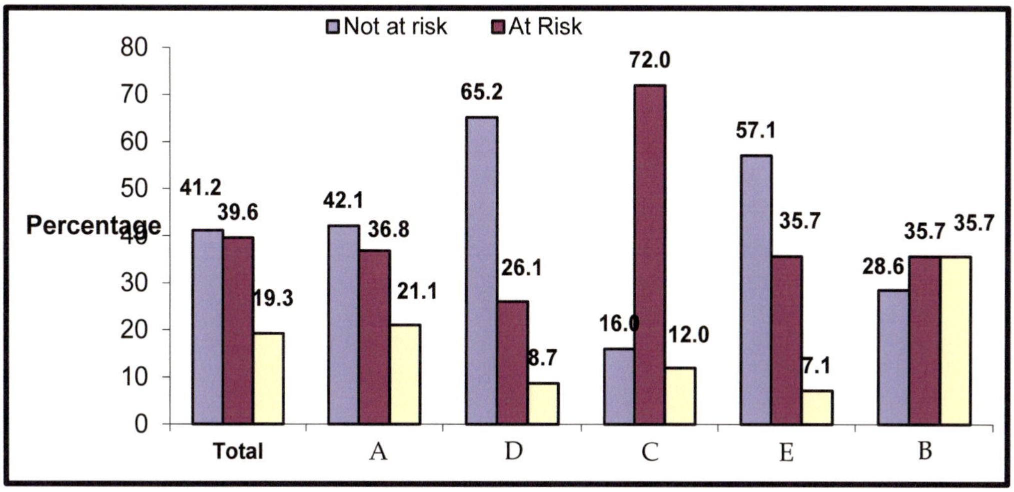

Fig. 5. Perceived risk of UNIFIL towards HIV infection on the total sample by nationality.

3.5 Condom use

More than half of the respondents (53%) did not consistently use condoms with casual sex partners. This fact denotes a high-risk behavior and a risk of HIV or other STDs. The partner respected the choice of condom use among 74% of the respondents. Among those who used condoms, reasons for using condoms included prevention of all STDs (86.4%), prevention of pregnancy (58.3%), and prevention of HIV specifically (53.4%). On the other hand, the reasons for not using condoms included; not being necessary (28%), dislike condoms (20%), unavailability and partner objection (15% each), and faithfulness (13%) of partner. A significant and gradual association was found between having a good comprehensive knowledge about HIV/AIDS and consistently using condoms with non-regular partners.

In fact, those who always used condoms had a prevalence rate of comprehensive knowledge on HIV/AIDS 1.6 times higher than that of those who never use condoms with casual sexual partners (68.7% vs. 43.6%). However, this trend was not consistent across all nationalities as it was only present among the (Bs), the (As), and the (Ds).

Use of condoms with non-regular partners varied significantly by nationality ($p<0.05$) as revealed in Fig. 6. The (Ds) had the highest rates of consistent condom use (71%), followed by the (As) (56%). However, the (Cs), (Bs), and (Es) reported the highest rates on inconsistent condom use (78%, 64% and 60%, respectively). The main reason for not using condoms among the (Cs) and (Bs) are "dislike", while believing that it is "unnecessary" was the most common reason reported by the Es (47%).

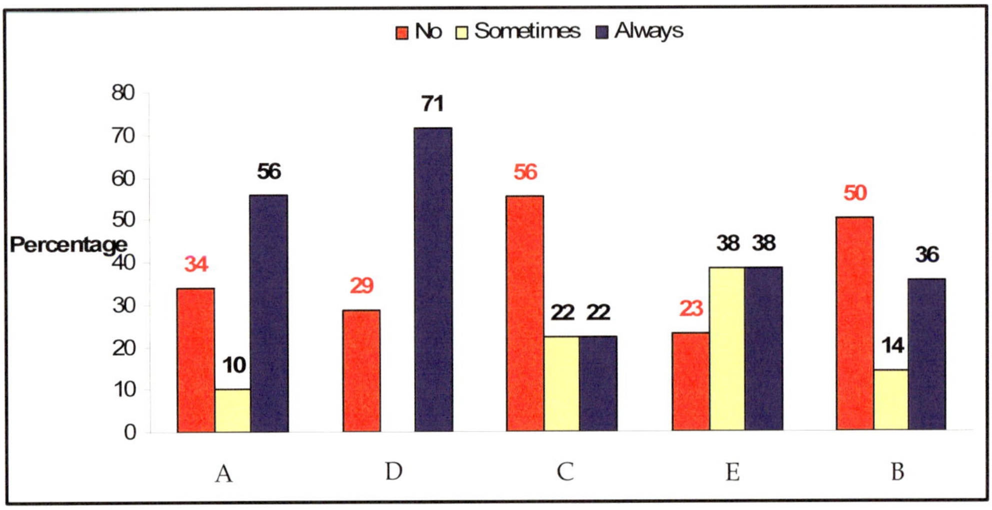

Fig. 6. Condom use with non-regular partners by nationality.

Although condom use was inconsistent, the majority (84%) of the respondents knew the location, as where to get condoms. The (Bs) had the lowest knowledge on the location of condoms as only 60% of the (Bs) respondents knew where to obtain condoms. Only 38% of the total respondents have ever seen a female condom with the highest rates reported by the (Ds) (70%), and the (As) (49%), and while the lowest rates by the (Bs) (3.6%), followed by the (Es) (14.3%), and the (Cs) (24%). Furthermore, only 16% of the study participants have ever been distributed female condoms, almost the number of women participants.

3.6 Alcohol and sexual relations

The majority of the study respondents drank alcohol with the exception of the (Bs), for religious reasons. More than one third of the study participants drank alcohol on a regular basis (weekly or daily). The (Cs) and (Es) had the highest rates of alcohol consumption as 71% and 57%, respectively; they drank alcohol at least on a weekly basis. In addition, more than half (56.5%) of the study participants reported engaging in sexual relations under alcohol influence; always 7%, on holidays 23% or rarely 26.3% (Fig. 7).

The (Cs) and (Es) had the highest rates of engaging in sexual relations under alcohol influence (Fig. 8) while the (Ds) reported the lowest rates of sexual relations under influence. It is worth noting that a significant correlation ($r=0.591$, $p<0.01$), and an increasing association were found between the amount/frequency of drinking alcohol and frequency of practicing sexual relations under alcohol influence, as 76% of those who always practice sex under influence, drink alcohol on a weekly or daily basis.

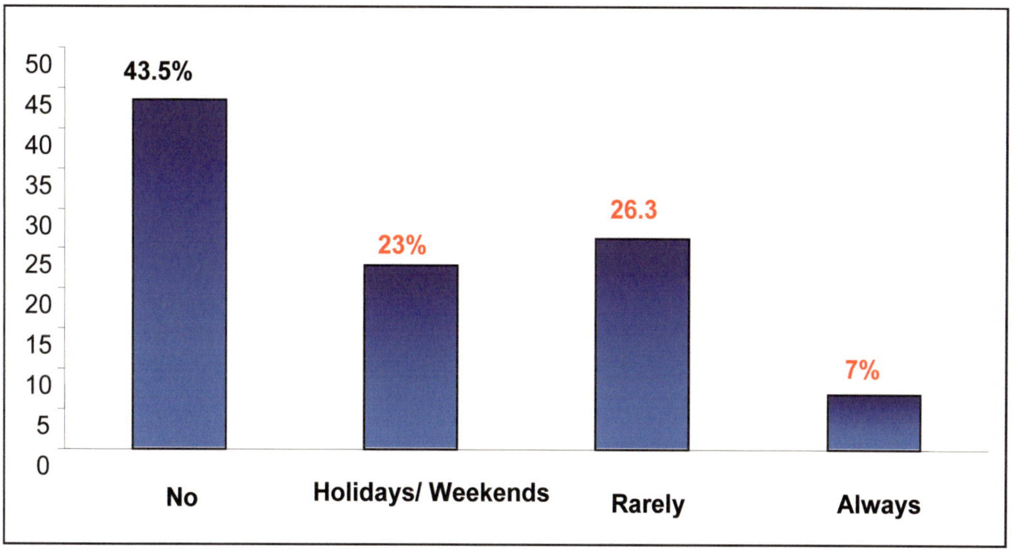

Fig. 7. Overall rates of sexual relations under alcohol influence (5) (%).

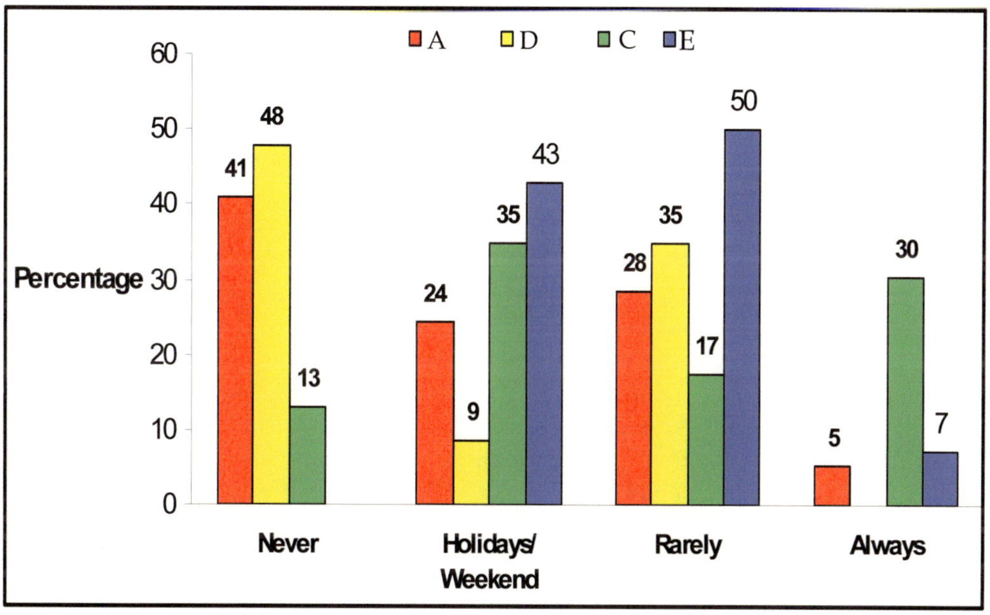

Fig. 8. Rates of sexual behavior under alcohol influence by nationality.

The vast majority of UNIFIL members (83.2%) would seek medical care in the UNIFIL clinic in case of a suspected STD (Table 5). The (Es) and the (Cs) had the highest appropriate health seeking behavior as more than 95% of them would consult a medical doctor in the battalion. Asking a colleague was considered an appropriate measure by a small but significant percentage of the respondents ranging from 0% to 14.3%.

This particular point highlights the importance of the availability of peer leaders among the soldiers in order to direct their friends for medical treatment. It is noteworthy that the (Bs) had the least appropriate health seeking behavior in case of a suspected STD as almost 11% would not seek any help or consultations, 14.3% would ask a colleague, and 75% would consult a health care professional.

	Total	A	D	E	C	B
Health seeking behaviour in case of suspected STD						
Nothing	3.8%	4.2%	0%	0%	0%	10.7%
Ask a colleague	8.6%	10.5%	4.3%	0%	4.2%	14.3%
Seek medical care	83.2%	82.1%	86.9%	100%	95.8%	75.0%
Other	4.3%	3.2%	8.8%	0%	0%	0%
Previous HIV testing (%yes)	49.5%	55.3%	65.2%	64.3%	40.0%	17.9%
Counselling during previous HIV test						
No	47.8%	38.5%	73.3%	66.7%	60.0%	20.0%
Yes, before the test	26.1%	30.8%	13.3%	0%	40.0%	40.0%
Yes, after the test	3.3%	1.9%	0%	22.2%	0%	0%
Yes, both before and after the test	22.8%	28.8%	13.3%	11.1%	0%	40.0%
Interested in counselling in this mission (% yes)	87.1%	92.6%	90.9%	100.0%	60.0%	82.1%
Interested in HIV test in this mission (% yes)	38.2%	37.2%	34.8%	71.4%	40.0%	28.6%

Table 5. Health seeking behaviour, counselling and testing for HIV by nationality.

Almost half of the respondents (49.5%) have been previously tested for HIV as depicted in Table 5, and the majority was tested within the past three years. The highest percentage of people tested was reported by the (Es) (64.3%) while the lowest was listed by the (Bs) (17.9%). Among those who had been tested for HIV, the majority (47.8%) did not receive any form of counseling either before or after the test, especially among the (Ds), (Es) and (Cs) respondents. Among the (A) respondents, 32/52 HIV tested individuals had some forms of counseling while 4/5 of (Bs) tested received counseling. It is notable that (Ds) had the highest rates of lack of counseling before or after an HIV test, while this test is mandatory for all individuals before deployment. Hence, there is a need to incorporate voluntary counseling and confidential testing (VCCT) as recommended by the UNAIDS, instead of only mandatory HIV testing (UNAIDS, 2010).

Almost 90% of respondents would be interested to go for counselling in case of suspected HIV infection, and 38.2% would be interested to have an HIV test done. The (Es) were the most interested in having an HIV test (71%), while the (Bs) were the least interested (28.6%). The main reasons for not going to counselling were fear that the counselling is not confidential (32.6%), fear to be discriminated, and afraid to hear the result (10.5% each). In addition, the lack of interest in having an HIV test was also due to the low perception of risk to catching HIV as 86% of those who are not interested to be tested in this mission reported that they do not consider themselves to be at risk.

3.8 Information sources on HIV/AIDS

There were wide disparities, ranging from 46.4% (B) to 84% (C), in reported levels of pre-deployment training on HIV/AIDS among the different nationalities. Overall, almost two thirds (65.2%) of the respondents had received some kind of information on HIV/AIDS before deployment. The majority of this information was provided by the battalion medical staff (62.5%) followed by peer educators (11.7%), and UN medical staff (6.7%). Other sources were either schools or special teams designated to give information on HIV/AIDS. However, the majority of the respondents (more than 90%) have never heard of the resolution 1308 on the need to incorporate HIV/AIDS training among peacekeeping forces. Those who did hear about this resolution reported reading about them during military training (7/189), in the media (11/189), or through self-study (2/189).

Currently, 76.4% of all the respondents would trust a trained peer for HIV/STD information (Table 6). Trust in peer leaders varied by country ranging between 92.3% with the (Es) and 71.4% with the (Bs). The other contingents had a trust rate close to the overall rate ranging between 72.8% and 81.8%. The main reasons for not trusting peer leaders was the misconception that they are not credible (43.2%). As for the best preferred sources of information on STDs including HIV, medical doctors were the preferred source for the majority of the contingents, followed by awareness materials including brochures, pamphlets, and cards, among others. This finding goes in hand with the trend that medical doctors are respected, trusted and considered to have the most credible knowledge on the disease which makes them the best source of information on any health issue. Peer educators are considered as good sources of information for almost one third of the (Cs) and 28% of the (Bs) and 23% of the (Es). However, the (As) had the least interest in peer educators for HIV information.

	Average	A	D	E	C	B
Trusts a Trained Peer Leader						
% Yes	76.4%	72.8%	81.8%	92.3%	80.0%	71.4%
Best sources of information on STIs						
Military medical doctors	71.7%	81.7%	69.6%	84.6%	56.0%	46.4%
Peer educators	16.3%	7.5%	17.4%	23.1%	32.0%	28.6%
Awareness material (Brochures, pamphlets)	36.4%	33.3%	34.8%	53.8%	56.0%	25.0%
Workshops	18.0%	18.5%	8.7%	0%	8.0%	42.9%

Table 6. Preferred sources of information on HIV/AIDS by nationality.

3.9 Gender and culturally sensitive issues

The majority of the respondents (87.6%) never heard of the UNSCR 1325 on the role of women in peace and security. The media and military training were the main sources of information on this resolution among those who heard about it. On the other hand, 28% of the respondents claimed to know the role of women in the local population; however, few could actually specify this role. Most of the respondents perceived the local women to be submissive to men and responsible mainly for the care of her children and family. Few of the respondents (13.5%) had been previously involved in a development intervention involving women. The (Cs) had the highest rates of involvement (40%) while the (Ds) reported the lowest rate (4.5%). Only 4/25 individuals who were involved in development interventions with women had communication problems with them. The main stated problem was the inability of women in the local population to talk to male soldiers due to cultural constraints.

Furthermore, almost 72% of the respondents were interested to learn more about the local population with the (Cs) and (Es) displaying the highest interest (88% and 86%, respectively) while the (Bs) had the lowest interest (57.1%) in knowing more about the culture, traditions or habits of the local population. The (As) and (Ds) had rates of interest, close to the overall rate. The majority of the (As) and the (Es) had been previously informed on the way to approach the local population (88.4% and 85.7%, respectively). In other contingents, almost 78% of the respondents had been told how to approach the local population.

4. Disscussion

4.1 Knowledge gap

Despite the fact that pre-deployment training on HIV/AIDS was relatively high, knowledge about HIV/AIDS was incomplete as only a third of the respondents could correctly list three prevention methods against HIV. In addition, there were high rates of misconceptions noted regarding HIV/AIDS transmission across all nationalities. Mother to child transmission was not known to the majority of the respondents, and the majority did not know that breastfeeding could transmit HIV. Another significant finding was the relatively high percentage of respondents who thought that there is a cure for HIV especially among the (Es) (43%). This gap in knowledge, in spite of previous training, illustrates a problem with the retention of information which has negative consequences on sexual behavior. It also highlights the need to consistently repeat information on HIV/AIDS during deployment. Peer leaders could be of significant value for this purpose as they will be reaching all age groups and genders. This is in line with what UNAIDS advocates for promoting peer Leadership within the uniformed services as a key measure to ensure ongoing awareness and sensitization that will impact, in the long term, on individual risk behaviors (UNAIDS, 2011).

Another interesting finding was that two thirds of the respondents did not know that women were vulnerable and at a high risk of exposure to HIV due to several physiological (e.g. higher concentration of the virus were in sperm, larger surface area of the genitals in women), social (e.g. rape, coercive sex, inability to negotiate condom use), and economical reasons (e.g. commercial sex workers). This fact requires to be highlighted for both men and women in future awareness campaigns.

Moreover, only few of the respondents (31%) knew that a UNIFIL soldier living with HIV could not be legally dismissed from his/her work. This denoted the importance of addressing the legal aspects towards people living with HIV among UNIFIL forces especially when providing pre-deployment training or screening. In general the attitudes towards people living with HIV among the UNIFIL were negative especially among the (Bs) whereby 85% of them believed that a person living with HIV should be dismissed from the UNIFIL. More sensitization and information for the soldiers on the topic of HIV could possibly change their negative attitudes. Furthermore, it is noteworthy that the majority of the respondents did not know about the situation and the prevalence of HIV/AIDS in Lebanon. This was important to underscore a common belief that Lebanon does not have a high HIV prevalence and hence, many soldiers would tend to engage in unprotected sexual relations. For this purpose, all soldiers deployed need to be informed on the situation and prevalence of certain diseases including STDs and HIV/AIDS in Lebanon.

4.2 Risky behavior

Although several respondents considered themselves to be at risk for HIV infection, these same respondents did not take any preventive measures to decrease this risk. For example, the (Cs) had the highest perception of being at risk to catch HIV, however, despite this awareness, they had the highest rates of inconsistent condom use with casual sexual partners, and the highest rates of engaging in sexual relations under alcohol influence. Moreover, condom use was highly inconsistent. In addition, the relation between alcohol and engaging in sexual relations under influence was another important problem. Alcohol not only increases sexual arousal but it also leads to forgetting to use condoms, or inappropriately using condoms as a result of breaking. Furthermore, alcohol was served, in general, in places where sex workers were usually available, which increased the risk of catching HIV (UNAIDS, 2010).

Despite the high risk sexual behavior, the majority reported a good health seeking behavior as 83.2% would seek help from the UNIFIL clinic in case they suspect a STD. Asking a colleague was another option which also denoted the importance of having well informed peer leaders among the soldiers to direct them to seek medical care in case of STD suspicion.

4.3 HIV testing and counseling

The study highlighted inconsistent implementation of testing policies (mandatory versus voluntary) within battalions and insufficient levels of counseling accompanying testing across all groups. There was a risk that in some cases a peacekeeper may assume that he/she has been tested as part of his/her pre-deployment medical and is HIV-negative, when in fact he/she has not undergone a test and may be positive. Counseling should be considered crucial so that individuals understand the relevance of the test result, and how to maintain an HIV-negative status, or look after themselves and their families, if the result were positive. Counseling both before and after a test should accompany all pre-deployment testing, and be carried out by contributing countries to peacekeeping operations.

The survey found significant levels (90%) of individuals who would be interested to go for counseling in this mission if available. Moreover, more than one third of the respondents would be interested to be tested for HIV in this mission, with significant variations by nationality as 71% of the (Es) would like to be tested. Therefore, availability of VCCT centers is needed in certain battalions where high risk behavior prevails.

4.4 Limitations of the study

There were a few limitations in this survey that needed to be addressed. First, the study findings could not be generalized to all UNIFIL forces in Lebanon as it only included few battalions which speak English, French or Arabic. Secondly, the questionnaire itself had several limitations due to deletion of some relevant questions by the UNIFIL project coordination team. It would have been of help to have information on the sexual practices of UNIFIL soldiers in Lebanon, similar to studies that were implemented in other countries

(Bazergan, 2006; Bing et al., 2008). Having such information would give a better understanding of the situation. Thirdly, questions related to STDs and their symptoms were also deleted by the UNIFIL. Such information could have also helped in assessing the risk of the respondents towards HIV, as STDs facilitate the transmission of HIV, and indicate that the person is engaging in high risk sexual behavior.

5. Conclusion

This survey, despite its limitations, depicted areas of weaknesses and gaps to manage, as well as elements of strength to build on. The results could constitute a basis to develop strategies and activities in line of the UN mandates regarding HIV/AIDS, STDs and gender sensitive issues. STDs are rooted in history and AIDS is clearly a long-wave pandemic with impacts taking various forms and unfolding over generations. However different groups and different countries are affected differently, including the military. It is very important to "know your epidemic" as declared by UNAIDS 2008, but it is equally important to know the social, economic, and political contexts. They can influence the direction of the HIV epidemic, which is based on individual behaviors. Taking the appropriate policy decisions is crucial to design and adopt the relevant strategies within a highly sensitive establishment like the military (Barnett & Prins, 2006).

Such strategies are becoming more crucial in light of the limited information on Lebanon concerning these health issues, and the expanding involvement of the UNIFIL forces in the life and development of the Lebanese. They are being conceived not only as peacekeepers but also as social actors in the development of the region through social interventions and projects in almost every village of the South. They deal frequently with locals; use their shops, their swimming pools among other things (Jurjus & Watfa, 2008).

In order to make resolutions and commitments realities, more efforts should be deployed. This is becoming of great importance in light of the increasing demand for peacekeeping forces worldwide reaching up to 15 missions from more than 115 countries with various HIV prevalence rates. In this context, the institution of mandatory pre-deployment HIV testing and STDs screening as well as health education activities, and counseling services, might constitute an essential basis for an effective prevention program. Such efforts and commitment to confront the HIV and STD spread, and the unfolding of their impact in terms of human lives lost, in the devastation of families, classes, civil societies, social organizations, business structures, and armed forces. The implementation of such a comprehensive approach should include gender sensitive issues, because of the increasing role of women in the military. Women are more likely to contract an STD than men. Without government policies and support for women's property rights, education, livelihoods, and access to healthcare, unsafe transactional sex can become one of the few alternatives for survival (Klot & Nguyen, 2009).

It is now well established that military personnel, both men and women, especially when deployed for extended periods, are among the most vulnerable populations to STDs and HIV. The resulting rates would go up to 2-5 times higher, maybe more than the civilian population. Such harsh realities need to be appropriately tackled with a complete package involving pre and post-deployment programs:

1. STD and HIV prevention programs should be conducted on a regular basis: before, during, and after deployment to reinforce health promoting behaviors and enhance the knowledge of HIV/AIDS prevention and transmission.
2. Educational programs should focus on changing perception of military personnel of risk for HIV/AIDS.
3. There should be policies covering the regular supply and distribution of male and female condoms. Condom promotion activities should be adapted to local, social, economic, and cultural sensitivities of the country.
4. Efforts should be made to ensure that STD symptoms are widely known and appropriately managed.
5. Pre and post-test counseling sites and services should be improved with high level assurance of confidentiality and job security.
6. More behavioral and biological studies are needed to determine prevalence of HIV/STDs in the UNIFIL and the military in general.
7. Further studies are needed to review the length of time military personnel are required to spend during peace keeping, so that healthy sexual and marital relationships can be promoted.

In brief, the interplay between sex work, injecting drug use and sex between men is accelerating the spread of HIV and HIV/STD co-infections in armies. Evaluations of the various programs implemented should be periodic and the ultimate aim should be to transform the peacekeepers into prevention actors rather than being transmission vectors (AIDS, Security and Conflict Initiative, 2009). In post-conflict countries with low HIV prevalence, like Lebanon, monitoring HIV-related behavior of military personnel could constitute an early warning signal to forecast the spread of the epidemic.

The HIV/AIDS pandemic needs to be under more control. The evolving landscape of demographic crises and conflicts throughout the world has reshaped the challenges and underscored the need to reinvigorate international commitments to achieve universal access to HIV/STD prevention, treatment, care and support for peacekeepers, their families and the communities they serve.

Ultimately, the goal is to provide a multidisciplinary framework that integrates the social science and biomedical paradigm, and acknowledges the potential for bidirectional interplay for effective control of these diseases, prevent their sequelae, and limit their costs to society.

6. Acknowledgments

The authors would like to thank the United Nations Population Fund for supporting this project and The UNIFIL commanders and medical team for facilitating the implementation of the survey.

7. References

Abu-Raddad L., Ayodeji F., Iris Semini et al. (2010), Characterization of the HIV/AIDS Epidemic in the Middle East and North Africa: Time for Strategic Action, World Bank Publications
http://www-wds.worldbank.org/external/default/WDSContentServer/

WDSP/IB/2010/06/04/000333038_20100604011533/Rendered/PDF/548890PUB0EPI11C10Dislosed061312010.pdf

Adib S., Akoum S., & Jurjus A. , (2002), Heterosexual awareness and practices among Lebanese male conscripts, *East Mediterr Health J.* 8 (6): 765-775

AIDS, Security and Conflict Initiative (2009), HIV/AIDS, security and conflict: new realities, new responses. New York, Social Science Research Council (SSRC) and the Netherlands Institute of International Relations, AIDS, Security and Conflict Initiative, accessed April 2011 http://asci.researchhub.ssrc.org/HIVAIDS%20Security%20and%20Conflict%20New%20Realities%20New%20Responses.pdf

AIDS, Security and Conflict Initiative (2011). New York, AIDS, Security and Conflict Initiative, accessed April 2011 http://asci.researchhub.ssrc.org

Ba O., O'Regan C., Nachega J. Cooper C. Anema A. & Rachlis B. (2008) Mills E. HIV/AIDS in African militaries: an ecological analysis, *Med Confl Surviv.* 24(2):88-100

Baliunas D., Rehm J., Irving H., & Shuper P. (2010), Alcohol consumption and risk of incident human immunodeficiency virus infection: a meta-analysis, *Int J Public Health,* 55(3):159-66

Barnett T. & Prins G. (2006), HIV/AIDS and security: fact, fiction and evidence; a report to UNAIDS, International Affairs, 82:359–368.

Bazergan R. (2006), HIV/AIDS Knowledge, Attitude and Practice survey: UN uniformed peacekeepers in Liberia, Peacekeeping Best Practices, United Nations.

Bing E., Ortiz D., & Ovalle-Bahamón R. Cheng K. Huang F. Ernesto F. Duan N. (2008) HIV/AIDS behavioral surveillance among Angolan military men, AIDS Behav. 12(4):578-84.

Bolan G. (2011), Lessons learned: STD awareness Month 2011, accessed August 2011 http://www.rhrealitycheck.org/blog/2011

Centers for Disease Control (CDC) (1981), Kaposi's sarcoma and Pneumocystis pneumonia among homosexual men--New York City and California, *MMWR Morb Mortal Wkly Rep.* 30(25):305-8

Centers for Disease Control and Prevention (2009), Sexually Transmitted Diseases: Sexually Transmitted Diseases Surveillance, accessed July 2011, http://www.cdc.gov/STD/stats09/toc.htm

De Waal A. (2010) HIV/AIDS and the challenges of security and conflict, *Lancet,* 375(9708):22-23

Ebrahim S., McKenna M., & Marks J. (2005), Sexual behavior: related adverse health burden in the United States, *Sex Transm Infect.* 81(1):38-40

Emerson L. (1997), Sexually transmitted disease control in the armed forces, past and present, *Mil Med.* 162(2):87-91

European Centre for Disease Prevention and Control and WHO Regional Office for Europe (2009), HIV/AIDS surveillance in Europe 2008, Stockholm, European Centre for Disease Prevention and Control

Family Health Services (2005), HIV/AIDS and the Uniformed Services.

Gaydos C., Quinn T., & Gaydos J. (2000), The Challenge of Sexually Transmitted Diseases for the Military: What has changed?, *Clinical Infectious Diseases,* 30: 719-722

Gilbert D., & Greenberg J., (1976), Vietnam: preventive medicine orientation. Mil Med. 132(10):769-90

Greenberg J. (1972), Venereal disease in the Armed Forces, *Med Clin North Am.* 56(5):1087-100

Jurjus A., & Watfa N., (2008), Working and at Risk Drop-out Children and HIV/AIDS in War-inflected Lebanon, International Labor Office- IPEC. ISBN 978-92-2-120983-6

Jurjus A., & Tohme R., (2008), HIV/AIDS in Lebanon: Situation and Recommendations, *Human & Health* (2): 33-37

Kahhaleh J., El Nakib M., &Jurjus A. (2009), Knowledge, attitudes, beliefs and practices in Lebanon concerning HIV/AIDS, 1996-2004, *East Mediterr Health J.* 15(4):920-33

Kampmeier R. (1982), Venereal disease in the United States Army: 1775-1900, *Sex Transm. Dis.* 9(2):100-10

Karam W., Bedran F., Tohme R., Moukarbel N., Abdallah I., Jurjus A., Jurjus R., Khairallah S., & Aftimos G. (2005), "Human Papilloma Virus Testing an Adjunct to Cytology Evaluation in Cervical Specimens of Selected and Consecutively Screened Lebanese Women: A Prospective Clinical Study.", *Lebanese Medical Journal*, 53(3): 132-138

Kershaw R. (2008), The impact of HIV/AIDS on the operational effectiveness of military forces. New York, AIDS, Security and Conflict Initiative, ASCI Research Report No. 4; accessed April 2011, http://asci.researchhub.rc.org/working-papers/Kershaw.pdf

Kim J. Y. (2002), HIV/AIDS in the Eastern Mediterranean: a false immunity, *East Mediterr Health J*, 8(6): 684-688

Klot J. & Nguyen VK. (2009), The Fourth Wave: Violence, Gender, Culture & HIV in the 21st Century, accessed June 2011, http://blogs.ssrc.org/fourthwave/

Lazenby G. (2011), Trichomonas vaginalis screening and prevention in order to impact the HIV pandemic: Isn't it time we take this infection seriously?, *Infectious disease Reports*, 3:12-14

Lowicki-Zucca M., Karmin S., & Dehne K-L. (2009), HIV among peacekeepers and its likely impact on prevalence on host countries' HIV epidemics, *International Peacekeeping*, 216:352–363.

Mokhbat J., Ibrahim N., Abdul-Karim F., Kuleilat-Shatila M., & Salem Z. (1985), "The Acquired Immunodeficiency Syndrome: Report of the First Case in Lebanon and Review of the Literature.", *Lebanese Medical Journal*, 35: 295-319

National AIDS Program: Report on HIV/AIDS in Lebanon, Beirut: NAP, 2011. http://www.moph.gov.lb/Prevention/AIDS/Pages/Background.aspx

Nwokoji U. & Ajuwon A. (2004), Knowledge of AIDS and HIV risk-related sexual behavior among Nigerian naval personnel, *BMC Public Health.* 4: 24.

Oriel J. (1994), The British Journal of Venereal Diseases and Genitourinary Medicine: the first 70 years, *Genitourin Med.* 70(4):235-9

Rasnake M., Conger N., McAllister K., Holmes K., & Tramont E. (2005), History of U.S. military contributions to the study of sexually transmitted diseases, *Mil Med.* 170 (4):61-5

Security Council sc/102 72 unanimously adopting 1983 Encourage Inclusion of HIV Prevention, Treatment, Care, Support in Implementing Peacekeeping Mandates, accessed June, 2011 (http://www.un.org/News/Press/docs/2011)

Shuper P., Joharchi N., Irving H., & Rehm J. (2009), Alcohol as a correlate of unprotected sexual behavior among people living with HIV/AIDS: review and meta-analysis, *AIDS Behav.* 13(6):1021-36.

Sing B. & BanerjeeA. (2006), HIV prevention in the Armed Forces; Perceptions and Attitudes of Regimental Officesrs, *MJAFI* 62:335-338

STD Statistics Worldwide (2011), STD, http://infertilityeggdonor.com/std_statistics_worldwide

Tawilah J., Tawil O., Bassiri S., & Ziady H. (2002), Information needs assessment for HIV/AIDS and STIs in the Eastern Mediterranean Region, *East Mediterr Health J.* 8(6):689-98

The Well Project (2009), Sexually Transmitted Diseases, accessed June, 2011 http://www.thewellproject.org/en_US/Diseases_and_Conditions/Other_Diseases_and_Conditions/STD.jsp

World Health Organization (2007), Sexually Transmitted Infections, Fact sheet number 110, October 2007

UNAIDS (2010), UNAIDS Global Report on the AIDS epidemic, Geneva, UNAIDS accessed July, 2011, http://www.unaids.org/globalreport

UNAIDS (2011), On the Frontline. A Review of programmes that address HIV among international peacekeepers and uniformed services, accessed July 2011 http://www.un.org/peacekeeping

UNAIDS and WHO (2008), "2008 AIDS Epidemic Update.", accessed 11 October 2009, (http://data.unaids.org/pub/EPISlides/2008/2008_epiupdate_en.pdf)

United Nations (2000), UN Security Council Resolution 1308 on the responsibility of the Security Council in the maintenance of international peace and security: HIV/AIDS and international peacekeeping operations, Retrieved on July, 2007 from: http://daccessdds.un.org/doc/UNDOC/GEN/N00/536/02/PDF/N0053602.pdf?OpenElement

United Nations (2000), UN Security Council Resolution 1325 on Women and Peace and Security, Retrieved on July 2007 from: http://daccessdds.un.org/doc/UNDOC/GEN/N00/720/18/PDF/N0072018.pdf?OpenElement

United Nations Development Programme (2010), Bringing HIV related issues into humanitarian instruments, New York, UNDP

United Nations Population Fund (2009), Working with uniformed services to promote reproductive health and prevent HIV: UNFPA experience, Fact sheet New York, UNFPA.

United Nations Population Fund (2009). Working with uniformed services to promote reproductive health and prevent HIV: UNFPA experience report, New York, UNFPA.

United Nations Population Fund (2010), Unified Budget and Work plan broad activity implementation - biennial report (2008-2009), New York, UNFPA.

United States Department of Defence HIV/AIDS Prevention Programme (2011), Department of Defence HIV/AIDS Prevention Programme (DHAPP) 2010 annual report.

Whiteside A., De Waal A., & Tensae G. (2006), AIDS, Security and the Military in Africa: A sober appraisal, *African Affairs*, 105(419): 201-218

WHO and Global coalition on Women and AIDS (2004), Intimate Partner violence and HIV/AIDS. Geneva, WHO, accessed April 2011, http://www.who.int/hac/techguidance/pht/InfoBulletinIntimatePartnerViolenceFinal.pdf

Worldstats.htm, accessed June 2011, http://www.avert.org//aidsnews.htm